D0291843

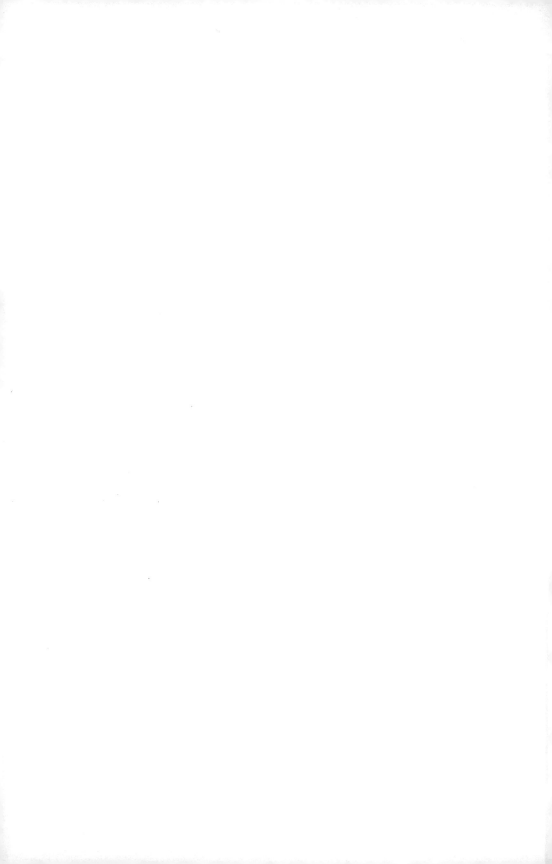

BEST CARE AT LOWER COST

The Path to Continuously Learning Health Care in America

Committee on the Learning Health Care System in America

Mark Smith, Robert Saunders, Leigh Stuckhardt, and J. Michael McGinnis,
Editors

INSTITUTE OF MEDICINE
OF THE NATIONAL ACADEMIES

THE NATIONAL ACADEMIES PRESS
Washington, D.C.
www.nap.edu

THE NATIONAL ACADEMIES PRESS   500 Fifth Street, NW   Washington, DC 20001

NOTICE: The project that is the subject of this report was approved by the Governing Board of the National Research Council, whose members are drawn from the councils of the National Academy of Sciences, the National Academy of Engineering, and the Institute of Medicine. The members of the committee responsible for the report were chosen for their special competences and with regard for appropriate balance.

Support for this report was provided by the Blue Shield of California Foundation; the Charina Endowment Fund; and the Robert Wood Johnson Foundation. Any opinions, findings, conclusions, or recommendations expressed in this publication are those of the author(s) and do not necessarily reflect the view of the organizations or agencies that provided support for this project.

Library of Congress Cataloging-in-Publication Data

Best care at lower cost : the path to continuously learning health care in America / Committee on the Learning Health Care System in America, The Institute of Medicine ; Mark Smith ... [et al.], editors.
    p. ; cm.
  Includes bibliographical references.
  ISBN 978-0-309-26073-2 (hardcover) — ISBN 978-0-309-26074-9 (pdf)
  I. Smith, Mark D., M.D. II. Institute of Medicine (U.S.). Committee on the Learning Health Care System in America.
  [DNLM: 1. Delivery of Health Care—economics—United States. 2. Costs and Cost Analysis—United States. 3. Efficiency, Organizational—economics—United States. 4. Quality of Health Care—economics—United States. W 84 AA1]

    368.38'200973—dc23
                            2012040484

Additional copies of this report are available from the National Academies Press, 500 Fifth Street, NW, Keck 360, Washington, DC 20001; (800) 624-6242 or (202) 334-3313; http://www.nap.edu.

For more information about the Institute of Medicine, visit the IOM home page at: **www.iom.edu.**

Printed in the United States of America

The serpent has been a symbol of long life, healing, and knowledge among almost all cultures and religions since the beginning of recorded history. The serpent adopted as a logotype by the Institute of Medicine is a relief carving from ancient Greece, now held by the Staatliche Museen in Berlin.

Suggested citation: IOM (Institute of Medicine). 2013. *Best care at lower cost: The path to continuously learning health care in America.* Washington, DC: The National Academies Press.

"Knowing is not enough; we must apply.
Willing is not enough; we must do."
—Goethe

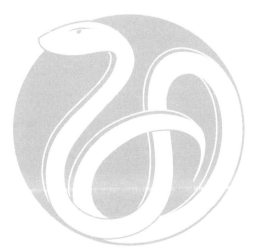

INSTITUTE OF MEDICINE
OF THE NATIONAL ACADEMIES

Advising the Nation. Improving Health.

THE NATIONAL ACADEMIES
Advisers to the Nation on Science, Engineering, and Medicine

The **National Academy of Sciences** is a private, nonprofit, self-perpetuating society of distinguished scholars engaged in scientific and engineering research, dedicated to the furtherance of science and technology and to their use for the general welfare. Upon the authority of the charter granted to it by the Congress in 1863, the Academy has a mandate that requires it to advise the federal government on scientific and technical matters. Dr. Ralph J. Cicerone is president of the National Academy of Sciences.

The **National Academy of Engineering** was established in 1964, under the charter of the National Academy of Sciences, as a parallel organization of outstanding engineers. It is autonomous in its administration and in the selection of its members, sharing with the National Academy of Sciences the responsibility for advising the federal government. The National Academy of Engineering also sponsors engineering programs aimed at meeting national needs, encourages education and research, and recognizes the superior achievements of engineers. Dr. Charles M. Vest is president of the National Academy of Engineering.

The **Institute of Medicine** was established in 1970 by the National Academy of Sciences to secure the services of eminent members of appropriate professions in the examination of policy matters pertaining to the health of the public. The Institute acts under the responsibility given to the National Academy of Sciences by its congressional charter to be an adviser to the federal government and, upon its own initiative, to identify issues of medical care, research, and education. Dr. Harvey V. Fineberg is president of the Institute of Medicine.

The **National Research Council** was organized by the National Academy of Sciences in 1916 to associate the broad community of science and technology with the Academy's purposes of furthering knowledge and advising the federal government. Functioning in accordance with general policies determined by the Academy, the Council has become the principal operating agency of both the National Academy of Sciences and the National Academy of Engineering in providing services to the government, the public, and the scientific and engineering communities. The Council is administered jointly by both Academies and the Institute of Medicine. Dr. Ralph J. Cicerone and Dr. Charles M. Vest are chair and vice chair, respectively, of the National Research Council.

www.national-academies.org

COMMITTEE ON THE LEARNING HEALTH
CARE SYSTEM IN AMERICA

IOM Staff

ROBERT SAUNDERS, Study Director
LEIGH STUCKHARDT, Program Associate
JULIA C. SANDERS, Senior Program Assistant
BRIAN W. POWERS, Senior Program Assistant (through July 2012)
VALERIE ROHRBACH, Senior Program Assistant
CLAUDIA GROSSMAN, Senior Program Officer
ISABELLE VON KOHORN, Program Officer
BARRET ZIMMERMANN, Program Assistant
J. MICHAEL McGINNIS, Senior Scholar

Consultants

RONA BRIERE, Briere Associates, Inc.
ALISA DECATUR, Briere Associates, Inc.

Reviewers

This report has been reviewed in draft form by individuals chosen for their diverse perspectives and technical expertise, in accordance with procedures approved by the National Research Council's Report Review Committee. The purpose of this independent review is to provide candid and critical comments that will assist the institution in making its published report as sound as possible and to ensure that the report meets institutional standards for objectivity, evidence, and responsiveness to the study charge. The review comments and draft manuscript remain confidential to protect the integrity of the deliberative process. We wish to thank the following individuals for their review of this report:

WYLIE BURKE, Professor and Chair, Department of Bioethics and Humanities, University of Washington, Seattle

MICHAEL CHERNEW, Professor of Health Care Policy, Harvard Medical School, Boston, MA

JANET CORRIGAN, Former President and Chief Executive Officer, National Quality Forum, Washington, DC

JOHN HALAMKA, Chief Information Officer, CareGroup Health System, Boston, MA

GEORGE ISHAM, Medical Director and Chief Health Officer, HealthPartners, Inc., Bloomington, MN

STEPHEN KIMMEL, Professor of Medicine, University of Pennsylvania School of Medicine, Philadelphia

ALLEN S. LICHTER, Chief Executive Officer, American Society of Clinical Oncology, Alexandria, VA

Although the reviewers listed above provided many constructive comments and suggestions, they were not asked to endorse the report's conclusions or recommendations, nor did they see the final draft of the report before its release. The review of this report was overseen by coordinator **Robert S. Galvin,** Chief Executive Officer, Equity Healthcare, The Blackstone Group, New York, NY, and monitor **Emmett B. Keeler,** Professor of Health Services, Pardee RAND Graduate School, University of California, Los Angeles, School of Public Health, Santa Monica, CA. Appointed by the National Research Council and Institute of Medicine, they were responsible for making certain that an independent examination of this report was carried out in accordance with institutional procedures and that all review comments were carefully considered. Responsibility for the final content of this report rests entirely with the authoring committee and the institution.

Foreword

Best Care at Lower Cost: The Path to Continuously Learning Health Care in America presents a vision of what is possible if the nation applies the resources and tools at hand by marshaling science, information technology, incentives, and care culture to transform the effectiveness and efficiency of care—to produce high-quality health care that continuously learns to be better.

More than a decade since the Institute of Medicine's (IOM's) *To Err Is Human: Building a Safer Health System* was published, the U.S. health care system continues to fall far short of its potential. Although *To Err Is Human* and other IOM reports, including the *Crossing the Quality Chasm* series, have helped spark numerous efforts to improve practices, persistent health care underperformance and high costs highlight the considerable challenge of bringing isolated successes to scale. The nation has yet to see the broad improvements in safety, accessibility, quality, or efficiency that the American people need and deserve.

Leaders from every sector that bears on health have a part to play in realizing such broad improvements. Recognizing the need for cross-sector collaboration, in 2006 the IOM organized the Roundtable on Value & Science-Driven Health Care. The Roundtable convenes leaders from across the health care system—including representatives of patients and consumers, providers, manufacturers, payers, research, and policy—to help make continuous improvement in performance an intrinsic part of U.S. health care.

Under the guidance of its membership, the Roundtable has developed and articulated a vision of this new system—a *learning health care system* that links personal and population data to researchers and practitioners, dramatically enhancing the knowledge base on effectiveness of interventions and providing real-time guidance for superior care in treating and preventing illness. A health care system that gains from continuous learning is a system that can provide Americans with superior care at lower cost.

The IOM Committee on the Learning Health Care System in America was convened to explore and advance this vision of continuously learning health care. The committee's report describes the key challenges faced by the health care system today—the mounting complexity of modern medicine, the rising cost of care, and the limited return on investment—and outlines how to harness new technologies, innovations, and approaches to overcome these challenges.

Importantly, the report demonstrates how a health care system that delivers the best care at lower cost is not only necessary, but also possible. The committee has articulated detailed strategies for incorporating continuous learning and improvement into all facets of health care. The report recognizes the multifaceted and integrative nature of the needed transformation and outlines the multiple and concerted actions necessary across all sectors to achieve that transformation. No one individual, organization, or sector alone can effect the scope and scale of transformative change necessary for a true learning system. Rather, leadership from all sectors working in concert will be required.

I would like to express my gratitude to the committee and staff who produced this report that sets forth a vision for a successful, sustainable health care system—one that continuously learns and improves. The insights, ideas, and recommendations offered here point the way to building a superior health care system for all Americans.

Harvey V. Fineberg, M.D., Ph.D.
President, Institute of Medicine

Preface

The tragic life of Dr. Ignaz Semmelweis offers an example of the challenges faced in building a truly learning health care system. The Hungarian physician observed that simply washing hands could drastically reduce high rates of maternal death during childbirth. But since he could not prove a connection between hand washing and the spread of infection, he was ridiculed and ignored. Hounded out of his profession, he died in a mental hospital. More than 165 years later, half of clinicians still do not regularly wash their hands before seeing patients.

The challenges today are in some ways that straightforward, and in many other ways significantly more complex. Narrow-minded rejection of scientific evidence is rarely encountered today in medicine, yet the American health care system imposes significant institutional, economic, and pedagogic barriers to learning and adapting.

For more than a decade, reports of the Institute of Medicine (IOM) have focused attention on a persistent set of problems within the American health care system that urgently need to be addressed, including poor quality; lax safety; high cost; questionable value; and the maldistribution of care based on income, race, and ethnicity. Each report has called for substantive transformation of the nation's health care system. Many have pointed out a disturbing paradox: the coexistence of overtreatment and undertreatment. The committee that authored this report found a similar situation: learning and adoption that are maddeningly slow—as with hand washing—coexisting with *overly* rapid adoption of some new techniques, devices, and drugs, with harmful results.

Exemplary efforts under way across the nation are working on these problems. Indeed, some members of this committee come from organizations that are pacesetters in continuous learning. But the pace of change is too slow, and adoption is too spotty; the system is not evolving quickly enough. The system needs to learn more rapidly, digest what does and does not work, and spread that knowledge in ways that can be broadly adapted and adopted. This report offers a roadmap for accomplishing this vision to benefit patients and society.

The committee identified two reasons for the above problems that grow more urgent every year. One is the increasingly unmanageable complexity of the science of health care. During the past half-century, there has been an explosion of biomedical and clinical knowledge, with even more dazzling clinical capabilities just over the horizon. However, the systems by which health care providers are trained, deployed, paid, and updated cannot usefully digest this deluge of information. Second is the ever-escalating cost of care, which is widely acknowledged to be wasteful and unsustainable. Unless ways are found to provide more efficient, lower-cost health care, more and more Americans will lose coverage of and access to care.

The committee also believes that opportunities exist for attacking these problems—opportunities that did not exist even a decade ago.

- Vast *computational power* (with associated sophistication of information technology) has become affordable and widely available. This capability makes it possible to harvest useful information from actual patient care (as opposed to one-time studies), something that previously was impossible.
- *Connectivity* allows that power to be accessed in real time virtually anywhere by professionals and patients, permitting unprecedented diffusion of information cheaply, quickly, and on demand.
- Progress in human and *organizational capabilities* and *management science* can improve the reliability and efficiency of care, permitting more scientific deployment of human and technical resources to match the complexity of systems and institutions.
- Increasing *empowerment of patients* unleashes the potential for their participation, in concert with clinicians, in the prevention and treatment of disease—tasks that increasingly depend on personal behavior change.

The committee recognizes that individual physicians, nurses, technicians, pharmacists, and others involved in patient care work diligently to provide high-quality, compassionate care to their patients. The problem is not that they are not working hard enough; it is that the system does not adequately support them in their work. The system lags in adjusting to new discoveries, disseminating data in real time, organizing and coordinating the enormous volume of research and recommendations, and providing incentives for choosing the smartest route to health, not just the newest, shiniest—and often most expensive—tool. These broader issues prevent clinicians from providing the best care to their patients and limit their ability to continuously learn and improve.

In completing its work, the committee solicited the views of more than 200 individuals, representing clinicians, patients, health care delivery leaders, clinical researchers, professional societies, life science industries, information technology developers, and government agencies. The information gleaned from these individuals enabled the committee to better understand the challenges to learning and improvement, as well as to learn from the experiences of those who have successfully incorporated learning and improvement into their regular work. In addition, the IOM staff provided excellent research, analysis, and writing support for this project and assisted the committee in its deliberative process.

Given the imperatives and opportunities outlined above, this is the right time for the vision proposed in this report to be realized. Developing a continuously learning health care system is critical for the future of health care, as well as for the future physical and financial health of the nation. There is no simple path forward; rather, actions need to be taken by every stakeholder if this vision is to become a reality. Such concerted action will enable the nation's health care system to evolve to one that continuously learns and improves, finally providing Americans with the best care at lower cost.

Mark D. Smith, *Chair*
Committee on the Learning Health Care System in America

Acknowledgments

Best Care at Lower Cost: The Path to Continuously Learning Health Care for America reflects the contributions of many people. The committee would like to acknowledge and express strong appreciation to those who so generously participated in the development of this report.

First, we would like to thank the sponsors of this project, the Blue Shield of California Foundation, the Charina Endowment Fund, and the Robert Wood Johnson Foundation, for their financial support.

The committee would also like to thank Lynn Etheredge for his assistance with this effort. He was a member of the committee from January 1, 2011, until August 2, 2011, and his contributions to the committee's early thinking are very much appreciated.

The committee's deliberations were informed by presentations and discussions at four meetings held between January 2011 and January 2012. Additional input was sought from numerous outside stakeholders, and we would like to thank the 137 organizations and individuals who provided their input on committee directives.

A number of Institute of Medicine (IOM) staff played instrumental roles in coordinating the committee meetings and the preparation of this report, including Leigh Stuckhardt, Julia Sanders, Claudia Grossmann, Brian Powers, Valerie Rohrbach, and Isabelle Von Kohorn. The committee would also like to thank Lauren Tobias, Laura Harbold DeStefano, and Sarah Ziegenhorn for helping to coordinate the various aspects of report review, production, and publication. Committee consultant Rona Briere, Briere Associates, Inc., made indispensable contributions to the report production and publication processes. Additionally, we would like to thank both Column Five Media and LeAnn Locher for their contributions to the graphic portrayal and cover of this report. The committee would especially like to thank Robert Saunders, study director, for his overall guidance and support. Finally, we would like to acknowledge the guidance and contributions of Michael McGinnis, IOM senior scholar, throughout the study process.

America has the potential to realize a transformative learning health care system that could revolutionize the way care is delivered and understood. While great strides have already been made with new policy, sturdy dedication and engagement will continue to be instrumental as health care delivery in the United States is restructured. We look forward to building upon the ideas that have emerged in this report and achieving a learning health care system.

Contents

Abstract

Health care in America presents a fundamental paradox. The past 50 years have seen an explosion in biomedical knowledge, dramatic innovation in therapies and surgical procedures, and management of conditions that previously were fatal, with ever more exciting clinical capabilities on the horizon. Yet, American health care is falling short on basic dimensions of quality, outcomes, costs, and equity. Available knowledge is too rarely applied to improve the care experience, and information generated by the care experience is too rarely gathered to improve the knowledge available. The traditional systems for transmitting new knowledge—the ways clinicians are educated, deployed, rewarded, and updated—can no longer keep pace with scientific advances. If unaddressed, the current shortfalls in the performance of the nation's health care system will deepen on both quality and cost dimensions, challenging the well-being of Americans now and potentially far into the future. Health care needs major improvements with respect to its ability to meet patients' specific needs, to offer choice, to adapt, to become more affordable, to improve—in short, to learn. Americans should be served by a health care system that consistently delivers reliable performance and constantly improves, systematically and seamlessly, with each care experience and transition.

In the face of these realities, the Institute of Medicine (IOM) convened the Committee on the Learning Health Care System in America to explore the most fundamental challenges to health care today and to propose actions that can be taken to achieve a health care system characterized by continuous learning and improvement. This report, *Best Care at Lower Cost: The Path to Continuously Learning Health Care in America*, explores

1

the imperatives for change, the emerging tools that make transformation possible, the vision for a continuously learning health care system, and the path for achieving this vision. The title of the report underscores that care that is based on the best available evidence, takes appropriate account of individual preferences, and is delivered reliably and efficiently—*best care*— is possible today, and also is generally less expensive than the less effective, less efficient care that is now too commonly provided.

The foundation for a learning health care system is continuous knowledge development, improvement, and application. Although unprecedented levels of information are available, patients and clinicians often lack access to guidance that is relevant, timely, and useful for the circumstances at hand. Overcoming this challenge will require applying computing capabilities and analytic approaches to develop real-time insights from routine patient care, disseminating knowledge using new technological tools, and addressing the regulatory challenges that can inhibit progress.

Engaged patients are central to an effective, efficient, and continuously learning system. Clinicians supply information and advice based on their scientific expertise in treatment and intervention options, along with potential outcomes, while patients, their families, and other caregivers bring personal knowledge on the suitability—or lack thereof—of different treatments for the patient's circumstances and preferences. Both perspectives are needed to select the right care option for the patient. Communication and collaboration among patients, their families, and care teams are needed to fully address the issues affecting patients.

Health care payment policies strongly influence how care is delivered, whether new scientific insights and knowledge about best care are diffused broadly, and whether improvement initiatives succeed. New models of paying for care and organizing care delivery are emerging to improve quality and value. While evidence is conflicting on which payment models might work best and under what circumstances, it is clear that high-value care requires structuring incentives to reward the best outcomes for patients.

Finally, the culture of health care is central to promoting learning at every level. Creating continuously learning organizations that generate and transfer knowledge from every patient interaction will require systematic problem solving; the application of systems engineering techniques; operational models that encourage and reward sustained quality and improved patient outcomes; transparency on cost and outcomes; and strong leadership and governance that define, disseminate, and support a vision of continuous improvement.

Achieving the vision of continuously learning health care will depend on broad action by the complex network of individuals and organizations that make up the current health care system. Missed opportunities for better health care have real human and economic impacts. If the care in every state were of the quality delivered by the highest-performing state, an estimated 75,000 fewer deaths would have occurred across the country in 2005. Current waste diverts resources from productive use, resulting in an estimated $750 billion loss in 2009. It is only through shared commitments, with a supportive policy environment, that the opportunities afforded by science and information technology can be captured to address the health care system's growing challenges and to ensure that the system reaches its full potential. The nation's health and economic futures—best care at lower cost—depend on the ability to steward the evolution of a continuously learning health care system.

Summary

Health care in America presents a fundamental paradox. The past 50 years have seen an explosion in biomedical knowledge, dramatic innovation in therapies and surgical procedures, and management of conditions that previously were fatal, with ever more exciting clinical capabilities on the horizon. Yet, American health care is falling short on basic dimensions of quality, outcomes, costs, and equity. Available knowledge is too rarely applied to improve the care experience, and information generated by the care experience is too rarely gathered to improve the knowledge available. The traditional systems for transmitting new knowledge—the ways clinicians are educated, deployed, rewarded, and updated—can no longer keep pace with scientific advances. If unaddressed, the current shortfalls in the performance of the nation's health care system will deepen on both quality and cost dimensions, challenging the well-being of Americans now and potentially far into the future.

Consider the impact on American services if other industries routinely operated in the same manner as many aspects of health care:

- If banking were like health care, automated teller machine (ATM) transactions would take not seconds but perhaps days or longer as a result of unavailable or misplaced records.
- If home building were like health care, carpenters, electricians, and plumbers each would work with different blueprints, with very little coordination.

- If shopping were like health care, product prices would not be posted, and the price charged would vary widely within the same store, depending on the source of payment.
- If automobile manufacturing were like health care, warranties for cars that require manufacturers to pay for defects would not exist. As a result, few factories would seek to monitor and improve production line performance and product quality.
- If airline travel were like health care, each pilot would be free to design his or her own preflight safety check, or not to perform one at all.

The point is not that health care can or should function in precisely the same way as all other sectors of people's lives—each is very different from the others, and every industry has room for improvement. Yet, if some of the transferable best practices from banking, construction, retailing, automobile manufacturing, flight safety, public utilities, and personal services were adopted as standard best practices in health care, the nation could see patient care in which

- records would be immediately updated and available for use by patients;
- care delivered would be proven reliable at the core and tailored at the margins;
- patient and family needs and preferences would be a central part of the decision process;
- all team members would be fully informed in real time about each other's activities;
- prices and total costs would be fully transparent to all participants;
- payment incentives were structured to reward outcomes and value, not volume;
- errors would be promptly identified and corrected; and
- results would be routinely captured and used for continuous improvement.

Unfortunately, these are not features that would describe much of health care in America today. Health care can lag behind many other sectors with respect to its ability to meet patients' specific needs, to offer choice, to adapt, to become more affordable, to improve—in short, to learn. Americans should be served by a health care system that consistently delivers reliable performance and constantly improves, systematically and seamlessly, with each care experience and transition.

In the face of these realities, the Institute of Medicine (IOM) convened the Committee on the Learning Health Care System in America to explore the most fundamental challenges to health care today and to propose actions that can be taken to achieve a health care system characterized by continuous learning and improvement. This study builds on earlier IOM studies on various aspects of the health care system, from *To Err Is Human: Building a Safer Health System* (1999), on patient safety; to *Crossing the Quality Chasm: A New Health System for the 21st Century* (2001a), on health care quality; to *Unequal Treatment: Confronting Racial and Ethnic Disparities in Health Care* (2003), on health care disparities. The study process was also facilitated and informed by the published summaries of workshops conducted under the auspices of the IOM Roundtable on Value & Science-Driven Health Care. Over the past 6 years, 11 workshop summaries have been produced, exploring various aspects of the challenges and opportunities in health care today, with a particular focus on the foundational elements of a learning health system.

Meeting the challenges discussed at those workshops has taken on great urgency as a result of two overarching imperatives:

- to manage the health care system's ever-increasing **complexity,** and
- to curb ever-escalating **costs.**

The convergence of these imperatives makes the status quo untenable. At the same time, however, opportunities exist to address these problems— opportunities that did not exist even a decade ago:

- vast **computational power** that is affordable and widely available;
- **connectivity** that allows information to be accessed in real time virtually anywhere;
- **human and organizational capabilities** that improve the reliability and efficiency of care processes; and
- the recognition that effective care must be delivered by **collaborations between teams of clinicians and patients,** each playing a vital role in the care process.

The committee undertook its work to consider how these opportunities for best care at lower cost can be leveraged to meet the challenges outlined above. The committee, whose work was supported by the Blue Shield of California Foundation, the Charina Endowment Fund, and the Robert Wood Johnson Foundation, was charged with (1) identifying how the effectiveness and efficiency of the current health care system can be transformed through tools and incentives for continuous assessment and improvement and (2) developing recommendations for actions that can be taken to that end. This report explores the imperatives for change, describes the emerging tools that make transformation possible, sets forth a vision for a continuously learning health care system, and delineates a path for achieving this vision. Detailed findings are presented throughout the report, together with the conclusions and recommendations they support, which are also highlighted in this summary.

The title of the report underscores that care that is based on the best available evidence, takes appropriate account of individual preferences, and is delivered reliably and efficiently—*best care*—is possible today. When such care is routinely implemented, moreover, it is generally less expensive than the less effective, less efficient care that is now too commonly provided. Moreover, the transition to best care envisioned in this report is urgently needed given the budgetary, economic, and health pressures facing the nation's health care system.

THE IMPERATIVES

Decades of rapid innovation and technological improvement have created an extraordinarily complex health care system. Clinicians and health care staff work tirelessly to care for their patients in an increasingly complex, inefficient, and stressful environment. Certain breakthrough innovations have benefited millions of patients, but the aggregate impact of the flood of new interventions has introduced challenges for both clinicians and patients in treating and managing health conditions. In addition to the challenge of complexity, and in part because of it, health care often falls short of its potential in the quality of care delivered and the patient outcomes achieved. These shortfalls are occurring even as costs are rising to unsustainable levels. Additionally, new opportunities emerging from technology, industry, and policy can be leveraged to help mold the system into one characterized by continuous learning and improvement. In this context, the committee identified three imperatives for achieving a continuously learning health care system that provides the best care at lower cost: (1) managing rapidly increasing complexity; (2) achieving greater value in health care; and (3) capturing opportunities from technology, industry, and policy.

Managing Rapidly Increasing Complexity

The complexity of health care has increased in multiple dimensions—in the ever-increasing treatment, diagnostic, and care management options available; in the rapidly rising levels of biomedical and clinical evidence; and in administrative complexities, from complicated workflows to fragmented financing. The complexity due to ever-increasing treatment options can be illustrated by the evolution of care for two common conditions— heart disease and cancer. During much of the twentieth century, heart attacks commonly were treated with weeks of bed rest. Today, advanced diagnostics allow for customized treatments for patients; interventions such as percutaneous coronary interventions and coronary artery bypass grafts can reopen blocked vessels and restore blood flow to the heart; and pharmaceutical therapies, such as thrombolytics and beta-blockers, improve survival and reduce the chances of subsequent heart attacks (Certo, 1985; Nabel and Braunwald, 2012). Similarly, five decades ago, breast cancer was detected from a physical exam, and mastectomy was the recommended treatment. Today, multiple imaging technologies exist for the detection and diagnosis of the disease, and once diagnosed, the cancer can be further classified and treated according to genetic characteristics and hormone receptor status (Harrison, 1962; IOM, 2001b; Kasper and Harrison, 2005).

As a result of improved scientific understanding, new treatments and interventions, and new diagnostic technologies, the U.S. health care system now is characterized by more to do, more to know, and more to manage than at any time in history. As one quantification of this increase, the volume of the biomedical and clinical knowledge base has rapidly expanded, with research publications having risen from more than 200,000 per year in 1970 to more than 750,000 in 2010 (see Figure S-1). The result is a

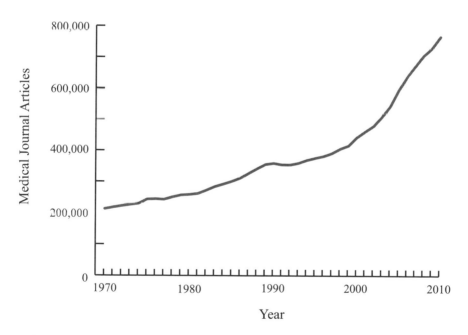

FIGURE S-1 Number of journal articles published on health care topics per year from 1970 to 2010. Publications have increased steadily over 40 years, with the rate of increase becoming more pronounced starting approximately in 2000.
SOURCE: Data obtained from online searches at PubMed: http://www.ncbi.nlm.nih.gov/pubmed/.

paradox: advances in science and technology have improved the ability of the health care system to treat diseases, yet the sheer volume of new discoveries stresses the capabilities of the system to effectively generate and manage knowledge and apply it to regular care. These advances have occurred at the same time as, and sometimes have contributed to, challenges in health care quality and value.

> *Conclusion: Diagnostic and treatment options are expanding and changing at an accelerating rate, placing new stresses on clinicians and patients, as well as potentially impacting the effectiveness and efficiency of care delivery.*

Beyond the increasing stores of biomedical and clinical knowledge, changes in disease prevalence and patient demographics have altered the landscape for care delivery. The prevalence of chronic conditions, for example, has increased over time. In 2000, 125 million people suffered from such conditions; by 2020, that number is projected to grow to an estimated 157 million (Anderson, 2010). The role of chronic diseases has changed as the demographics of the population have shifted. In general, the population has gotten older; in the past decade, the portion of the population over age 65 has increased at 1.5 times the rate of the rest of the population (Howden and Meyer, 2011). Almost half of those over 65 receive treatment for at least one chronic disease, and more than 20 percent receive treatment for multiple chronic diseases (Schneider et al., 2009); fully 75 million people in the United States have multiple chronic conditions (Parekh and Barton, 2010).

Managing these multiple conditions requires a holistic approach, because the use of various clinical practice guidelines developed for single diseases may have adverse effects (Boyd et al., 2005a; Parekh and Barton, 2010; Tinetti et al., 2004). For example, existing clinical practice guidelines would suggest that a hypothetical 79-year-old woman with osteoporosis, osteoarthritis, type 2 diabetes, hypertension, and chronic obstructive pulmonary disease should take as many as 19 doses of medication per day. Such guidelines might also make conflicting recommendations for the woman's care. If she had peripheral neuropathy, guidelines for osteoporosis would recommend that she perform weight-bearing exercise, while guidelines for diabetes would recommend that she avoid such exercise (Boyd et al., 2005a). These situations create uncertainty for clinicians and patients as to the best course of action to pursue as they attempt to manage the treatments for multiple conditions.

> *Conclusion: Chronic diseases and comorbid conditions are increasing, exacerbating the clinical, logistical, decision-making, and economic challenges faced by patients and clinicians.*

Care delivery also has become increasingly demanding. It would take an estimated 21 hours per day for individual primary care physicians to provide all of the care recommended to meet their patients' acute, preventive, and chronic disease management needs (Yarnall et al., 2009). Clinicians in intensive care units, who care for the sickest patients in a hospital, must manage in the range of 180 activities per patient per day—from replacing intravenous fluids, to administering drugs, to monitoring patients' vital signs (Donchin et al., 2003). In addition, rising administrative burdens and inefficient workflows mean that hospital nurses spend only about 30 percent of their time in direct patient care (Hendrich et al., 2008; Hendrickson et al., 1990; Tucker and Spear, 2006). These pressures are not limited to clinicians; patients often find the health care system uncoordinated, opaque, and stressful to navigate. One study found that for 1 of every 14 tests, either the patient was not informed of a clinically significant abnormal test result, or the clinician failed to record reporting the result to the patient (Casalino et al., 2009).

With specialization, moreover, clinicians must coordinate with multiple other providers; for their health care, Medicare patients now see an average of seven physicians, including five specialists, split among four different practices (Pham et al., 2007). One study found that in a single year, a typical primary care physician coordinated with an average of 229 other physicians in 117 different practices just for Medicare patients (Pham et al., 2009). The involvement of multiple providers tends to blur accountability. One survey found that 75 percent of hospital patients were unable to identify the clinician in charge of their care (Arora et al., 2009).

Conclusion: Care delivery has become increasingly fragmented, leading to coordination and communication challenges for patients and clinicians.

Achieving Greater Value In Health Care

In addition to, and sometimes as a result of, the challenge of complexity, health care quality and outcomes often fall short of their potential. A decade after the IOM (1999) estimated that 44,000 to 98,000 patients died each year from preventable medical errors, recent studies have reported that as many as one-third of hospitalized patients may experience harm or an adverse event, often from preventable errors (Classen et al., 2011; Landrigan et al., 2010; Levinson, 2010). While infections and complications once were viewed as routine consequences of medical care, it is now recognized that strategies and evidence-based interventions exist that can significantly reduce the incidence and severity of such events.

Similarly, medical care often is guided insufficiently by evidence, with Americans receiving only about half of the preventive, acute, and chronic care recommended by current research and evidence-based guidelines (McGlynn et al., 2003). Sometimes this occurs because available evidence is not applied to clinical care, while in other cases evidence is not available.

As a result of all of these factors, the nature and quality of health care vary considerably among states, with serious health and economic consequences. If all states could provide care of the quality delivered by the highest-performing state, an estimated 75,000 fewer deaths would have occurred across the country in 2005 (McCarthy et al., 2009; Schoenbaum et al., 2011).

> *Conclusion: Health care safety, quality, and outcomes for Americans fall substantially short of their potential and vary significantly for different populations of Americans.*

These deficiencies in care quality have occurred even as expenses have risen significantly. Health care costs[1] have increased at a greater rate than the economy as a whole for 31 of the past 40 years, and now constitute 18 percent of the nation's gross domestic product (CMS, 2012; Keehan et al., 2011). The growth in health care costs has contributed to stagnation in real income for American families. Although income has increased by 30 percent over the past decade, these gains have effectively been eliminated by a 76 percent increase in health care costs (Auerbach and Kellermann, 2011). These high costs have strained families' budgets and put health insurance coverage out of reach for many, contributing to the 50 million Americans without coverage (DeNavas-Walt et al., 2011).

In addition to unsustainable cost growth, there is evidence that a substantial proportion of health care expenditures is wasted, leading to little improvement in health or in the quality of care. Estimates vary on waste and excess health care costs, but they are large. The IOM workshop summary *The Healthcare Imperative: Lowering Costs and Improving Outcomes* contains estimates of excess costs in six domains: unnecessary services, services inefficiently delivered, prices that are too high, excess administrative costs, missed prevention opportunities, and medical fraud (IOM, 2010). These estimates, presented by workshop speakers with respect to their areas of expertise and based on assumptions from limited observations, suggest the

---

[1] In this report, *price* refers to the amount charged for a given health care service or product. It is important to note that there are frequently multiple prices for the same service or product, depending on the patient's insurance status and payer, as well as other factors. *Cost* is the total sum of money spent at a given level (episodes, patients, organizations, state, national), or price multiplied by the volume of services or products used.

substantial contribution of each domain to excessive health care costs (see Table S-1).

Although these estimates have unknown overlap, the sum of the individual estimates—$765 billion—suggests the significant scale of waste in the system. Two other independent and differing analytic approaches—considering regional variation in costs and comparing costs across countries—produce similar estimates, with total excess costs approaching $750 billion in 2009 (Farrell et al., 2008; IOM, 2010; Wennberg et al., 2002).

TABLE S-1 Estimated Sources of Excess Costs in Health Care (2009)

Category	Sources	Estimate of Excess Costs
Unnecessary Services	• Overuse—beyond evidence-established levels • Discretionary use beyond benchmarks • Unnecessary choice of higher-cost services	$210 billion
Inefficiently Delivered Services	• Mistakes—errors, preventable complications • Care fragmentation • Unnecessary use of higher-cost providers • Operational inefficiencies at care delivery sites	$130 billion
Excess Administrative Costs	• Insurance paperwork costs beyond benchmarks • Insurers' administrative inefficiencies • Inefficiencies due to care documentation requirements	$190 billion
Prices That Are Too High	• Service prices beyond competitive benchmarks • Product prices beyond competitive benchmarks	$105 billion
Missed Prevention Opportunities	• Primary prevention • Secondary prevention • Tertiary prevention	$55 billion
Fraud	• All sources—payers, clinicians, patients	$75 billion

SOURCE: Adapted with permission from IOM, 2010.

While there are methodological issues with each method for estimating excess costs, the consistently large figures produced by each signal the potential for reducing health care costs while improving quality and health outcomes.

At this level, unnecessary health care costs and waste exceed the 2009 budget for the Department of Defense by more than $100 billion (OMB, 2010). Health care waste also amounts to more than 1.5 times the nation's total infrastructure investment in 2004, including roads, railroads, aviation, drinking water, telecommunications, and other structures.[2] To put these estimates in the context of health care expenditures, the estimated redirected funds could provide health insurance coverage for more than 150 million workers (including both employer and employee contributions), which exceeds the 2009 civilian labor force.[3] And the total projected amounts could pay the salaries of all of the nation's first response personnel, including firefighters, police officers, and emergency medical technicians, for more than 12 years.[4]

> *Conclusion: The growth rate of health care expenditures is unsustainable, with waste that diverts major resources from necessary care and other priorities at every level—individual, family, community, state, and national.*

In sum, as illustrated in Figure S-2, each stage in the processes that shape the health care received—knowledge development, translation into medical evidence, application of evidence-based care—has prominent shortcomings and inefficiencies that contribute to a large reservoir of missed opportunities, waste, and harm. The threats to the health and economic security of Americans are clear, present, and compelling.

---

[2]The Department of Defense budget was calculated from the fiscal year 2009 outlays listed in the Fiscal Year 2011 U.S. Government Budget (OMB, 2010); the comparison of health care waste with the national infrastructure investment was drawn from a Congressional Budget Office analysis, with inflation adjusted according to the Consumer Price Index (CPI) (Congressional Budget Office, 2008).

[3]The average premiums for a single worker were calculated using the Kaiser Family Foundation's 2009 Employer Health Benefits survey, with the size of the civilian labor force drawn from Bureau of Labor Statistics estimates for 2009 (Kaiser Family Foundation and Health Research & Educational Trust, 2009; U.S. Bureau of Labor Statistics, 2012).

[4]The comparison with expenditures on first responders was calculated from the annual salary data for firefighters, police officers, and emergency medical technicians provided in the 2009 National Compensation Survey, while the total number of individuals in those occupations was drawn from the 2009 Occupational Employment Statistics (U.S. Bureau of Labor Statistics, 2010a,b).

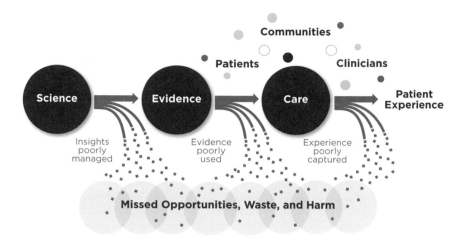

FIGURE S-2 Schematic of the health care system today.

Capturing Opportunities from Technology, Industry, and Policy

As noted earlier, new opportunities exist to address the challenges outlined above. Just as the information revolution has transformed many other fields, growing stores of data and computational abilities hold the same promise for improving clinical research, clinical practice, and clinical decision making. In the past three decades, for example, computer processing speed has grown by 60 percent per year on average, while the capacity to share information over telecommunications networks has risen by an average of 30 percent per year (Hilbert and López, 2011). These advances in computing and connectivity have the potential to improve health care by expanding the reach of knowledge, increasing access to clinical information when and where needed, and assisting patients and providers in managing chronic diseases. Studies also have found that using such electronic systems can improve safety—one study reported a 41 percent reduction in potential adverse drug events following the implementation of a computerized patient management system (computerized physician order entry, or CPOE), while another estimated that overall medication error rates dropped by 81 percent (Bates et al., 1998, 1999; Potts et al., 2004). Projections are for 90 percent of office-based physicians to have access to fully operational electronic health records by 2019, up from 34 percent in 2011 (Congressional Budget Office, 2009; Hsiao et al., 2011). Because these capacities are relatively early in their development in the health care arena, there is substantial room for progress as they are implemented in the field. However, multiple nontechnological developments, such as supportive care processes, governance, and patient and public engagement, will be necessary if these technologies are to reach their full potential.

> *Conclusion: Advances in computing, information science, and connectivity can improve patient-clinician communication, point-of-care guidance, the capture of experience, population surveillance, planning and evaluation, and the generation of real-time knowledge—features of a continuously learning health care system.*

In addition to advances in computing and connectivity, new organizational capabilities have been developed in diverse industries to improve safety, quality, reliability, and value. Advances in safety alone, for instance, enabled domestic commercial commuter airlines to report no fatalities from 2007 to 2010 (Bureau of Transportation Statistics, 2011). New capabilities in systems engineering, operations management, and production can be adapted to health care settings to improve performance. In one study, the use of checklists inspired by the aviation industry eliminated catheter-related bloodstream infections in the intensive care units of most hospitals in the study and resulted in an 80 percent decrease in infections per catheter-day (Pronovost et al., 2006, 2009). Commercial strategies to improve the reliability of the delivery of goods and services have potential applicability to health care as well. A pharmacy unit, for example, undertook systematic problem solving and reduced the time spent searching for medications by 30 percent and the frequency of out-of-stock medications by 85 percent (Spear, 2005).

> *Conclusion: Systematic, evidence-based process improvement methods applied in various sectors to achieve often striking results in safety, quality, reliability, and value can be similarly transformative for health care.*

Across the United States, moreover, there is growing momentum to implement novel partnerships and collaborations to test delivery system innovations aimed at high-value, high-quality health care. In many settings, stakeholders at all levels—federal, state, and local governments; public and private insurers; health care delivery organizations; employers; patients and consumers; and others—are working together with the shared objectives of controlling health care costs and improving health care quality. States ranging from Massachusetts to Utah to Vermont have introduced new initiatives aimed at expanding health insurance coverage, improving care quality and value, and advancing the overall health of their residents. Multiple initiatives by employers, specialty societies, patient and consumer groups, health care delivery organizations, health plans, and others—such as the American Board of Internal Medicine (ABIM) Foundation's Choosing Wisely® campaign and the Good Stewardship project—are focused on improving the health care system. Other initiatives currently under way range from the Patient-Centered Primary Care Collaborative, which seeks to spread patient-centered medical homes; to community-based initiatives, such as the Aligning Forces for Quality program and the Chartered Value Exchange project; to all-payer databases being established in various states around the country. And drawing on their experiences in improving outcomes and lowering costs through initiatives in their own institutions, a group of health care delivery leaders has developed "A CEO Checklist for High-Value Health Care," which describes system-change approaches that can be adopted in most health care settings to improve outcomes and reduce costs of care (Cosgrove et al., 2012) (see Appendix B). The convergence of these novel partnerships, a changing health care landscape, and investments in knowledge infrastructure has created a unique opportunity to achieve continuously learning health care.

> *Conclusion: Innovative public- and private-sector health system improvement initiatives, if adopted broadly, could support many elements of the transformation necessary to achieve a continuously learning health care system.*

THE VISION

The committee believes that achieving a learning health care system—one in which science and informatics, patient-clinician partnerships, incentives, and culture are aligned to promote and enable continuous and real-time improvement in both the effectiveness and efficiency of care—is both necessary and possible for the nation. Table S-2 lists the fundamental characteristics of such a system, according to the major dimensions in play.

There are challenges to implementing this vision in real-world clinical environments. Clinicians routinely report moderate or high levels of stress, feel there is not enough time to meet their patients' needs, and find their work environment chaotic (Burdi and Baker, 1999; Linzer et al., 2009; Trude, 2003). Furthermore, they struggle to deliver care while confronting inefficient workflows, administrative burdens, and uncoordinated systems. These time pressures, stresses, and inefficiencies prevent clinicians from focusing on additional tasks and initiatives, even those that have important goals for improving care. Similarly, professionals working in health care organizations are overwhelmed by the sheer volume of initiatives currently under way to improve various aspects of the care process, initiatives that appear to be unconnected with the organization's priorities. Often, these

TABLE S-2 Characteristics of a Continuously Learning Health Care System

Science and Informatics
  Real-time access to knowledge—A learning health care system continuously and reliably captures, curates, and delivers the best available evidence to guide, support, tailor, and improve clinical decision making and care safety and quality.
  Digital capture of the care experience—A learning health care system captures the care experience on digital platforms for real-time generation and application of knowledge for care improvement.

Patient-Clinician Partnerships
  Engaged, empowered patients—A learning health care system is anchored on patient needs and perspectives and promotes the inclusion of patients, families, and other caregivers as vital members of the continuously learning care team.

Incentives
  Incentives aligned for value—A learning health care system has incentives actively aligned to encourage continuous improvement, identify and reduce waste, and reward high-value care.

  Full transparency—A learning health care system systematically monitors the safety, quality, processes, prices, costs, and outcomes of care, and makes information available for care improvement and informed choices and decision making by clinicians, patients, and their families.

Continuous Learning Culture
  Leadership-instilled culture of learning—A learning health care system is stewarded by leadership committed to a culture of teamwork, collaboration, and adaptability in support of continuous learning as a core aim.

  Supportive system competencies—A learning health care system constantly refines complex care operations and processes through ongoing team training and skill building, systems analysis and information development, and creation of the feedback loops for continuous learning and system improvement.

initiatives may be successful in one setting yet may not translate to other parts of the same organization.

Given such real-world impediments, initiatives that focus merely on incremental improvements and add to a clinician's daily workload are unlikely to succeed. Just as the quantity of clinical information now available exceeds the capacity of any individual to absorb and apply it, the number of tasks needed for regular care outstrips the capabilities of any individual. Significant change can occur only if the environment, context, and systems in which these professionals practice are reconfigured so that the entire health care infrastructure and culture support learning and improvement.

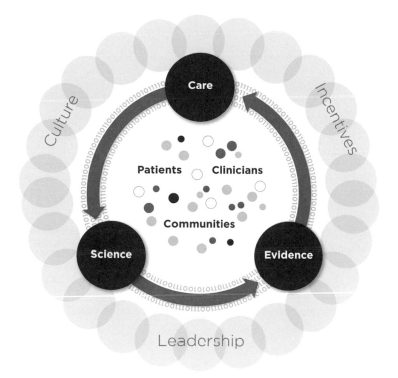

FIGURE S-3 Schematic of the continuously learning health care system.

Figure S-3 illustrates the committee's vision of how systematically capturing and translating information generated by clinical research and care delivery can close now open-ended learning loops.

THE PATH

The path to achieving the vision of a learning health care system entails generating and using real-time knowledge to improve outcomes; engaging patients, families, and communities; achieving and rewarding high-value care; and creating a new culture of care.

Generating and Using Real-Time Knowledge to Improve Outcomes

Although unprecedented and increasing levels of information are available in journals, guidelines, and other sources, patients and clinicians often lack practical access to guidance that is relevant, timely, and useful for the circumstances at hand. For example, fewer than half of the clinical guidelines for the nine most common chronic conditions consider older patients with multiple comorbid chronic conditions, even though, as noted earlier, 75 million Americans fall in that category (Boyd et al., 2005b; Parekh and Barton, 2010). In the case of localized prostate cancer, for instance, which treatment works best for a given patient—from watchful waiting, to radical prostatectomy, to radiation and chemotherapy—is unknown. Furthermore, the evidence base for clinical guidelines and recommendations needs to be strengthened. In some cases, 40 to 50 percent of the recommendations made in guidelines are based on expert opinion, case studies, or standards of care rather than on more systematic trials and studies (Chauhan et al., 2006; IOM, 2008, 2011a; Tricoci et al., 2009).

New methods are needed to address current limitations in clinical research. The cost of current clinical research methods averages $15-$20 million for larger studies—and much more for some—yet there are concerns about generalizing study results to all practice conditions and patient populations (Holve and Pittman, 2009, 2011). Given the increasing number of new medical treatments and technologies, the complexity of managing multiple chronic diseases, and the growing personalization of treatments and diagnostics, the challenge is to produce and deliver practical evidence that clinicians and patients can apply to clinical questions.

Conclusion: Despite the accelerating pace of scientific discovery, the current clinical research enterprise does not sufficiently address pressing clinical questions. The result is decisions by both patients and clinicians that are inadequately informed by evidence.

Meeting this challenge will require new approaches for generating clinical evidence that reduce the expense and effort of conducting research and improve the clinical applicability of research findings while retaining the rigorous reliability of the process. The issue is not determining which research method is best for a particular condition, but which method provides the information most appropriate to a particular clinical need. Each study must be well tailored to provide useful, practical, and reliable results for the condition at hand.

Opportunities for achieving these aims leverage the expanded capacity of the digital infrastructure along with new statistical and research techniques. Computational capabilities present promising, as yet unrealized, opportunities for care improvement, while advances in statistical analysis, simulation, and modeling can supplement traditional methods for conducting trials. The application of computing capacity and new analytic approaches enables the development of real-time research insights from patient populations. For example, one study found that real-time analysis of clinical data from electronic health records could have identified the increased risk of heart attack associated with one diabetes drug within 18 months of its introduction, as opposed to the 7-8 years between the medication's introduction and the point at which concerns were raised publicly (Brownstein et al., 2010). Computational capabilities also hold promise for hastening the derivation of important new insights from the care experience. A comprehensive disease registry for heart attack patients in Sweden, for example, has contributed to a 65 percent reduction in 30-day mortality and a 49 percent decrease in 1-year mortality from heart attacks (Larsson et al., 2012).

> *Conclusion: Growing computational capabilities to generate, communicate, and apply new knowledge create the potential to build a clinical data infrastructure to support continuous learning and improvement in health care.*

Harnessing this potential for care improvement will require systematic approaches that address the regulatory, commercial, communications, and technological challenges involved. Results of surveys of health researchers suggest that the current formulation and interpretation of privacy rules have increased the cost and time to conduct research, impeded collaboration, and hampered the recruiting of subjects (IOM, 2009; Ness, 2007). Privacy is a highly important societal and personal value, but the current rules, with their inconsistent interpretation, offer a relatively limited security advantage to patients while impeding the pace and scope of new insights from health research and care improvement.

> *Conclusion: Regulations governing the collection and use of clinical data often create unnecessary and unintended barriers to the effectiveness and improvement of care and the derivation of research insights.*

The current system for capturing and using new knowledge is already flawed and, absent change, is likely to be overwhelmed by the pace of knowledge growth. The diffusion of new evidence can take considerable time; in the case of thrombolytic drugs for heart attack treatment, for example, 13 years elapsed between when they were shown to be effective and when most experts recommended the treatment (Antman et al., 1992). Substantial work is required to identify high-quality evidence that minimizes the risk of contradiction by later studies and is sufficiently robust to provide insight on application to a particular patient's clinical circumstances. This is time-consuming work, which goes on while clinical patterns are being formed.

Realizing the prospect of faster, deeper knowledge bases will require parallel advances in the approaches to gathering and assessing evidence, making evidence-based recommendations, translating those recommendations to practice, and reinforcing their use through relevant policies. Computing capacity can help with assessment as well as dissemination. Technological tools, such as decision support tools that can be broadly embedded in electronic health records, hold promise for improving the application of evidence. One study found that digital decision support tools helped clinicians apply clinical guidelines, improving health outcomes for diabetics by 15 percent (Cebul et al., 2011).

Conclusion: *As the pace of knowledge generation accelerates, new approaches are needed to deliver the right information, in a clear and understandable format, to patients and clinicians as they partner to make clinical decisions.*

Engaging Patients, Families, and Communities[5]

The structure, incentives, and culture of the health care system are poorly aligned to engage patients and respond to their needs. While clinicians supply information and advice based on their scientific expertise in treatment and intervention options, as well as potential outcomes, patients, their families, and other caregivers bring personal knowledge regarding the suitability—or lack thereof—of different treatments for the patient's circumstances and preferences. Information from *both* sources is needed to select the right care option, particularly because studies have found that patients and clinicians have differing views on the importance of different health goals and health care risks (Lee et al., 2010a,b). At the same time, it is important to note that patient-centered care does not mean simply agreeing to every patient request. Rather, it entails meaningful awareness, discussion, and engagement among patient, family, and clinician on the evidence, risks and benefits, options, and decisions in play.

Currently, patients often are insufficiently involved in their care decisions. Even when they are encouraged to play a role in decisions about their care, they often lack understandable, reliable information—from evidence on the efficacy and risks of different treatment options to information on the quality of different providers and health care organizations—that is customized to their needs, preferences, and health goals. Fewer than half

---

[5] While the term *patients* is used in this report for brevity, it always refers to patients, families and other caregivers, and the public. Similarly, the term *communities* includes all forms of community, such as those defined by geography, culture, disease or condition, occupation, and workplace.

of patients receive clear information on the benefits and trade-offs of treatments for their condition, and fewer than half are satisfied with their level of control in medical decision making (Degner et al., 1997; Fagerlin et al., 2010; IOM, 2011b; Lee et al., 2011, 2012; Sepucha et al., 2010).

To improve patients' involvement in their care decisions, communication tools need to be developed and customized to patient circumstances. Given the complexity of health care, even highly educated people may have difficulty finding and understanding health information and applying it to their own care or that of their loved ones (IOM, 2004), and those who produce health care information need to consider how that information will be received and used by patients (Maurer et al., 2012). Technology offers opportunities for clinicians to engage patients by meeting with them where they are. These opportunities include improving communications outside of traditional clinical visits by providing new venues for care; assisting patients in managing their own health; and explaining options for shared clinical decisions, a capability that highlights health professionals' need to assume new roles in partnering with patients in the use of reliable online sources of health information (Brach et al., 2012).

Patient-centered care takes on increasing importance in light of research linking such care to better health outcomes, lower costs, an enhanced care experience, better quality of life, and other benefits. Patient and family involvement in health care decisions has been associated in primary care settings with reduced pain and discomfort, faster recovery in physical health, and improvements in emotional health (Stewart et al., 2000). Well-informed patients also often choose less aggressive and costly therapies. For example, it has been reported that informed patients are up to 20 percent less likely than other patients to choose elective surgery (O'Connor et al., 2009; Stacey et al., 2011). Similarly, patient-centered communication in primary care visits has been correlated with fewer diagnostic tests and referrals (Epstein et al., 2005; Stewart et al., 2000), as well as with annual charges in the range of 33 percent lower (Bertakis and Azari, 2011a,b).

Not all care delivered in the name of patient-centeredness reduces costs or improves outcomes. For example, one study found that patient-centeredness was associated with better outcomes but also higher costs (Bechel et al., 2000). Other studies have yielded mixed results with respect to cost, quality, and value for care models that aim to implement different aspects of patient-centeredness, such as disease management and care coordination programs (Nelson, 2012; Peikes et al., 2009). This may be related in part to the difficulty of identifying what truly constitutes patient-centered care, with well-meaning but poorly informed efforts producing changes that are superficial and adding little value to the experience. In the name of patient-centeredness, for example, some health care organizations have adopted luxury, hotel-like amenities or renovated their facilities. Although some of these initiatives may appeal to patient tastes, they do not achieve the true goals of patient-centered care and may increase costs while not directly addressing the patient's needs, preferences, or goals most important to improving quality, health, and value.

This report builds on the definition of patient-centered care offered in *Crossing the Quality Chasm*: "providing care that is respectful of and responsive to individual patient preferences, needs, and values and ensuring that patient values guide all decisions" (IOM, 2001a). The concept encompasses multiple dimensions, including respect for patients' values, preferences, and needs; coordination and integration of care; information, communication, and education; physical comfort; emotional support; and involvement of family and friends. This definition provides a framework for care to be fully patient-centered.

> *Conclusion: Improved patient engagement is associated with better patient experience, health, and quality of life and better economic outcomes, yet patient and family participation in care decisions remains limited.*

Given the increasing incidence of chronic diseases, the complexity of modern health care, and the multiple determinants of health, the challenges facing the health care system cannot be met by any individual or organization acting alone. Yet care often is poorly coordinated among clinicians both within and across settings. In one survey, roughly 25 percent of patients noted that a test had to be repeated, often because the results had not been shared by another provider (Stremikis et al., 2011). This inadequate, sometimes absent, continuity of care endangers patients and contributes to system waste. For example, almost one-fifth of Medicare patients are rehospitalized within 30 days, often without seeing their primary care provider in the interim (Jencks et al., 2009). Comprehensive health care also requires accounting for factors typically outside of the traditional health care system. Most determinants of the health status of individuals and populations lie not in health care—medical care accounts for only 10 to 20 percent of overall health prospects—but in such factors as behavior, social circumstances, and environment. Thus, close clinical-community coordination is required to protect and improve health (McGinnis et al., 2002).

> *Conclusion: Coordination and integration of patient services currently are poor. Improvement in this area will require strong and sustained avenues of communication and cooperation between and among clinical and community stewards of services.*

Achieving and Rewarding High-Value Care

Health care payment policies strongly influence how care is delivered, whether new scientific insights and knowledge about best care are diffused broadly, and whether improvement initiatives succeed. Clinicians reimbursed for each service tend to recommend more visits and services than clinicians who are reimbursed under other payment methods. In one study, initiation of encounter- and procedure-based reimbursement for primary care led to an increased number of encounters and procedures, with visits increasing from 11 to 61 percent depending on the specialty (Helmchen and Lo Sasso, 2010). As with most aspects of health care, a variety of financial incentives and payment models currently are in use. However, most of these models tend to pay clinicians and health care organizations without a specific focus on patient health and value, which has contributed to waste and inefficiency. One study found, on average, only a 4.3 percent correlation between the quality of care delivered and the price of the medical service, with higher prices often being associated with lower quality (Office of the Attorney General of Massachusetts, 2011).

Conclusion: The prevailing approach to paying for health care, based predominantly on individual services and products, encourages wasteful and ineffective care.

Given the clear need for change, several health care organizations and health insurers across the nation have been testing new models of paying for care and organizing care delivery. While many individual initiatives have demonstrated success, evidence is conflicting on which payment models might work best and under what circumstances. Yet, it is clear that high-value care—the best care for the patient, with the optimal result for the circumstances, delivered at the right price—requires that payment and practice incentives be structured to reward the best outcomes for the patient.

To transition to a health care payment system that rewards value, assessment techniques are needed to identify and encourage high-value care. In part, this is a clinical effectiveness issue. Unnecessary and marginal treatments and tests have the potential for side effects and harm. But at its core, health care value is a basic representation of the efficient use of individual and societal resources—time, money—for individual and societal benefit. Because measures of value must fundamentally balance the results of care with the costs required to achieve the results, accurate information is needed on the various dimensions of cost, as well as the various dimensions of health—health status, quality of life, quality of care, satisfaction, and population health.

organization's operational model can incentivize continuous learning, help control variability and waste that do not contribute to quality care, recoup savings to invest in improving care processes and patient health, and make improvement sustainable.

> *Conclusion: Realizing the potential of a continuously learning health care system will require a sustained commitment to improvement, optimized operations, concomitant culture change, aligned incentives, and strong leadership within and across organizations.*

ACTIONS FOR CONTINUOUS LEARNING, BEST CARE, AND LOWER COSTS

Based on the findings and conclusions derived in the course of its work, the committee offers recommendations for specific actions that would accelerate progress toward continuous learning, best care, and lower costs. As displayed in Box S-1, these recommendations can be grouped into three categories: foundational elements, care improvement targets, and a supportive policy environment.

Following are the committee's recommendations, which are supported by the material presented in the full report; also identified are the stakeholders whose engagement is necessary for the implementation of each recommendation. Each recommendation describes the core improvement aim for the area, followed by specific strategies representing initial steps that stakeholders should take in acting on the recommendation. Additional activities will have to be undertaken by numerous stakeholder groups to sustain and advance the continuous improvement required.

Foundational Elements

Recommendation 1: The Digital Infrastructure

Improve the capacity to capture clinical, care delivery process, and financial data for better care, system improvement, and the generation of new knowledge. Data generated in the course of care delivery should be digitally collected, compiled, and protected as a reliable and accessible resource for care management, process improvement, public health, and the generation of new knowledge.

Strategies for progress toward this goal:

- *Health care delivery organizations* and *clinicians* should fully and effectively employ digital systems that capture patient care

---

BOX S-1
Categories of the Committee's Recommendations

Foundational Elements

Recommendation 1: *The digital infrastructure.* Improve the capacity to capture clinical, care delivery process, and financial data for better care, system improvement, and the generation of new knowledge.
Recommendation 2: *The data utility.* Streamline and revise research regulations to improve care, promote the capture of clinical data, and generate knowledge.

Care Improvement Targets

Recommendation 3: *Clinical decision support.* Accelerate integration of the best clinical knowledge into care decisions.
Recommendation 4: *Patient-centered care.* Involve patients and families in decisions regarding health and health care, tailored to fit their preferences.
Recommendation 5: *Community links.* Promote community-clinical partnerships and services aimed at managing and improving health at the community level.
Recommendation 6: *Care continuity.* Improve coordination and communication within and across organizations.
Recommendation 7: *Optimized operations.* Continuously improve health care operations to reduce waste, streamline care delivery, and focus on activities that improve patient health.

Supportive Policy Environment

Recommendation 8: *Financial incentives.* Structure payment to reward continuous learning and improvement in the provision of best care at lower cost.
Recommendation 9: *Performance transparency.* Increase transparency on health care system performance.
Recommendation 10: *Broad leadership.* Expand commitment to the goals of a continuously learning health care system.

---

experiences reliably and consistently, and implement standards and practices that advance the interoperability of data systems.

- *The National Coordinator for Health Information Technology, digital technology developers,* and *standards organizations* should ensure that the digital infrastructure captures and delivers the core data elements and interoperability needed to support better care, system improvement, and the generation of new knowledge.
- *Payers, health care delivery organizations,* and *medical product companies* should contribute data to research and analytic consortia to support expanded use of care data to generate new insights.

- *Patients* should participate in the development of a robust data utility; use new clinical communication tools, such as personal portals, for self-management and care activities; and be involved in building new knowledge, such as through patient-reported outcomes and other knowledge processes.
- The *Secretary of Health and Human Services* should encourage the development of distributed data research networks and expand the availability of departmental health data resources for translation into accessible knowledge that can be used for improving care, lowering costs, and enhancing public health.
- *Research funding agencies and organizations*, such as the *National Institutes of Health*, the *Agency for Healthcare Research and Quality*, the *Veterans Health Administration*, the *Department of Defense*, and the *Patient-Centered Outcomes Research Institute*, should promote research designs and methods that draw naturally on existing care processes and that also support ongoing quality improvement efforts.

Recommendation 2: The Data Utility

Streamline and revise research regulations to improve care, promote the capture of clinical data, and generate knowledge. Regulatory agencies should clarify and improve regulations governing the collection and use of clinical data to ensure patient privacy but also the seamless use of clinical data for better care coordination and management, improved care, and knowledge enhancement.

Strategies for progress toward this goal:

- The *Secretary of Health and Human Services* should accelerate and expand the review of the Health Insurance Portability and Accountability Act (HIPAA) and institutional review board (IRB) policies with respect to actual or perceived regulatory impediments to the protected use of clinical data, and clarify regulations and their interpretation to support the use of clinical data as a resource for advancing science and care improvement.
- *Patient and consumer groups, clinicians, professional specialty societies, health care delivery organizations, voluntary organizations, researchers,* and *grantmakers* should develop strategies and outreach to improve understanding of the benefits and importance of accelerating the use of clinical data to improve care and health outcomes.

Care Improvement Targets

Recommendation 3: Clinical Decision Support

Accelerate integration of the best clinical knowledge into care decisions. Decision support tools and knowledge management systems should be routine features of health care delivery to ensure that decisions made by clinicians and patients are informed by current best evidence.

Strategies for progress toward this goal:

- *Clinicians* and *health care organizations* should adopt tools that deliver reliable, current clinical knowledge to the point of care, and organizations should adopt incentives that encourage the use of these tools.
- *Research organizations, advocacy organizations, professional specialty societies,* and *care delivery organizations* should facilitate the development, accessibility, and use of evidence-based and harmonized clinical practice guidelines.
- *Public and private payers* should promote the adoption of decision support tools, knowledge management systems, and evidence-based clinical practice guidelines by structuring payment and contracting policies to reward effective, evidence-based care that improves patient health.
- *Health professional education programs* should teach new methods for accessing, managing, and applying evidence; engaging in lifelong learning; understanding human behavior and social science; and delivering safe care in an interdisciplinary environment.
- *Research funding agencies and organizations* should promote research into the barriers and systematic challenges to the dissemination and use of evidence at the point of care, and support research to develop strategies and methods that can improve the usefulness and accessibility of patient outcome data and scientific evidence for clinicians and patients.

Recommendation 4: Patient-Centered Care

Involve patients and families in decisions regarding health and health care, tailored to fit their preferences. Patients and families should be given the opportunity to be fully engaged participants at all levels, including individual care decisions, health system learning and improvement activities, and community-based interventions to promote health.

Strategies for progress toward this goal:

- *Patients and families* should expect to be offered full participation in their own care and health and encouraged to partner, according to their preference, with clinicians in fulfilling those expectations.
- *Clinicians* should employ high-quality, reliable tools and skills for informed shared decision making with patients and families, tailored to clinical needs, patient goals, social circumstances, and the degree of control patients prefer.
- *Health care delivery organizations,* including programs operated by the *Department of Defense,* the *Veterans Health Administration,* and the *Health Resources and Services Administration,* should monitor and assess patient perspectives and use the insights thus gained to improve care processes; establish patient portals to facilitate data sharing and communication among clinicians, patients, and families; and make high-quality, reliable tools available for shared decision making with patients at different levels of health literacy.
- The *Agency for Healthcare Research and Quality,* partnering with the *Centers for Medicare & Medicaid Services, other payers,* and *stakeholder organizations,* should support the development and testing of an accurate and reliable core set of measures of patient-centeredness for consistent use across the health care system.
- The *Centers for Medicare & Medicaid Services* and *other public and private payers* should promote and measure patient-centered care through payment models, contracting policies, and public reporting programs.
- *Digital technology developers* and *health product innovators* should develop tools to assist individuals in managing their health and health care, in addition to providing patient supports in new forms of communities.

Recommendation 5: Community Links

Promote community-clinical partnerships and services aimed at managing and improving health at the community level. Care delivery and community-based organizations and agencies should partner with each other to develop cooperative strategies for the design, implementation, and accountability of services aimed at improving individual and population health.

Strategies for progress toward this goal:

- *Health care delivery organizations* and *clinicians* should partner with *community-based organizations* and *public health agencies* to leverage and coordinate prevention, health promotion, and community-based interventions to improve health outcomes, including strategies related to the assessment and use of Web-based tools.
- *Public and private payers* should incorporate population health improvement into their health care payment and contracting policies and accountability measures.
- *Health economists, health service researchers, professional specialty societies,* and *measure development organizations* should continue to improve measures that can readily be applied to assess performance on both individual and population health.

Recommendation 6: Care Continuity

Improve coordination and communication within and across organizations. Payers should structure payment and contracting to reward effective communication and coordination between and among members of a patient's care team.

Strategies for progress toward this goal:

- *Health care delivery organizations* and *clinicians*, partnering with *patients, families,* and *community organizations*, should develop coordination and transition processes, data sharing capabilities, and communication tools to ensure safe, seamless patient care.
- *Health economists, health service researchers, professional specialty societies,* and *measure development organizations* should develop and test metrics with which to monitor and evaluate the effectiveness of care transitions in improving patient health outcomes.
- *Public and private payers* should promote effective care transitions that improve patient health through their payment and contracting policies.

Recommendation 7: Optimized Operations

Continuously improve health care operations to reduce waste, streamline care delivery, and focus on activities that improve patient health. Care delivery organizations should apply systems engineering tools and process improvement methods to improve operations and care delivery processes.

Strategies for progress toward this goal:

- *Health care delivery organizations* should utilize systems engineering tools and process improvement methods to eliminate inefficiencies, remove unnecessary burdens on clinicians and staff, enhance patient experience, and improve patient health outcomes.
- The *Centers for Medicare & Medicaid Services, the Agency for Healthcare Research and Quality, the Patient-Centered Outcomes Research Institute, quality improvement organizations,* and *process improvement leaders* should develop a learning consortium aimed at accelerating training, technical assistance, and the collection and validation of lessons learned about ways to transform the effectiveness and efficiency of care through continuous improvement programs and initiatives.

Supportive Policy Environment

Recommendation 8: Financial Incentives

Structure payment to reward continuous learning and improvement in the provision of best care at lower cost. Payers should structure payment models, contracting policies, and benefit designs to reward care that is effective and efficient and continuously learns and improves.

Strategies for progress toward this goal:

- *Public and private payers* should reward continuous learning and improvement through outcome- and value-oriented payment models, contracting policies, and benefit designs. Payment models should adequately incentivize and support high-quality team-based care focused on the needs and goals of patients and families.
- *Health care delivery organizations* should reward continuous learning and improvement through the use of internal practice incentives.
- *Health economists, health service researchers, professional specialty societies,* and *measure development organizations* should partner with *public and private payers* to develop and evaluate metrics, payment models, contracting policies, and benefit designs that reward high-value care that improves health outcomes.

Recommendation 9: Performance Transparency

Increase transparency on health care system performance. Health care delivery organizations, clinicians, and payers should increase the availability of information on the quality, prices and cost, and outcomes of care to help inform care decisions and guide improvement efforts.

Strategies for progress toward this goal:

- *Health care delivery organizations* should collect and expand the availability of information on the safety, quality, prices and cost, and health outcomes of care.
- *Professional specialty societies* should encourage transparency on the quality, value, and outcomes of the care provided by their members.
- *Public and private payers* should promote transparency in quality, value, and outcomes to aid plan members in their care decision making.
- *Consumer and patient organizations* should disseminate this information to facilitate discussion, informed decision making, and care improvement.

Recommendation 10: Broad Leadership

Expand commitment to the goals of a continuously learning health care system. Continuous learning and improvement should be a core and constant priority for all participants in health care—patients, families, clinicians, care leaders, and those involved in supporting their work.

Strategies for progress toward this goal:

- *Health care delivery organizations* should develop organizational cultures that support and encourage continuous improvement, the use of best practices, transparency, open communication, staff empowerment, coordination, teamwork, and mutual respect and align rewards accordingly.
- *Leaders* of these organizations should define, disseminate, support, and commit to a vision of continuous improvement; focus attention, training, and resources on continuous learning; and build an operational model that incentivizes continuous improvement and ensures its sustainability.
- *Governing boards of health care delivery organizations* should support and actively participate in fostering a culture of continuous

improvement, request continuous feedback on the progress being made toward the adoption of such a culture, and align leadership incentive structures accordingly.

- *Clinical professional specialty societies, health professional education programs, health professions specialty boards, licensing boards,* and *accreditation organizations* should incorporate basic concepts and specialized applications of continuous learning and improvement into health professions education; continuing education; and licensing, certification, and accreditation requirements.

Given the interconnected nature of the problems to be solved, it will be important to take the actions identified above in concert. To elevate the quantity of evidence available to inform clinical decisions, for example, it is necessary to increase the supply of evidence by expanding the clinical research base; make the evidence easily accessible by embedding it in clinical technological tools, such as clinical decision support; encourage use of the evidence through appropriate payment, contracting, and regulatory policies and cultural factors; and assess progress toward the goal using reliable metrics and appropriate transparency. The absence of any one of these factors will substantially limit overall improvement. To guide success, progress on the recommendations in this report should be monitored continuously.

ACHIEVING THE VISION

Implementing the actions detailed above and achieving the vision of continuous learning and improvement will depend on the exercise of broad leadership by the complex network of decentralized and loosely associated individuals and organizations that make up the health care system. Given the complexity of the system and the interconnectedness of its different actors and sectors, no one actor or sector alone can bring about the scope and scale of transformative change necessary to develop a system that continuously learns and improves. Each stakeholder brings different strengths, skills, needs, and expertise to the task of improving the system, faces unique challenges, and is accountable for different aspects of the system's success. There is a distinct need for collaboration between and among stakeholders to produce effective and sustainable change.

As the end users of all health care services, patients are central to the success of any improvement initiative. Any large-scale change will require the participation of patients as partners, with the system building trust on every dimension. Patients can promote learning and improvement by engaging in their own care; setting high expectations for their care in terms of quality, value, and the use of scientific evidence and selecting clinicians, organizations, and plans that meet those expectations; sharing decision making with their clinicians; and, with the help of their caregivers, directly applying evidence to their self-care and self-management on an ongoing basis.

Partnering with patients are the health care professionals who deliver care. Physicians, nurses, pharmacists, and other health professionals represent the front lines of health care delivery and the primary interface for patients and consumers. Expanding the supply of clinical information, promoting the use of evidence, and better involving patients in their care are all contingent upon the engagement and teaming of health professionals.

By convening their constituent professionals and providing a forum for action, professional societies have important roles in achieving the vision of a learning health care system. Through guidelines, performance measures, quality improvement initiatives, and data infrastructures for assessing performance with respect to specific procedures or conditions, these societies can take a leadership role in improving quality, safety, and efficiency.

Health care delivery organizations, because of their size and care capacities, have several levers by which they can steward progress toward a continuously improving system, such as using new practice methods, setting standards, and sharing resources and information with other care delivery organizations. Furthermore, through investments in health information technology, these organizations can build their capacity to perform near-real-time research, speeding the generation of practical evidence and its translation to the bedside.

Those who finance care also have opportunities to leverage their unique position to improve the quality and efficiency of care. As organizations that interact directly with patients, public and private payers can support patients as they seek to maintain healthy behaviors and access quality health care services, while their payment and contracting policies have a strong influence on how clinicians practice. Similarly, employers can support efforts to improve quality and value by using their purchasing power to drive improvement efforts through contracts with providers and insurers, the design of benefit plans, and the provision of incentives and information for employees.

Digital technology developers, health product innovators, and regulators are additional stakeholders that need to be engaged in achieving the vision of a learning health care system. Digital technology developers create the products and infrastructure necessary to meet the growing demand for capturing, storing, retrieving, and sharing information in virtually every aspect of health care. Continuous improvement in diagnostic and treatment options is contingent on a safe and innovative product development enterprise. Health product innovators, by conducting clinical research and devising new treatments and interventions, can develop novel products for diagnosis and treatment. Essential partners in this arena are regulators, including the Food and Drug Administration, who can work to develop streamlined methods for ensuring that safe, effective products are brought to market without delay.

A learning health care system depends on evidence to promote improvements in care delivery processes and patient care and overall system improvement. Consequently, health researchers are critical partners in generating knowledge on the effectiveness and value of interventions and care protocols. A commitment to practical and efficient research methods across the spectrum of the research enterprise—the design and operation of clinical trials, the development of clinical registries and clinical databases, the creation of standards and metrics, modeling and simulation studies, studies of health services and care delivery processes, and the aggregation of study results into systematic reviews and clinical guidelines—is foundational for a learning system. Through their programmatic and funding activities, private philanthropies, as well as agencies and organizations such as the Agency for Healthcare Research and Quality, the National Institutes of Health, and the Patient-Centered Outcomes Research Institute have a central role to play in the stewardship and strategic direction of these activities.

Missed opportunities for better health care have real human and economic impacts. If the care in every state was at the quality delivered by the highest performing state, there would have been an estimated 75,000 fewer deaths across the country in 2005 (McCarthy et al., 2009; Schoenbaum et al., 2011). Current waste diverts resources from productive use—an estimated $750 billion lost (IOM, 2010). It is only through shared commitments, in alignment with a supportive policy environment, that the opportunities offered by science and information technology can be captured to address the health care system's growing challenges and to ensure that it reaches its full potential to provide the best care for each patient. The nation's health and economic futures—best care at lower cost—depend on the ability to steward the evolution of a continuously learning health care system.

REFERENCES

Anderson, G. F. 2010. *Chronic care: Making the case for ongoing care.* Princeton, NJ: Robert Wood Johnson Foundation.

Antman, E. M., J. Lau, B. Kupelnick, F. Mosteller, and T. C. Chalmers. 1992. A comparison of results of meta-analyses of randomized control trials and recommendations of clinical experts. Treatments for myocardial infarction. *Journal of the American Medical Association* 268(2):240-248.

Arora, V., S. Gangireddy, A. Mehrotra, R. Ginde, M. Tormey, and D. Meltzer. 2009. Ability of hospitalized patients to identify their in-hospital physicians. *Archives of Internal Medicine* 169(2):199-201.

Auerbach, D. I., and A. L. Kellermann. 2011. A decade of health care cost growth has wiped out real income gains for an average US family. *Health Affairs* 30(9):1630-1636.

Bates, D. W., L. L. Leape, D. J. Cullen, N. Laird, L. A. Petersen, J. M. Teich, E. Burdick, M. Hickey, S. Kleefield, B. Shea, M. Vander Vliet, and D. L. Seger. 1998. Effect of computerized physician order entry and a team intervention on prevention of serious medication errors. *Journal of the American Medical Association* 280(15):1311-1316.

Bates, D. W., J. M. Teich, J. Lee, D. Seger, G. J. Kuperman, N. Ma'Luf, D. Boyle, and L. Leape. 1999. The impact of computerized physician order entry on medication error prevention. *Journal of the American Medical Informatics Association* 6(4):313-321.

Bechel, D. L., W. A. Myers, and D. G. Smith. 2000. Does patient-centered care pay off? *Joint Commission Journal on Quality Improvement* 26(7):400-409.

Bertakis, K. D., and R. Azari. 2011a. Determinants and outcomes of patient-centered care. *Patient Education and Counseling* 85(1):46-52.

Bertakis, K. D., and R. Azari. 2011b. Patient-centered care is associated with decreased health care utilization. *Journal of the American Board of Family Medicine* 24(3):229-239.

Boyd, C. M., J. Darer, C. Boult, L. P. Fried, L. Boult, and A. W. Wu. 2005a. Clinical practice guidelines and quality of care for older patients with multiple comorbid diseases. *Journal of the American Medical Association* 294(6):716.

Boyd, C. M., J. Darer, C. Boult, L. P. Fried, L. Boult, and A. W. Wu. 2005b. Clinical practice guidelines and quality of care for older patients with multiple comorbid diseases: Implications for pay for performance. *Journal of the American Medical Association* 294(6):716-724.

Brach, C., B. Dreyer, P. Schyve, L. M. Hernandez, C. Baur, A. J. Lemerise, and R. Parker. 2012. *Attributes of a health literate organization*. Discussion Paper, Institute of Medicine, Washington, DC. http://www.iom.edu/Global/Perspectives/2012/Attributes.aspx (accessed May 27, 2012).

Brownstein, J. S., S. N. Murphy, A. B. Goldfine, R. W. Grant, M. Sordo, V. Gainer, J. A. Colecchi, A. Dubey, D. M. Nathan, J. P. Glaser, and I. S. Kohane. 2010. Rapid identification of myocardial infarction risk associated with diabetes medications using electronic medical records. *Diabetes Care* 33(3):526-531.

Burdi, M. D., and L. C. Baker. 1999. Physicians' perceptions of autonomy and satisfaction in California. *Health Affairs* 18(4):134.

Bureau of Transportation Statistics. 2011. *National transportation statistics*. Washington, DC: Research and Innovation Technology Administration, U.S. Department of Transportation.

Casalino, L. P., D. Dunham, M. H. Chin, R. Bielang, E. O. Kistner, T. G. Karrison, M. K. Ong, U. Sarkar, M. A. McLaughlin, and D. O. Meltzer. 2009. Frequency of failure to inform patients of clinically significant outpatient test results. *Archives of Internal Medicine* 169(12):1123-1129.

Cebul, R. D., T. E. Love, A. K. Jain, and C. J. Hebert. 2011. Electronic health records and quality of diabetes care. *New England Journal of Medicine* 365(9):825-833.

Certo, C. M. 1985. History of cardiac rehabilitation. *Physical Therapy* 65(12):1793-1795.

Chauhan, S. P., V. Berghella, M. Sanderson, E. F. Magann, and J. C. Morrison. 2006. American College of Obstetricians and Gynecologists practice bulletins: An overview. *American Journal of Obstetrics and Gynecology* 194(6):1564-1572.

Chernew, M. E., R. E. Mechanic, B. E. Landon, and D. G. Safran. 2011. Private-payer innovation in Massachusetts: The "alternative quality contract." *Health Affairs (Millwood)* 30(1):51-61.

Classen, D. C., R. Resar, F. Griffin, F. Federico, T. Frankel, N. Kimmel, J. C. Whittington, A. Frankel, A. Seger, and B. C. James. 2011. "Global trigger tool" shows that adverse events in hospitals may be ten times greater than previously measured. *Health Affairs (Millwood)* 30(4):581-589.

CMS (Centers for Medicare & Medicaid Services). 2012. *National health expenditures summary and GDP: Calendar years 1960-2010.* http://www.cms.gov/Research-Statistics-Data-and-Systems/Statistics-Trends-and-Reports/NationalHealthExpendData/downloads/tables.pdf (accessed August 31, 2012).

Congressional Budget Office. 2008. *Issues and options in infrastructure investment.* Washington, DC: Congressional Budget Office.

Congressional Budget Office. 2009. *Health Information Technology for Economic and Clinical Health Act.* Washington, DC: Congressional Budget Office.

Cosgrove, D., M. Fisher, P. Gabow, G. Gottlieb, G. C. Halvorson, B. James, G. Kaplan, J. Perlin, R. Petzel, G. Steele, and J. Toussaint. 2012. *A CEO checklist for high-value health care.* Discussion Paper, Institute of Medicine, Washington, DC. http://www.iom.edu/CEOChecklist (accessed August 31, 2012).

Curry, L. A., E. Spatz, E. Cherlin, J. W. Thompson, D. Berg, H. H. Ting, C. Decker, H. M. Krumholz, and E. H. Bradley. 2011. What distinguishes top-performing hospitals in acute myocardial infarction mortality rates? A qualitative study. *Annals of Internal Medicine* 154(6):384-390.

Degner, L. F., L. J. Kristjanson, D. Bowman, J. A. Sloan, K. C. Carriere, J. O'Neil, B. Bilodeau, P. Watson, and B. Mueller. 1997. Information needs and decisional preferences in women with breast cancer. *Journal of the American Medical Association* 277(18):1485-1492.

DeNavas-Walt, C., B. D. Proctor, and J. C. Smith. 2011. *Income, poverty, and health insurance coverage in the United States: 2010.* Washington, DC: U.S. Census Bureau.

Donchin, Y., D. Gopher, M. Olin, Y. Badihi, M. Biesky, C. L. Sprung, R. Pizov, and S. Cotev. 2003. A look into the nature and causes of human errors in the intensive care unit. *Quality & Safety in Health Care* 12(2):143-147.

Epstein, R. M., P. Franks, C. G. Shields, S. C. Meldrum, K. N. Miller, T. L. Campbell, and K. Fiscella. 2005. Patient-centered communication and diagnostic testing. *Annals of Family Medicine* 3(5):415-421.

Fagerlin, A., K. R. Sepucha, M. P. Couper, C. A. Levin, E. Singer, and B. J. Zikmund-Fisher. 2010. Patients' knowledge about 9 common health conditions: The decisions survey. *Medical Decision Making* 30(Suppl. 5):S35-S52.

Farrell, D., E. Jensen, B. Kocher, N. Lovegrove, F. Melhem, L. Mendonca, and B. Parish. 2008. *Accounting for the cost of US health care: A new look at why Americans spend more.* Washington, DC: McKinsey Global Institute.

Harrison, T. R. 1962. *Principles of internal medicine.* 4th ed. New York: Blakiston Division, McGraw-Hill.

Helmchen, L. A., and A. T. Lo Sasso. 2010. How sensitive is physician performance to alternative compensation schedules? Evidence from a large network of primary care clinics. *Health Economics* 19(11):1300-1317.

Hendrich, A., M. P. Chow, B. A. Skierczynski, and Z. Lu. 2008. A 36-hospital time and motion study: How do medical-surgical nurses spend their time? *The Permanente Journal* 12(3):25-34.

Hendrickson, G., T. M. Doddato, and C. T. Kovner. 1990. How do nurses use their time? *Journal of Nursing Administration* 20(3):31-37.

Hilbert, M., and P. López. 2011. The world's technological capacity to store, communicate, and compute information. *Science* 332(6025):60-65.

Holve, E., and P. Pittman. 2009. *A first look at the volume and cost of comparative effectiveness research in the United States.* Washington, DC: AcademyHealth.

Holve, E., and P. Pittman. 2011. The cost and volume of comparative effectiveness research. In *Learning what works: Infrastructure required for comparative effectiveness research: Workshop summary.* Institute of Medicine. Washington, DC: The National Academies Press. Pp. 89-96.

Howden, L. M., and J. A. Meyer. 2011. *Age and sex composition: 2010.* Washington, DC: U.S. Census Bureau, U.S. Department of Commerce.

Hsiao, C.-J., E. Hing, T. C. Socey, and B. Cai. 2011. *Electronic health record systems and intent to apply for meaningful use incentives among office-based physician practices: United States, 2001-2011.* Hyattsville, MD: National Center for Health Statistics.

IOM (Institute of Medicine). 1999. *To err is human: Building a safer health system.* Washington, DC: National Academy Press.

IOM. 2001a. *Crossing the quality chasm: A new health system for the 21st century.* Washington, DC: National Academy Press.

IOM. 2001b. *Mammography and beyond: Developing technologies for the early detection of breast cancer.* Washington, DC: National Academy Press.

IOM. 2003. *Unequal treatment: Confronting racial and ethnic disparities in health care.* Washington, DC: The National Academies Press.

IOM. 2004. *Health literacy: A prescription to end confusion.* Washington, DC: The National Academies Press.

IOM. 2008. *Knowing what works in health care: A roadmap for the nation.* Washington, DC: The National Academies Press.

IOM. 2009. *Beyond the HIPAA privacy rule: Enhancing privacy, improving health through research.* Washington, DC: The National Academies Press.

IOM. 2010. *The healthcare imperative: Lowering costs and improving outcomes: Workshop series summary, Learning health system series.* Washington, DC: The National Academies Press.

IOM. 2011a. *Clinical practice guidelines we can trust.* Washington, DC: The National Academies Press.

IOM. 2011b. *Patients charting the course: Citizen engagement in the learning health system: Workshop summary.* Washington, DC: The National Academies Press.

Jencks, S. F., M. V. Williams, and E. A. Coleman. 2009. Rehospitalizations among patients in the Medicare fee-for-service program. *New England Journal of Medicine* 360(14):1418-1428.

Joint Commission. 2011. *Improving America's hospitals: The Joint Commission's annual report on quality and safety.* http://www.jointcommission.org/assets/1/6/IJC_Annual_Report_2011_9_13_11_.pdf (accessed September 25, 2011).

Kaiser Family Foundation and Health Research & Educational Trust. 2009. *Employer health benefits: 2009 annual survey.* Menlo Park, CA: Kaiser Family Foundation and Health Research & Educational Trust.

Kasper, D. L., and T. R. Harrison. 2005. *Harrison's principles of internal medicine.* 16th ed., 2 vols. New York: McGraw-Hill, Medical Publications Division.

Keehan, S. P., A. M. Sisko, C. J. Truffer, J. A. Poisal, G. A. Cuckler, A. J. Madison, J. M. Lizonitz, and S. D. Smith. 2011. National health spending projections through 2020: Economic recovery and reform drive faster spending growth. *Health Affairs (Millwood)* 30(8):1594-1605.

Landrigan, C. P., G. J. Parry, C. B. Bones, A. D. Hackbarth, D. A. Goldmann, and P. J. Sharek. 2010. Temporal trends in rates of patient harm resulting from medical care. *New England Journal of Medicine* 363(22):2124-2134.

Larsson, S., P. Lawyer, G. Garellick, B. Lindahl, and M. Lundström. 2012. Use of 13 disease registries in 5 countries demonstrates the potential to use outcome data to improve health care's value. *Health Affairs (Millwood)* 31(1):220-227.

Lee, C. N., R. Dominik, C. A. Levin, M. J. Barry, C. Cosenza, A. M. O'Connor, A. G. Mulley, Jr., and K. R. Sepucha. 2010a. Development of instruments to measure the quality of breast cancer treatment decisions. *Health Expectations* 13(3):258-272.

Lee, C. N., C. S. Hultman, and K. Sepucha. 2010b. Do patients and providers agree about the most important facts and goals for breast reconstruction decisions? *Annals of Plastic Surgery* 64(5):563-566.

Lee, C. N., J. Belkora, Y. Chang, B. Moy, A. Partridge, and K. Sepucha. 2011. Are patients making high-quality decisions about breast reconstruction after mastectomy? *Plastic and Reconstructive Surgery* 127(1):18-26.

Lee, C. N., Y. Chang, N. Adimorah, J. K. Belkora, B. Moy, A. H. Partridge, D. W. Ollila, and K. R. Sepucha. 2012. Decision making about surgery for early-stage breast cancer. *Journal of the American College of Surgeons* 214(1):1-10.

Levinson, D. R. 2010. *Adverse events in hospitals: National incidence among Medicare beneficiaries.* Washington, DC: U.S. Department of Health and Human Services, Office of Inspector General.

Linzer, M., L. B. Manwell, E. S. Williams, J. A. Bobula, R. L. Brown, A. B. Varkey, B. Man, J. E. McMurray, A. Maguire, B. Horner-Ibler, M. D. Schwartz, and MEMO (Minimizing Error, Maximizing Outcome) Investigators. 2009. Working conditions in primary care: Physician reactions and care quality. *Annals of Internal Medicine* 151(1):28-36, W26-W29.

Maurer, M., P. Dardess, K. L. Carman, K. Frazier, and L. Smeeding. 2012. *Guide to patient and family engagement: Environmental scan report.* Rockville, MD: Agency for Healthcare Research and Quality.

McCarthy, D., S. How, C. Schoen, J. Cantor, and D. Belloff. 2009. *Aiming higher: Results from a state scorecard on health system performance.* New York: Commonwealth Fund Commission on a High Performance Health System.

McGinnis, J. M., P. Williams-Russo, and J. R. Knickman. 2002. The case for more active policy attention to health promotion. *Health Affairs (Millwood)* 21(2):78-93.

McGlynn, E. A., S. M. Asch, J. Adams, J. Keesey, J. Hicks, A. DeCristofaro, and E. A. Kerr. 2003. The quality of health care delivered to adults in the United States. *New England Journal of Medicine* 348(26):2635-2645.

Mechanic, R. E., P. Santos, B. E. Landon, and M. E. Chernew. 2011. Medical group responses to global payment: Early lessons from the "alternative quality contract" in Massachusetts. *Health Affairs (Millwood)* 30(9):1734-1742.

Nabel, E. G., and E. Braunwald. 2012. A tale of coronary artery disease and myocardial infarction. *New England Journal of Medicine* 366(1):54-63.

Neily, J., P. D. Mills, Y. Young-Xu, B. T. Carney, P. West, D. H. Berger, L. M. Mazzia, D. E. Paull, and J. P. Bagian. 2010. Association between implementation of a medical team training program and surgical mortality. *Journal of the American Medical Association* 304(15):1693-1700.

Neily, J., P. D. Mills, N. Eldridge, B. T. Carney, D. Pfeffer, J. R. Turner, Y. Young-Xu, W. Gunnar, and J. P. Bagian. 2011. Incorrect surgical procedures within and outside of the operating room: A follow-up report. *Archives of Surgery* 146(11):1235-1239.

Nelson, L. 2012. *Lessons from Medicare's demonstration projects on disease management and care coordination.* Washington, DC: Congressional Budget Office.

Ness, R. B. 2007. Influence of the HIPAA privacy rule on health research. *Journal of the American Medical Association* 298(18):2164-2170.

O'Connor, A. M., C. L. Bennett, D. Stacey, M. Barry, N. F. Col, K. B. Eden, V. A. Entwistle, V. Fiset, M. Holmes-Rovner, S. Khangura, H. Llewellyn-Thomas, and D. Rovner. 2009. Decision aids for people facing health treatment or screening decisions. *Cochrane Database of Systematic Reviews* (3):CD001431.

Office of the Attorney General of Massachusetts. 2011. *Examination of health care cost trends and cost drivers pursuant to G.L. c. 118g, § 6½(b).* http://www.mass.gov/ago/docs/healthcare/2011-hcctd-full.pdf (accessed August 30, 2012).

OMB (Office of Management and Budget). 2010. *Fiscal year 2011 budget of the U.S. government.* Washington, DC: OMB.

Parekh, A. K., and M. B. Barton. 2010. The challenge of multiple comorbidity for the US health care system. *Journal of the American Medical Association* 303(13):1303-1304.

Peikes, D., A. Chen, J. Schore, and R. Brown. 2009. Effects of care coordination on hospitalization, quality of care, and health care expenditures among Medicare beneficiaries: 15 randomized trials. *Journal of the American Medical Association* 301(6):603-618.

Pham, H. H., D. Schrag, A. S. O'Malley, B. Wu, and P. B. Bach. 2007. Care patterns in Medicare and their implications for pay for performance. *New England Journal of Medicine* 356(11):1130-1139.

Pham, H. H., A. S. O'Malley, P. B. Bach, C. Saiontz-Martinez, and D. Schrag. 2009. Primary care physicians' links to other physicians through Medicare patients: The scope of care coordination. *Annals of Internal Medicine* 150(4):236-242.

Potts, A. L., F. E. Barr, D. F. Gregory, L. Wright, and N. R. Patel. 2004. Computerized physician order entry and medication errors in a pediatric critical care unit. *Pediatrics* 113(1 Pt. 1):59-63.

Pronovost, P., D. Needham, S. Berenholtz, D. Sinopoli, H. T. Chu, S. Cosgrove, B. Sexton, R. Hyzy, R. Welsh, G. Roth, J. Bander, J. Kepros, and C. Goeschel. 2006. An intervention to decrease catheter-related bloodstream infections in the ICU. *New England Journal of Medicine* 355(26):2725-2732.

Pronovost, P. J., C. A. Goeschel, K. L. Olsen, J. C. Pham, M. R. Miller, S. M. Berenholtz, J. B. Sexton, J. A. Marsteller, L. L. Morlock, A. W. Wu, J. M. Loeb, and C. M. Clancy. 2009. Reducing health care hazards: Lessons from the commercial aviation safety team. *Health Affairs (Millwood)* 28(3):w479-w489.

Schneider, K. M., B. E. O'Donnell, and D. Dean. 2009. Prevalence of multiple chronic conditions in the United States' Medicare population. *Health and Quality of Life Outcomes* 7:82.

Schoenbaum, S. C., C. Schoen, J. L. Nicholson, and J. C. Cantor. 2011. Mortality amenable to health care in the United States: The roles of demographics and health systems performance. *Journal of Public Health Policy* 32(4):407-429.

Sepucha, K. R., A. Fagerlin, M. P. Couper, C. A. Levin, E. Singer, and B. J. Zikmund-Fisher. 2010. How does feeling informed relate to being informed? The decisions survey. *Medical Decision Making* 30(Suppl. 5):S77-S84.

Song, Z., D. G. Safran, B. E. Landon, Y. He, R. P. Ellis, R. E. Mechanic, M. P. Day, and M. E. Chernew. 2011. Health care spending and quality in year 1 of the alternative quality contract. *New England Journal of Medicine* 65(10):909-918.

Spear, S. J. 2005. Fixing health care from the inside, today. *Harvard Business Review* 83(9):78.

Stacey, D., C. L. Bennett, M. J. Barry, N. F. Col, K. B. Eden, M. Holmes-Rovner, H. Llewellyn-Thomas, A. Lyddiatt, F. Legare, and R. Thomson. 2011. Decision aids for people facing health treatment or screening decisions. *Cochrane Database of Systematic Reviews* (10):CD001431.

Stewart, M., J. B. Brown, A. Donner, I. R. McWhinney, J. Oates, W. W. Weston, and J. Jordan. 2000. The impact of patient-centered care on outcomes. *Journal of Family Practice* 49(9):796-804.

Stremikis, K., C. Schoen, and A.-K. Fryer. 2011. *A call for change: The 2011 Commonwealth Fund survey of public views of the U.S. health system.* New York: Commonwealth Fund.

Tinetti, M. E., S. T. Bogardus, and J. V. Agostini. 2004. Potential pitfalls of disease-specific guidelines for patients with multiple conditions. *New England Journal of Medicine* 351(27):2870-2874.

Tricoci, P., J. M. Allen, J. M. Kramer, R. M. Califf, and S. C. Smith, Jr. 2009. Scientific evidence underlying the ACC/AHA clinical practice guidelines. *Journal of the American Medical Association* 301(8):831-841.

Trude, S. 2003. So much to do, so little time: Physician capacity constraints, 1997-2001. *Tracking report/Center for Studying Health System Change* (8):1.

Tucker, A. L., and S. J. Spear. 2006. Operational failures and interruptions in hospital nursing. *Health Services Research* 41(3 Pt. 1):643-662.

U.S. Bureau of Labor Statistics. 2010a. *May 2009 national occupational employment and wage estimates.* http://www.bls.gov/oes/2009/may/oes_nat.htm (accessed May 22, 2012).

U.S. Bureau of Labor Statistics. 2010b. *National compensation survey: Occupational earnings in the United States, 2009.* http://www.bls.gov/ncs/ocs/sp/nctb1346.pdf (accessed May 22, 2012).

U.S. Bureau of Labor Statistics. 2012. *Labor force statistics from the current population survey.* http://data.bls.gov/pdq/SurveyOutputServlet?request_action=wh&graph_name=LN_cpsbref1 (accessed May 23, 2012).

Wennberg, J. E., E. S. Fisher, and J. S. Skinner. 2002. Geography and the debate over Medicare reform. *Health Affairs (Millwood)* (Suppl. Web Exclusives):W96-W114.

Yarnall, K. S. H., K. Krause, K. Pollak, M. Gradison, and J. Michener. 2009. Family physicians as team leaders: "Time" to share the care. *Preventing Chronic Disease* 6(2).

Part I

The Imperatives

1

Introduction and Overview

Health care in America presents a fundamental paradox. The past 50 years have seen an explosion in biomedical knowledge, dramatic innovation in therapies and surgical procedures, and management of conditions that previously were fatal, with ever more exciting clinical capabilities on the horizon. Yet, American health care is falling short on basic dimensions of quality, outcomes, costs, and equity. Available knowledge is too rarely applied to improve the care experience, and information generated by the care experience is too rarely gathered to improve the knowledge available. The traditional systems for transmitting new knowledge—the ways clinicians are educated, deployed, rewarded, and updated—can no longer keep pace with scientific advances. If unaddressed, the current shortfalls in the performance of the nation's health care system will deepen on both quality and cost dimensions, challenging the well-being of Americans now and potentially far into the future.

Consider the impact on American services if other industries routinely operated in the same manner as many aspects of health care:

- If banking were like health care, automated teller machine (ATM) transactions would take not seconds but perhaps days or longer as a result of unavailable or misplaced records.
- If home building were like health care, carpenters, electricians, and plumbers each would work with different blueprints, with very little coordination.

- If shopping were like health care, product prices would not be posted, and the price charged would vary widely within the same store, depending on the source of payment.
- If automobile manufacturing were like health care, warranties for cars that require manufacturers to pay for defects would not exist. As a result, few factories would seek to monitor and improve production line performance and product quality.
- If airline travel were like health care, each pilot would be free to design his or her own preflight safety check, or not to perform one at all.

The point is not that health care can or should function in precisely the same way as all other sectors—each is very different from the others, and every industry has room for improvement. Yet, if some of the transferable best practices from banking, construction, retailing, automobile manufacturing, flight safety, public utilities, and personal services were adopted as standard best practices in health care, the nation could see patient care in which:

- records were immediately updated and available for use by patients;
- care delivered were proven reliable at the core and tailored at the margins;
- patient and family needs and preferences were a central part of the decision process;
- all team members were fully informed in real time about each other's activities;
- prices and total costs were fully transparent to all participants;
- payment incentives were structured to reward outcomes and value, not volume;
- errors were promptly identified and corrected; and
- results were routinely captured and used for continuous improvement.

Unfortunately, these are not features that would describe much of health care in America today. Health care can lag behind many other sectors with respect to its ability to meet patients' specific needs, to offer choice, to adapt, to become more affordable, to improve—in short, to learn. Americans should be served by a health care system that consistently delivers reliable performance and constantly improves, systematically and seamlessly, with each care experience and transition.

THE NEED FOR A CONTINUOUSLY
LEARNING HEALTH CARE SYSTEM

Decades of rapid innovation and technological improvement have created a health care system that is extraordinarily complex. The discovery of penicillin, which could treat many previously incurable bacterial diseases quickly and completely, heralded the advent of widespread antibiotic treatments for many communicable diseases. The development of insulin therapy has allowed diabetics to control their blood sugar and manage their condition effectively. Imaging systems, from computed tomography (CT) scans to magnetic resonance imaging (MRI), have allowed clinicians to view the inside of the body in extraordinary detail. These and other innovations have benefited millions of patients, but they also have introduced new challenges for both clinicians and patients in treating and managing health conditions.

Today in health care, there is more to know, more to manage, and more to do than ever before. The rate at which new scientific knowledge is being produced outstrips the cognitive capacity of even the most adroit clinician to monitor and evaluate effectively. Physicians specialize and subspecialize to manage the growing stores of health care knowledge, and patients now visit multiple providers for most conditions. New developments promise to accelerate this trend and further challenge the ability of clinicians to remain current on the state of the field. New research in genetics, epigenetics, proteomics, and related molecular biology topics, for example, is adding myriad factors to what clinicians may have to consider when helping patients choose the most appropriate treatment for their circumstances.

Most physicians, nurses, and other health care professionals work diligently to care for their patients, but they often are contending with the challenges of a system that is poorly configured for the current complexity of treatments, technologies, and clinical science. These difficulties are exacerbated by administrative and organizational complexity that requires time that could be spent with patients.

The growing complexity of health care challenges not only providers but also patients. Increasing specialization has made it difficult for patients to navigate the system and find the right care for their conditions. Furthermore, as patients move among providers and settings, they often encounter communication and coordination problems that can result in treatment errors, duplicative services, and fragmented care. Improving the quality of care, patient health outcomes, and the value of care is possible, but will require broad changes in the culture, incentives, administration, and information supports that govern the current health care environment.

Absent such change, the very solvency of the system is threatened, because the cost of health care continues to rise relentlessly. In 2012, the United States will spend an estimated $2.8 trillion on the health care

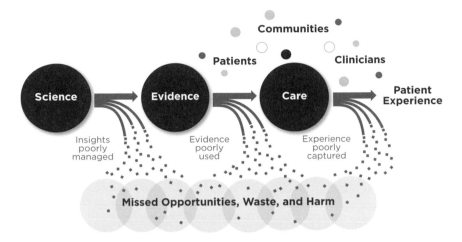

FIGURE 1-1 Schematic of the health care system today.

system, or about 18 percent of gross domestic product (CMS, 2012; Keehan et al., 2011). For 31 of the past 40 years, health care costs have increased at a greater rate than the rest of the economy, and the cumulative increase over that time has been 2.5 times the economy's growth (BEA, 2011; CMS, 2011). If this level of expenditure produced extraordinary results, it could be justified. On the contrary, however, assessments show that much of this investment is wasted on care activities that do little to improve patients' health or quality of life.

In sum, as illustrated in Figure 1-1, each stage in the processes that shape the health care received—knowledge development, translation into medical evidence, application of evidence-based care—has prominent short-comings and inefficiencies that contribute to a large reservoir of missed opportunities, waste, and harm. The threats to the health and economic security of Americans are clear, present, and compelling. What is needed—and possible—to transform care is a system that leverages the growing scientific evidence base, knowledge from other sectors on how to design reliable processes, and advances in information systems to enable continuous improvement in care, consistent implementation of best practices, and the ability to draw on knowledge generated every day through clinical care.

STUDY CONTEXT

In the face of these realities, the Institute of Medicine (IOM) convened the Committee on the Learning Health Care System in America to explore the most fundamental challenges to health care today and to propose actions that can be taken to achieve a health care system characterized by continuous learning and improvement. This study builds on earlier IOM studies on various aspects of the health care system, from *To Err Is Human: Building a Safer Health System* (1999), on patient safety; to *Crossing the Quality Chasm: A New Health System for the 21st Century* (2001), on health care quality; to *Unequal Treatment: Confronting Racial and Ethnic Disparities in Health Care* (2003b), on health care disparities. The study process also was facilitated and informed by published summaries of workshops conducted under the auspices of the IOM Roundtable on Value & Science-Driven Health Care. Over the past 6 years, 11 workshop summaries have been produced, exploring various aspects of the challenges and opportunities in health care today, with a particular focus on the foundational elements of a learning health system.

While examples of progress exist, many of the problems documented by these reports persist. Medical errors are far too common, different patient populations receive different intensities of services for the same conditions, and health care quality remains uneven. The lack of widespread progress on these now well-documented dimensions of care highlights the need for a substantially new approach. In some cases, successful pilot projects have been undertaken, yet their results have not been disseminated. In other cases, the problem may lie in the need to help clinicians manage the flow of knowledge and apply relevant information to their practice. In still other cases, the difficulty may occur because clinicians and front line staff do not have at their disposal the tools needed to answer the questions they encounter. These problems point to the need for a transformation in how the health care enterprise generates, processes, and applies information to further patient care.

Meeting the challenges outlined in the above IOM reports has taken on great urgency as a result of two overarching imperatives:

- to manage the health care system's ever-increasing **complexity**, and
- to curb ever-escalating **costs**.

The convergence of these imperatives makes the status quo untenable. At the same time, however, opportunities exist to address these problems— opportunities that did not exist even a decade ago:

- vast **computational power** that is affordable and widely available;
- **connectivity** that allows information to be accessed in real time virtually anywhere;
- **human and organizational capabilities** that improve the reliability and efficiency of care processes; and

- the recognition that effective care must be delivered by **collaborations between teams of clinicians and patients,** each playing a vital
role in the care process.

This report presents a vision for a continuously learning health care
system that can leverage these opportunities and recommends priority actions that can be taken to accelerate progress toward that vision.

This study entailed identifying the principal structural, economic, and
cultural obstacles to improving health care; reviewing strategies that have
been successful to date in transforming care; and assessing the potential
consequences of inaction. The actions required will be notable, substantial,
and highly disruptive. If these changes do not occur, however, the health
care system will continue on its current path. Some patients will receive
excellent, world-class care, while too many others will experience unnecessary harm and poor quality. The stress placed on physicians will grow as
modern health care becomes ever more complex. At the system level, costs
and waste will continue to increase, further taxing national, state, and
family budgets. The choice, then, is not whether or when the necessary
transformation should be initiated—it is how.

Related Assessments of Others

The scale of actions needed to transform the health care system will
require concerted effort on the part of numerous individuals and organizations. Indeed, a variety of organizations have devoted substantial effort to
initiatives aimed at improving the safety, effectiveness, patient-centeredness,
quality, and value of the health care enterprise. This report is intended to
build on this important contextual work. This section highlights several
notable examples of these prior initiatives; further examples are noted
throughout the report.

One notable initiative aimed at revitalizing the health care system is the
Commission on a High Performance Health System, sponsored by the Commonwealth Fund. The goal of this effort is "to promote a high-performing
health system that provides Americans with affordable access to high-
quality, safe care while maximizing efficiency in its delivery and administration" (The Commonwealth Fund, 2012). Major accomplishments of the
Commission include measuring health system performance, highlighting
areas for improvement, and recommending strategies for addressing those
gaps. A number of the policy options advanced by the Commission are
being implemented, in part under provisions of the Affordable Care Act
(ACA) of 2010 (The Commonwealth Fund, 2012).

The Robert Wood Johnson Foundation's Aligning Forces for Quality initiative is an effort to "improve health care quality in targeted communities,

reduce racial and ethnic disparities in care, and provide models for national reform" (Robert Wood Johnson Foundation, 2012). A goal is to build multistakeholder alliances to focus on common areas for progress at the local level. These alliances include physicians, nurses, patients, consumers and consumer groups, purchasers, hospitals, health plans, safety-net providers, and others. The Aligning Forces initiative has spread to 16 communities in different geographic areas with various demographic and economic profiles. Communities involved in the initiative have assisted providers seeking to improve the care they offer, increased the measurement and reporting of care performance, and expanded the ability of patients and consumers to recognize and demand high-quality care (Robert Wood Johnson Foundation, 2012).

The Brookings Institution's Engelberg Center for Health Care Reform seeks to develop data-driven, practical policy solutions that promote broad access to high-quality, affordable, and innovative care. The Center pursues this goal by conducting research, making policy recommendations, facilitating consensus around key issues, and providing technical support to stakeholders implementing new solutions. Specific projects in which the Center has been involved include the Accountable Care Organization (ACO) Learning Network, a member-driven network that provides participating organizations the tools necessary to implement accountable care successfully; the Quality Alliance Steering Committee, a collaborative effort aimed at implementing measures to improve the quality and efficiency of health care; and the Medicare Payment Reform Project, which is developing policy proposals to reward providers for improving the efficiency, quality, and coordination of care by moving toward greater accountability and support for overall quality and value (The Brookings Institution, 2012; Quality Alliance Steering Committee, 2012).

These examples highlight the diversity of initiatives that are under way, as well as the energy available for transformative action. They are part of a large body of work on which this report draws in exploring what is needed to move toward a health care system that continuously learns and improves.

Related Work of the Institute of Medicine

With a dedicated commitment to improving the quality of care delivered in the United States, the IOM has produced a number of highly influential reports—such as *To Err Is Human: Building a Safer Health System* (1999), *Crossing the Quality Chasm: A New Health System for the 21st Century* (2001), *Building a Better Delivery System: A New Engineering/ Health Care Partnership* (2005), *Knowing What Works in Health Care: A Roadmap for the Nation* (2008b), and *Initial National Priorities for Comparative Effectiveness Research* (2009a). These reports have drawn attention to key shortfalls in the performance of the health care system, have led to demonstrable changes in policy, and have helped identify priorities for improving the care delivery system.

More than a decade ago, the IOM released its groundbreaking report *To Err Is Human*. According to that report, at least 44,000 and perhaps as many as 98,000 people die in hospitals each year as a result of preventable medical errors (IOM, 1999). The report notes that individual error is not the main cause of adverse events; rather, most medical errors are caused by poorly designed systems and processes that fail to prevent adverse events. This report was followed soon after by *Crossing the Quality Chasm* (IOM, 2001), which highlights the gap between the care that is possible given advances in science and medical knowledge and the care that is routinely received by patients. The report identifies six aims for the health care system: care should be safe, effective, patient-centered, timely, efficient, and equitable (Box 1-1).

Following up on the *Quality Chasm* report, the IOM conducted a summit on health professions education, releasing the results of this summit in the 2003 report *Health Professions Education: A Bridge to Quality*. This report cites the need for major changes in health professions education to keep pace with shifts in the nation's patient population and health care delivery environment and a rapidly expanding evidence base (IOM, 2003a).

In 2004, the IOM launched the Redesigning Health Insurance Performance Measures, Payment, and Performance Improvement Project, which

---

BOX 1-1
Six Aims of Health Care Improvement

- *Safe*—avoiding injuries to patients from the care that is intended to help them.
- *Effective*—providing services based on scientific knowledge to all who could benefit and refraining from providing services to those not likely to benefit.
- *Patient-centered*—providing care that is respectful of and responsive to individual patient preferences, needs, and values and ensuring that patient values guide all clinical decisions.
- *Timely*—reducing waits and sometimes harmful delays for both those who receive and those who give care.
- *Efficient*—avoiding waste, in particular waste of equipment, supplies, ideas, and energy.
- *Equitable*—providing care that does not vary in quality because of personal characteristics such as gender, ethnicity, geographic location, and socioeconomic status.

SOURCE: IOM, 2001, pp. 39-40.

produced the *Pathways to Quality Health Care* series of reports. Each report in this series addresses a different aspect of health care quality, including measuring and reporting performance data, designing payment incentives, and structuring quality improvement initiatives. *Performance Measurement: Accelerating Improvement* reviews the performance measures then available and highlights the need to develop improved measures that are longitudinal, comprehensive, population based, and patient-centered (IOM, 2006b). *Medicare's Quality Improvement Organization Program: Maximizing Potential* considers the Quality Improvement Organization program and the need for technical assistance to aid providers undertaking improvement initiatives (IOM, 2006a). The final publication in the series, *Rewarding Provider Performance: Aligning Incentives in Medicare*, explores the potential of pay-for-performance systems and payment incentives to improve value in health care, especially in the context of the Medicare program (IOM, 2007b).

Most recently, the IOM Roundtable on Value & Science-Driven Health Care has marshaled the insights of the nation's leading experts to explore in detail the prospects, and the imperative, for transformational change in the fundamental elements of health and health care. The result has been the *Learning Health System* series of publications, which summarize 15 public workshops held to identify and consider the foundational elements of a learning health system. Brief synopses of the 11 volumes of the series are presented below:

- **Vision**—*The Learning Healthcare System*, the first in the series, explores the various dimensions—evidence development and standards, care culture, system design and operation, health data, clinical research, information technology, value—on which emerging insights and scientific advances can be applied to achieve health care in which both the development and application of evidence flow seamlessly and continuously in the course of care (IOM, 2007a).
- **Care Complexity**—*Evidence-Based Medicine and the Changing Nature of Health Care* considers the forces, such as genetic insights and increasing care complexity, driving the need for better medical evidence; the challenges with which patients and providers must contend; the need to transform the speed and reliability of new medical evidence; and the legislative and policy changes that could enable the evolution of an evidence-based, learning system (IOM, 2008a).
- **Effectiveness Research**—*Redesigning the Clinical Effectiveness Research Paradigm: Innovation and Evidence-Based Approaches* reviews the growing scope and scale of the need for clinical

effectiveness research alternatives, the limits of current approaches, the potential for emerging research and data networks, innovative study designs, and new methods of analysis and modeling (IOM, 2010b).

- **The Data Utility**—*Clinical Data as the Basic Staple of Health Learning: Creating and Protecting a Public Good* identifies the transformational prospects for large interoperable clinical and administrative data sets to allow real-time discovery on issues ranging from disease etiology to personalized diagnosis and treatment. It also explores the key priorities for data stewardship if clinical data are to be a carefully nurtured resource for continuous learning and better care (IOM, 2011a).

- **Evidence**—*Learning What Works: Infrastructure Required for Comparative Effectiveness Research* assesses the nature and magnitude of needed capacity for new knowledge and evidence about what care works best under different circumstances, including the necessary skills and workforce, data linkage and improvement, study coordination and dissemination of results, and innovation in research methods (IOM, 2011c).

- **Digital Platform**—*Digital Infrastructure for the Learning Health System: The Foundation for Continuous Improvement in Health and Health Care* explores current efforts and opportunities to accelerate progress in improving health and health care through information technology systems. The publication presents summary overviews and priority follow-up action targets in four important cross-cutting dimensions: technical innovation, data and research insights, patient and public engagement, and stewardship and governance (IOM, 2011b).

- **Systems Engineering**—*Engineering a Learning Healthcare System: A Look at the Future* reviews lessons from the systems and operations engineering sciences applicable to improving the organization, structure, and function of the delivery, monitoring, and change processes in health care—in effect, engineering approaches to continuous feedback and improvement on quality, safety, knowledge, and value in health care (IOM and NAE, 2011).

- **Patients and the Public**—*Patients Charting the Course: Citizen Engagement and the Learning Health System* assesses the prospects for improving health and lowering costs by advancing patient involvement in the elements of a learning health system. It underscores the centrality of communication strategies that account for and engage individual perspectives, needs, preferences, and understanding and the support necessary to mobilize change (IOM, 2011d).

- **Cost and Outcomes**—*The Healthcare Imperative: Lowering Costs and Improving Outcomes* presents a six-domain framework for understanding and estimating excessive health care costs: unnecessary services, inefficiently delivered services, excessive administrative costs, prices that are too high, missed prevention opportunities, and medical fraud. Additionally, it summarizes estimates of the excessive costs, reviews approaches to their control, and considers ways to reduce health expenditures by 10 percent within 10 years without compromising health status or valued innovation (IOM, 2010a).
- **Value**—*Value in Health Care: Accounting for Cost, Quality, Safety, Outcomes, and Innovation* explores alternative perspectives and approaches for defining, estimating, and attaining value in health care. It includes case studies on value-enhancing strategies in development, such as value-based insurance design and ACOs, and emphasizes the basic need for broad transparency on cost, quality, and outcomes in care (IOM, 2010c).
- **Leadership**—*Leadership Commitments to Improve Value in Health Care: Finding Common Ground* presents discussions of opportunity statements from those in key health stakeholder sectors—patients, clinicians, health organizations, insurers, product manufacturers, employers, government, information technology, and researchers—on priority actions they can and will undertake cooperatively to transform quality and value in health care (IOM, 2009b).

STATEMENT OF TASK, SCOPE, AND METHODS

As the above discussion makes clear, the work of the IOM Committee on the Learning Health Care System in America was undertaken as the health care system confronts these very real challenges in order to consider ways of leveraging undeniable opportunities for best care at lower cost. The committee, whose work was supported by the Blue Shield of California Foundation, the Charina Endowment Fund, and the Robert Wood Johnson Foundation, was charged with (1) identifying how the effectiveness and efficiency of the current health care system can be transformed through tools and incentives for continuous assessment and improvement and (2) developing recommendations for actions that can be taken to that end (see Box 1-2). This transformation has the potential to improve the entire health care system, leading to progress in patient safety, health care quality, and value for patients.

The enormity of the challenges currently facing the health care system can be overwhelming to the professionals seeking to improve the health of patients and the public. The learning health care system provides an

BOX 1-2
Charge to the IOM Committee on the
Learning Health Care System in America

An ad hoc Committee will consider the urgent and longer-term actions necessary to foster the development of a continuously learning health care system. Building on recent related work of the Institute of Medicine, particularly that undertaken to inform the dialogue and discussions of the Roundtable on Value & Science-Driven Health Care, the Committee will conduct a study and make recommendations that can help transform the current health care delivery system into one of continuous assessment and improvement for both the effectiveness and efficiency of health care.

Effectiveness. The Committee will define the foundational elements of a learning system for health care that is effective and continuously improving—that marshals the best and most appropriate evidence for application at the point of decision; accounts for patient circumstances and preferences; employs information systems that can accurately record and exchange information on care processes and results; is designed to capture information from the care experience in order to improve care through real-time insights, learning, and evidence development; accelerates the dissemination of innovation through processes, such as regulations, business models, and economic approaches, that also assure safety and value; and ensures continuous feedback for all decision levels.

Efficiency. The Committee will define the foundational characteristics of a health care system that is efficient, delivers increased value, and is continuously innovating and improving in its ability to deliver high value to patients—that has agreed-upon key elements and analytic methods for assessing the value proposition in health care; is fully transparent as to costs and outcomes in care; continuously assesses the effectiveness of health care delivered; accelerates exploration of alternatives; accounts appropriately for differences in patient circumstances and preferences; and appropriately assesses opportunity costs.

Based on this work, the Committee will prepare its Report with findings on major opportunities, deficiencies, and their consequences; identify the key pressure points; and propose policy initiatives and priorities for government and other stakeholders to accelerate progress for continuous improvement in the value of health care delivered to Americans.

organizing conceptual framework for addressing these challenges. The goal is not to create an ideal system that overcomes all of today's challenges. Because of the ever-changing nature of health care and the complexity of the enterprise, the goal is to transition to a system that can adapt—that is, continuously learn how to improve, manage new challenges, and take advantage of opportunities. Changes recommended by the committee should not be viewed as individual actions, but as means of achieving this overarching aim of continuous learning and improvement.

The committee's charge was broad, because the dramatic improvements needed in health care will require coordinated and systemwide change. Accordingly, the IOM assembled a committee comprising a diverse group of 18 individuals that included experts in health economics, health care delivery, information technology, systems, education, operations management, and patient safety, as well as individuals who understand the perspectives of employers, insurers, clinicians, researchers, and patients. Brief biographies of the committee members are presented in Appendix D.

Recognizing that achieving a continuously learning health care system will require concerted actions on the part of all stakeholders in the system, the committee designed an ambitious outreach strategy to gather feedback. Staff contacted 248 health care leaders from 215 organizations to solicit their thoughts on the current state of learning and improvement in the health care system and strategies for increasing learning among health care organizations and professionals. The committee received comments and suggestions from 137 individuals, who outlined the issues and challenges and highlighted successful strategies for moving forward. This feedback informed the committee's deliberations by providing a wide range of perspectives on the current functioning of the health care system and its potential for improvement.

The committee deliberated during four in-person meetings and several conference calls between January 2010 and March 2012. Its initial deliberations focused on clarifying the scope of the study, while later meetings focused on developing recommendations for moving the system forward. To accelerate its efforts, the committee drew on related IOM work, particularly that undertaken to inform the dialogue and discussions of the Roundtable on Value & Science-Driven Health Care. Staff and committee members reviewed the relevant literature in the field and investigated case studies of organizations in different stages of their journey toward adopting learning practices.

ORGANIZATION OF THE REPORT

This report explores in detail the imperatives of managing complexity, achieving greater value, and capturing opportunities from emerging tools and technologies and from a changing health policy landscape; the vision and foundation of a continuously learning health care system; the path to its accomplishment through transformations in clinical research, patient engagement, cost and outcomes, transparency, and care teamwork and continuity; and the critical need for stakeholder leadership. Detailed findings are highlighted throughout the report, with attendant conclusions and recommendations. Each recommendation describes the core improvement aim for the area, followed by specific strategies representing initial steps that stakeholders should take in acting on the recommendation. Additional activities will have to be undertaken by numerous stakeholders to sustain and advance the continuous improvement required.

The title of the report underscores that care that is based on the best available evidence, takes appropriate account of individual preferences, and is delivered reliably and efficiently—*best care*—is possible today. When such care is routinely implemented, moreover, it is generally less expensive than the less effective, less efficient care that is now too commonly provided. Moreover, the transition to best care envisioned in this report is urgently needed given the budgetary, economic, and health pressures facing the nation's health care system.

This report is divided into three parts. Part I builds the case for a continuously learning health care system, considering the challenges of managing complexity (Chapter 2), achieving greater value in health care (Chapter 3), and capturing opportunities that now make achievement of such a system possible (Chapter 4). Part II outlines a vision for the system, highlighting the key aims for improvement and the foundational elements of performance (Chapter 5). Part III outlines a path for achieving this vision, including new methods for generating and disseminating health care knowledge (Chapter 6); patient, family, and community engagement (Chapter 7); approaches for increasing the value achieved by the system (Chapter 8); and creation of a new culture of care (Chapter 9). Each of these chapters provides a framework for progress on its specific focus, outlining goals and recommendations for improvement, along with specific strategies that stakeholders can undertake to achieve these goals. Finally, Chapter 10 summarizes the actions recommended for each stakeholder to achieve the committee's vision of a learning health care system based on the conclusions and recommendations presented in prior chapters.

REFERENCES

BEA (Bureau of Economic Analysis). 2011. *National economic accounts data.* http://www.bea. gov/national/index.htm#gdp (accessed April 18, 2012).

The Brookings Institution. 2012. *Engelberg Center for Health Care Reform: About us.* http:// www.brookings.edu/health/About-Us.aspx (accessed April 12, 2012).

CMS (Centers for Medicare & Medicaid Services). 2011. *National health expenditure data.* https://www.cms.gov/NationalHealthExpendData/01_Overview.asp (accessed April 18, 2012).

CMS. 2012. *National health expenditures summary and GDP: Calendar years 1960-2010.* http://www.cms.gov/Research-Statistics-Data-and-Systems/Statistics-Trends-and-Reports/ NationalHealthExpendData/downloads/tables.pdf (accessed August 31, 2012).

The Commonwealth Fund. 2012. *Commission on a high performance health system.* http:// www.commonwealthfund.org/Program-Areas/Health-Reform-Policy/Commission-on-a-High-Performance-Health-System.aspx (accessed April 12, 2012).

IOM (Institute of Medicine). 1999. *To err is human: Building a safer health system.* Washington, DC: National Academy Press.

IOM. 2001. *Crossing the quality chasm: A new health system for the 21st century.* Washington, DC: National Academy Press.

IOM. 2003a. *Health professions education: A bridge to quality.* Washington, DC: The National Academies Press.

IOM. 2003b. *Unequal treatment: Confronting racial and ethnic disparities in health care.* Washington, DC: The National Academies Press.

IOM. 2005. *Building a better delivery system: A new engineering/health care partnership.* Washington, DC: The National Academies Press.

IOM. 2006a. *Medicare's quality improvement organization program: Maximizing potential.* Washington, DC: The National Academies Press.

IOM. 2006b. *Performance measurement: Accelerating improvement.* Washington, DC: The National Academies Press.

IOM. 2007a. *The learning healthcare system: Workshop summary.* Washington, DC: The National Academies Press.

IOM. 2007b. *Rewarding provider performance: Aligning incentives in Medicare.* Washington, DC: The National Academies Press.

IOM. 2008a. *Evidence-based medicine and the changing nature of health care: 2007 IOM annual meeting summary.* Washington, DC: The National Academies Press.

IOM. 2008b. *Knowing what works in health care: A roadmap for the nation.* Washington, DC: The National Academies Press.

IOM. 2009a. *Initial national priorities for comparative effectiveness research.* Washington, DC: The National Academies Press.

IOM. 2009b. *Leadership commitments to improve value in health care: Finding common ground: Workshop summary.* Washington, DC: The National Academies Press.

IOM. 2010a. *The healthcare imperative: Lowering costs and improving outcomes: Workshop series summary.* Washington, DC: The National Academies Press.

IOM. 2010b. *Redesigning the clinical effectiveness research paradigm: Innovation and practice-based approaches: Workshop summary.* Washington, DC: The National Academies Press.

IOM. 2010c. *Value in health care: Accounting for cost, quality, safety, outcomes, and innovation: Workshop summary.* Washington, DC: The National Academies Press.

IOM. 2011a. *Clinical data as the basic staple of health learning: Workshop summary.* Washington, DC: The National Academies Press.

IOM. 2011b. *Digital infrastructure for the learning health system: The foundation for continuous improvement in health and health care: A workshop summary.* Washington, DC: The National Academies Press.

IOM. 2011c. *Learning what works: Infrastructure required for comparative effectiveness research: Workshop summary.* Washington, DC: The National Academies Press.

IOM. 2011d. *Patients charting the course: Citizen engagement in the learning health system: Workshop summary.* Washington, DC: The National Academies Press.

IOM and NAE (National Academy of Engineering). 2011. *Engineering a learning healthcare system a look at the future: Workshop summary.* Washington, DC: The National Academies Press.

Keehan, S. P., A. M. Sisko, C. J. Truffer, J. A. Poisal, G. A. Cuckler, A. J. Madison, J. M. Lizonitz, and S. D. Smith. 2011. National health spending projections through 2020: Economic recovery and reform drive faster spending growth. *Health Affairs (Millwood)* 30(8):1594-1605.

Quality Alliance Steering Committee. 2012. *About QASC.* http://www.healthqualityalliance.org/ (accessed May 11, 2012).

Robert Wood Johnson Foundation. 2012. *Aligning forces for quality.* http://forces4quality.org/ (accessed April 12, 2012).

2

Imperative: Managing Rapidly Increasing Complexity

Dr. Charles Bennett, an academic oncologist whose clinical practice has been devoted solely to prostate cancer for 25 years, was diagnosed with prostate cancer in 2006. Upon examining his own biopsy results under the microscope, he was confronted with the same decision so many of his patients had faced before: surgery, radiation, or active surveillance? In an effort to be an informed patient, Dr. Bennett pursued opinions from medical, surgical, and radiation oncologists, and eventually chose to undergo a radical prostatectomy, convinced that his risks were small and the benefits would be great. Five years later, he remains cancer-free, but his right arm and leg are permanently weak, a dysfunction that appeared immediately after the surgery. Looking back, Dr. Bennett would have made a different decision. Prostatectomy provides the benefit of high prostate cancer–specific 20-year survival rates; even when performed by skilled surgeons, however, it carries significant risks of sexual, bladder, and bowel dysfunction, along with less common side effects such as Dr. Bennett's. Active surveillance, coupled with regular screening tests and physical examinations, is associated with much lower rates of these effects and allows for appropriate identification of when to switch from surveillance to treatment. Knowing what he now knows, Dr. Bennett would have opted for active surveillance, proving that even the most informed members of the health care system have difficulty making informed medical decisions as patients (Bennett, 2012).

Over the past century, the health of the U.S. population has improved dramatically. Life expectancy has increased by almost 60 percent, maternal mortality has declined by almost 99 percent, and infant mortality has dropped by more than 90 percent (Guyer et al., 2000). While these increases in survival have been due to many factors, such as public health efforts (CDC, 1999, 2011b), technical improvements in health care have played an increasingly significant role. The health care field today has a better understanding of the causes of individual diseases, as well as new techniques, treatments, and interventions for managing these diseases.

At the same time, the resulting complexity has implications for both patients and providers. The complexity of different health care options—in terms of treatments, diagnostics, and care management—increases the difficulty of the care decisions patients face. When making these decisions, patients often lack clear and understandable information on their options, the risks and benefits of each, and the actions they can take in managing their condition. For those working in the health care enterprise, the current complexity of clinical decision making challenges human cognitive capacity to manage information. One notable example of this complexity is advances in genetics, which offer unprecedented opportunities for personalized treatments but add to the already expansive array of clinical considerations for patients and providers. Moreover, administrative complexities, from complicated workflows to fragmented financing, add inefficiency and waste at the system level and prevent health care from centering its efforts on the patients it serves.

CLINICAL COMPLEXITY

Advances in clinical knowledge have allowed for dramatic improvements in the health of the U.S. population. One area in which these improvements are notable is the treatment of heart attack, or myocardial infarction. During most of the twentieth century, little could be done for a patient who had just suffered a heart attack. The most common intervention was to prescribe weeks of bed rest in the hope that the patient would heal on his or her own. Some patients did heal, but many lost skeletal muscle mass and the ability to care for themselves after the prolonged time in bed (Certo, 1985).

Recent decades have seen a transformation in cardiac care. Today, diagnostics recognize the different types of heart attacks, allowing for customized treatments for patients. Pharmaceutical therapies, such as beta-blockers and thrombolytics, improve survival and reduce the chances of subsequent heart attacks for many groups of patients. Finally, interventions such as percutaneous coronary intervention (PCI) and coronary artery bypass grafting (CABG) can reopen or bypass blockages in blood vessels and restore blood flow to the heart (Antman et al., 2004, 2008; Braunwald et al., 2000, 2002).

As illustrated in Figure 2-1, the research in cardiovascular disease has allowed for better understanding of the disease and new options in cardiac care (Nabel and Braunwald, 2012). These improvements in care, along with improvements in prevention, have contributed to decades-long declines in both acute and long-term mortality from heart attack (Heidenreich and McClellan, 2001; Rogers et al., 2008). For example, one study found that improvements in medications and interventions over the past three decades were associated with better hospital survival rates, which increased from 81 percent in 1975 to 91 percent in 2005 (Floyd et al., 2009). Similarly, another assessment found that in-hospital fatalities for heart attack patients dropped by almost two-thirds from 1979 to 2005 (Fang et al., 2010).

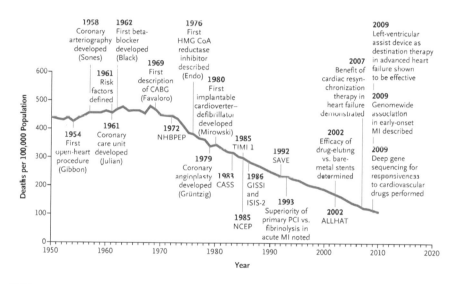

FIGURE 2-1 Timeline of advances in cardiac care, highlighting how improvements in care, prevention, and reduction in risk factors have contributed to declines in cardiovascular mortality over the same time frame.
NOTE: ALLHAT = Antihypertensive and Lipid-Lowering Treatment to Prevent Heart Attack Trial; CASS = Coronary Artery Surgery Study; GISSI = Italian Group for the Study of Survival in Myocardial Infarction; HMG-CoA = key enzyme for cholesterol synthesis; ISIS-2 = Second International Study of Infarct Survival; MI = myocardial infarction; NCEP = National Cholesterol Education Program; NHBPEP = National High Blood Pressure Education Program; PCI = percutaneous coronary intervention; SAVE = Survival and Ventricular Englargement; TIMI 1 = Thrombolysis in Myocardial Infarction trial 1.
SOURCE: Reprinted with permission from Nabel and Braunwald, 2012.

Comparable advances have been achieved in the treatment of many other diseases. One notable example is in care for HIV/AIDS, as summarized in Figure 2-2. In the three decades since this disease was first documented, 35 medications have been introduced for its treatment, sensitive tests have been developed to diagnose the disease at even earlier stages, and other tests have been developed to allow clinicians to identify specific genetic characteristics of the virus in a given patient (Fauci, 2003; FDA, 2011a; Fischl et al., 1987; Simon et al., 2006). These advances have transformed HIV from an almost entirely fatal disease to a chronic condition. At the same time, this remarkable achievement brings new complexity to clinical care. Clinicians must understand the resistance profiles of patients, tailoring the combination of therapies accordingly. They must monitor the patient's viral load to ensure that the treatment continues to work, assess over the course of treatment whether it is causing any adverse effects, and seek to prevent interactions between the patient's HIV drugs and treatments for other health conditions (from antacids to cardiac medications). Further, the pace of treatment advances, as well as mutations in the virus found in the general population, requires that clinicians who work in this

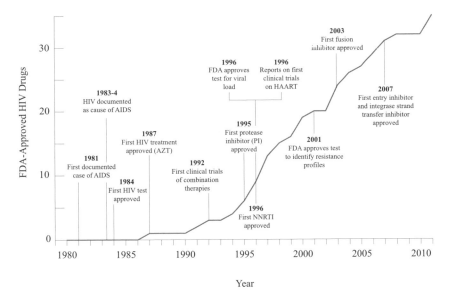

FIGURE 2-2 Timeline of advances in HIV treatment, highlighting increases in Food and Drug Administration (FDA)-approved HIV drugs in the same time frame.
NOTE: HAART = highly active antiretroviral therapy; NNRTI = non-nucleotide reverse transcriptase inhibitor.
SOURCE: Data derived from Fauci, 2003; FDA, 2011a,b; Fischl et al., 1987; Simon et al., 2006.

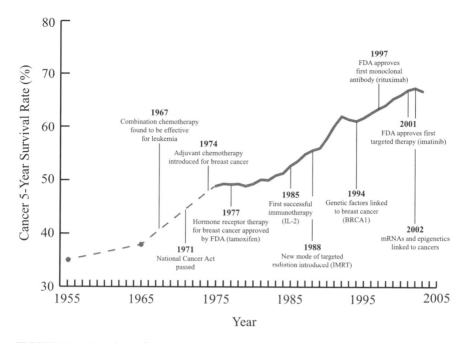

FIGURE 2-3 Timeline of advances in cancer care, highlighting improvements in the 5-year survival rate in the same time frame.
NOTE: BRCAI = breast cancer susceptibility gene 1; FDA = Food and Drug Administration; IL-2 = interleukin-2; IMRT = intensity modulated radiation therapy; mRNA = messenger ribonucleic acid.
SOURCE: Data derived from DeVita and Chu, 2008, DeVita and Rosenberg, 2012.

area constantly update the way they practice care (Panel on Antiretroviral Guidelines for Adults and Adolescents, 2011).

Such advances are not limited to these two diseases but are widespread, as illustrated for the example of cancer care in Figure 2-3. As a result of improved scientific understanding, new treatments and interventions, and new diagnostic technologies, the U.S. health care system now is characterized by more to do, more to know, and more to manage than at any time in history. The result is a paradox: advances in science and technology have improved the ability of the health care system to treat diseases, yet the sheer volume of new discoveries stresses the capabilities of the system to effectively generate and manage knowledge and apply it to regular care. As discussed in Chapter 3, these advances have occurred at the same time as, and sometimes have contributed to, challenges of health care quality and value.

Implications of Complexity for Clinical Decision Making

The complexity of the U.S. health care system means that patients and clinicians have more information to consider and more decisions to make than ever before. Often, these decisions are neither easy nor straightforward, and they include varying options, trade-offs, benefits, and risks. Further complicating matters, patients often lack the information they need to make decisions. Fewer than half of patients receive clear information on the benefits and trade-offs of the treatments for their condition (Fagerlin et al., 2010; Sepucha et al., 2010; Zikmund-Fisher et al., 2010).

As the description of Dr. Bennett's case at the beginning of this chapter demonstrates, one condition that entails difficult decisions is prostate cancer. Prostate cancer is common, developed by one in six men during their lifetime. In at least 80 percent of cases, it is diagnosed at a stage when it is still localized to the prostate gland (Howlader et al., 2011). Patients receiving a diagnosis of localized prostate cancer then must decide what course of action to take. They may choose either to wait and monitor the cancer for any changes (watchful waiting) or to treat it immediately. If they choose to treat it, they have a number of options to consider, including surgery to remove the prostate gland (traditional, laparoscopic, and robotic-assisted versions), various forms of radiation treatment (such as intensity modulated radiation therapy [IMRT], brachytherapy, and proton beam therapy), freezing of the prostate (cryotherapy), and hormone treatment (androgen deprivation therapy) (Institute for Clinical and Economic Review, 2010; Wilt et al., 2008b).

The difficulty of this decision is that localized prostate cancer generally is slow-growing and often causes no harm during the patient's lifetime. In addition, there is a distinct lack of evidence on which treatment works best for a given patient with localized cancer. This absence of evidence is acutely felt for emerging technologies, such as IMRT, proton beam therapy, laparoscopic and robotic-assisted prostatectomy, and cryotherapy, which nevertheless are increasingly being used (Hegarty et al., 2010; Institute for Clinical and Economic Review, 2010; Makarov et al., 2011; Wilt et al., 2008a,b). All treatments for this disease have varying, potentially long-lasting side effects, including sexual, urinary, and bowel problems. While it is unknown which treatment option is the right choice for a given patient, the cost of the treatments varies widely. For example, the Medicare reimbursement for traditional surgical removal of the prostate is approximately $10,000, while the first-year costs for proton beam therapy are nearly $40,000 (Institute for Clinical and Economic Review, 2010).

Increasing Occurrence of Multiple Chronic Conditions

Prostate cancer is not a unique case. For many conditions, patients and clinicians are presented with many diagnostic and treatment options but lack the evidence to know which option would be most effective. This situation is particularly prevalent for patients with chronic conditions. The prevalence of chronic conditions has increased over time. In 2000, 125 million people suffered from chronic conditions; by 2020, that number is projected to grow to an estimated 157 million (Anderson et al., 2010). Today one such condition, diabetes, affects almost 10 percent of the U.S. population (CDC, 2011a). Furthermore, approximately 75 million people in the United States have multiple, concurrent chronic conditions (Parekh and Barton, 2010). The costs of treating chronic conditions are high, with one study estimating that the care of patients with these conditions constitutes almost 80 percent of health care costs (Anderson and Horvath, 2004). A related finding illustrates the importance of caring for patients with serious health needs. An analysis of health care expenditures found that while patients with the highest health care costs represent just 5 percent of the total U.S. population, their care consumes 50 percent of total health care resources (Cohen and Yu, 2011).

The role of chronic conditions has changed as the demographics of the population have shifted. In general, the population has gotten older, with the portion of the population over the age of 65 having increased at 1.5 times the rate of the rest of the population in the past decade (Howden and Meyer, 2011). Almost half of the individuals in this population receive treatment for at least one chronic condition (Schneider et al., 2009); one-quarter are affected by just one of those conditions, diabetes (CDC, 2011a; Schneider et al., 2009). Furthermore, more than 20 percent of the elderly are receiving treatment for multiple chronic conditions (Schneider et al., 2009).

The complexity of care is particularly acute for patients with multiple chronic conditions. Treating these patients requires a holistic approach, because the use of multiple clinical practice guidelines developed for single diseases may have adverse effects (Boyd et al., 2005; Parekh and Barton, 2010; Tinetti et al., 2004). For example, various existing clinical practice guidelines would suggest that a hypothetical 79-year-old woman with osteoporosis, osteoarthritis, type 2 diabetes, hypertension, and chronic obstructive pulmonary disease should take as many as 19 doses of medication per day. Adherence to five separate sets of clinical practice guidelines for the woman's five diseases could result in adverse interactions between her medications, or a medication for one disease could exacerbate the symptoms of another (see Table 2-1 for potential treatment interactions). Such guidelines might also make conflicting recommendations for the woman's

TABLE 2-1 Potential Treatment Interactions for a Hypothetical 79-Year-Old Woman with Multiple Chronic Diseases

Disease	Type of Interaction		
	Medications with Potential Interactions	Medication and Other Disease	Medications for Different Diseases
Hypertension	Hydrochlorothiazide, lisinopril	Diabetes: diuretics increase serum glucose and lipids	• Diabetes medications: hydrochlorothiazide may decrease the effectiveness of glyburide
Diabetes	Glyburide, metformin, aspirin, atorvastatin	None known	• Osteoarthritis medications: NSAIDs plus aspirin increase the risk of bleeding • Diabetes medications: glyburide plus aspirin increase the risk of hypoglycemia; aspirin may decrease the effectiveness of lisinopril
Osteoarthritis	Nonsteroidal anti inflammatory drugs (NSAIDs)	Hypertension: NSAIDs raise blood pressure; NSAIDs plus hypertension increase risk of renal failure	• Diabetes medications: NSAIDs in combination with aspirin increase the risk of bleeding • Hypertension medications: NSAIDs decrease the efficacy of diuretics
Osteoporosis	Calcium, alendronate	None known	• Diabetes medications: calcium may decrease the efficacy of aspirin; aspirin plus alendronate can cause upset stomach • Osteoporosis medications: calcium may lower serum alendronate level
Chronic Obstructive Pulmonary Disease	Short-acting β-agonists	None known	• None known

SOURCE: Reprinted with permission from Boyd et al., 2005. Copyright © (2005) American Medical Association. All rights reserved.

care. If she had peripheral neuropathy, guidelines for osteoporosis would recommend that she perform weight-bearing exercise, while guidelines for diabetes would recommend that she avoid such exercise (Boyd et al., 2005). These situations create uncertainty for clinicians and patients as to the best course of action to pursue as they attempt to manage the treatments for multiple conditions.

A Strain on Human Capacity

As clinicians endeavor to provide the best and most appropriate care for their patients, they also struggle with the cognitive complexities inherent in making care decisions. In the clinical setting, providers begin the decision-making process from the moment they set eyes on their patients. For example, an emergency medicine clinician must make decisions on clinical factors such as the patient's medical history, test ordering, interpretation of laboratory results, diagnosis, treatment, and patient preferences, as well as nonclinical factors such as cost, allocation of resources, and administrative considerations (Croskerry, 2002).

Like the emergency department, the intensive care unit (ICU) is a particularly difficult environment for clinicians. These specialized units help the sickest and most fragile patients, who could not survive without the support of specialized technologies and equipment. The price of these new capabilities is extraordinary complexity that stresses the capabilities of individual clinicians. One observational study found that clinicians in ICUs perform in the range of 180 activities per patient per day, from replacing intravenous fluids, to calibrating a transducer, to administering drugs (Donchin et al., 2003). With new monitoring technologies, clinicians are able to observe the patient's health status precisely. For example, a patient who enters the ICU with acute respiratory distress is monitored with more than 20 vital sign parameters. With 6 to 12 patients in a typical ICU, a provider must monitor and act on up to 240 vital sign inputs, which stresses any individual provider's cognitive capabilities (Donchin and Seagull, 2002).

The growth in complexity is not limited to hospital environments. Physicians, nurses, physician assistants, and other health care professionals in outpatient settings are managing a great number of conditions and interventions. Quantifying the range of conditions managed by clinicians, a 2008 study of a large multispecialty practice in Massachusetts found that the practice managed more than 5,600 unique primary diagnoses and 6,400 unique secondary diagnoses, or almost half of all known identified diagnoses. Each clinician managed a median of approximately 250 unique primary diagnoses, 280 unique medications, and 130 unique laboratory tests. These figures were even higher for those clinicians in primary care fields, such as internal medicine, who managed a median of 370 unique primary diagnoses, 600 unique medications, and approximately 150 unique laboratory tests (Semel et al., 2010). These findings highlight the variety of needs clinicians now address, along with the variety of interventions and diagnostic tests they must manage.

Further, physicians often feel as though they do not have enough time to meet their patients' care needs (Burdi and Baker, 1999; Trude, 2003). Among primary care physicians responding to one survey, 30 percent reported not having adequate time to spend with their patients during a typical visit (Center for Studying Health System Change, 2004-2005), and a similar percentage of patients reported concerns about the amount of time their providers have to spend with them (AHRQ, 2010)—this despite evidence that the average length of a primary care visit has actually increased in recent years (Mechanic et al., 2001). Evidence suggests, however, that clinicians' perceptions are warranted. One study found that meeting a standard patient panel's acute, preventive, and chronic disease management needs would require more than 21 hours a day, as shown in Figure 2-4 (Yarnall et al., 2009).

As outlined above, the complexity of modern health care is reaching levels that challenge human cognitive capacity. Research in several areas has found that complexity can have negative effects on people's ability to make decisions (Simon, 1979, 1990; Weick and Sutcliffe, 2001). Complexity can cause people to defer making a decision, choose the default option, make no decision at all, or make an incorrect decision (Dhar, 1997; Shafir and Tversky, 1992; Shafir et al., 1993). As one example, when confronted with highly complex situations, people tend to use mental shortcuts, or heuristics, to manage the volume of evidence (Berner and Graber, 2008; Bullen and Sacks, 2003; Kampmann and Sterman, 1998; Payne et al., 1993;

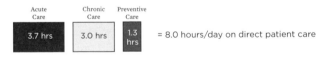

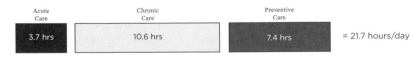

FIGURE 2-4 Time requirements for a primary care physician to treat a standard patient panel.
SOURCE: Data derived from Yarnall et al., 2009.

TABLE 2-2 Common Cognitive Errors in Clinical Decision Making

Error Type	Definition
Anchoring	Relying on initial impressions too early in the diagnostic process; failing to adjust initial impressions in light of new information
Availability	Judging a situation as being more likely or frequent if it easily comes to mind; judging based on the ease of recalling past cases
Framing bias	Tending to be swayed by subtleties in how a situation is presented (e.g., description of the risks and benefits of treatment options)
Premature closure	Accepting a diagnosis before it has been fully verified; believing in a single explanation of a situation without investigating other possibilities
Reliance on authority	Relying unduly on authority or technology

SOURCE: Reprinted with permission from Redelmeier, 2005.

Timmermans, 1993; Tversky and Kahneman, 1973, 1974). These mental shortcuts range from overrelying on memorable past experiences to accepting data that confirm preexisting expectations and ignoring data that do not (see Table 2-2 for a summary of five of the most common cognitive errors). Several studies suggest that heuristics are used in health care settings and can have real impacts on patient care (Gandhi et al., 2006; Graber et al., 2005).

In most cases, the shortcut works well to solve the problem at hand (Redelmeier, 2005). Precisely because these shortcuts usually produce the desired outcome, however, most people are unaware of their own susceptibility to cognitive errors. While strategies to overcome cognitive errors in clinical decision making are beginning to be identified (Croskerry, 2002, 2003; Redelmeier, 2005), time and resource constraints, increasing stress among providers, and growing complexity are all barriers to overcoming the risks of these errors.

The volume of biomedical and clinical knowledge being produced has increased steadily over the past few decades. The number of journal articles in biomedical and clinical research fields has quadrupled since 1970, rising from more than 200,000 a year in 1970 to more than 750,000 in 2010 (see Figure 2-5).[1] The pace of research now averages 75 trials and

---

[1]The number of peer-reviewed journal publications was determined from searches of PubMed for MEDLINE articles published during a given year using the following MeSH terms: Guideline [V02.515], Journal Article [V02.600], Review [V02.912], Technical Report [V02.989] (National Library of Medicine; http://www.ncbi.nlm.nih.gov/pubmed/).

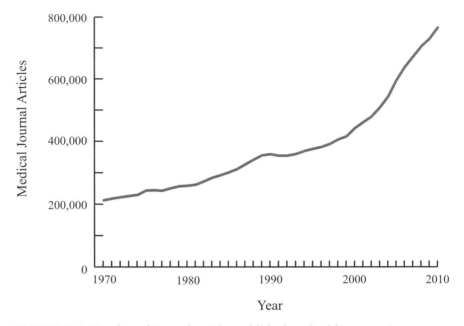

FIGURE 2-5 Number of journal articles published on health care topics per year from 1970 to 2010. Publications have increased steadily over 40 years, with the rate of increase becoming more pronounced starting approximately in 2000.
SOURCE: Data obtained from online searches at PubMed: http://www.ncbi.nlm. nih.gov/pubmed/.

11 systematic reviews of trials per day (Bastian et al., 2010). The pace at which new knowledge is produced outstrips the ability of any individual clinician to read, remember, and manage information that could inform clinical practice. A survey of faculty at one academic medical center found that they each read up to 322 papers per year (Tenopir et al., 2004). Given the almost 450,000 papers published in 2000, this amounts to less than 0.1 percent of the medical literature produced during the initial year in which the survey was conducted. Even within a narrow specialty, it is impossible for a clinician to keep pace with the published medical literature. If a clinician training in cardiac imaging read 40 papers a day for 5 days a week, then it would take more than 11 years for that clinician to become up to date in the field. By that time, however, another 82,000 potentially relevant papers would have been published, which would require another 8 years of reading. These figures assume that the clinician needs to know only about cardiac imaging and need not remain current in any other area of medical knowledge (Fraser and Dunstan, 2010).

The ever-increasing volume of evidence makes it difficult for clinicians to maintain a working knowledge of new clinical information. Even after identifying relevant information for a given condition, clinicians and their patients still must ensure that the information is of high quality. Clinicians must consider the quality of a study to minimize the possibility that the evidence will be contradicted by later studies, and ensure that the research is free of conflicts of interest and applies to their particular patient's clinical circumstances (Ioannidis, 2005; Prasad et al., 2011).

Uneven Diffusion of Knowledge

Although the supply of knowledge is increasing, there are lags in the time it takes to translate promising evidence into clinical practice. It is estimated that the results of a landmark study will take 15-16 years to be widely implemented following the study's publication (Balas and Boren, 2000). For example, it took 13 years for most experts to recommend thrombolytic drugs for heart attack treatment after their first positive clinical trial (Antman et al., 1992). Similarly, the results of major clinical trials often are not implemented in regular clinical practice, as was the case for the Occluded Artery Trial (OAT) on the timing of coronary angioplasty after heart attack (Deyell et al., 2011; Redberg, 2011), the Antihypertensive and Lipid-Lowering Treatment to Prevent Heart Attack Trial (ALLHAT) on effective treatments for high blood pressure (Avorn, 2010; Stafford et al., 2010), and the Clinical Outcomes Utilizing Revascularization and Aggressive Drug Evaluation (COURAGE) study on coronary angioplasty versus medical therapy (Borden et al., 2011). As a result of this slow diffusion of knowledge and other factors, Americans receive only half of the preventive, acute, and chronic care recommended by clinical guidelines (McGlynn et al., 2003) and approximately 60 percent of recommended pharmaceutical treatments (Shrank et al., 2006).

Implications of Advances in Genetics

The accelerating pace of research has led to striking prospects for individualized diagnoses and treatments. Although the potential is still largely unrealized, ongoing developments offer promise to accelerate this progress. For example, the cost of sequencing the whole genome has decreased from $2.7 billion, the cost when the first human genome was sequenced, to $10,000 in 2010 and may fall to as little as $1,000 in the foreseeable future (Samani et al., 2010). Between 2005 and 2008, more than 100 genetic variants associated with nearly 40 complex diseases and traits were identified and replicated using genomewide scans, and in 2008, genetic tests for more than 1,200 clinical conditions were available (Genetics and Public Policy

TABLE 2-3 Genetic Variants Used for Disease Diagnosis and Treatment

Disease/Condition	Genetic Factor
Hyperlipidemia susceptibility	LDL receptor gene mutation
Breast/ovarian cancer susceptibility	BRCA1/BRCA2 mutation
Lung cancer treatment	KRAS, EGFR, EML4-ALK, HER2, BRAF, MET, AKT1, MAP2K1, PIKCA mutations
Maturity-onset diabetes of the young classification	chromosome 7, glucokinase, chromosome 12, hepatic nuclear factor 1-alpha, etc., mutations

SOURCE: Data derived from IOM, 2011.

Center, 2008; Manolio, 2010; Pearson and Manolio, 2008). The genetic factors associated with a variety of diseases are now known and can be used in diagnosis and treatment (see Table 2-3) (IOM, 2011). These new discoveries highlight the magnitude of individual variation, adding numerous factors that clinicians may have to consider when evaluating the utility of different treatments and interventions.

One area in which advances in genetics have led to a more sophisticated understanding of disease is the ability to distinguish among different types of lung cancers. Traditionally, lung cancers were divided into types—small-cell and non-small-cell—based on the tumor's histological appearance. However, genetic discoveries have allowed histological classification to be replaced by classification based on the cancer cells' genetic profile, and more specifically, the genetic mutations that are the molecular drivers of cancer cell proliferation (see Figure 2-6). In 1987, one driver mutation, KRAS, was discovered, and another, EGFR, was discovered in 2004. Since then, knowledge of the molecular drivers of non-small-cell lung cancer has increased dramatically; by 2009, nine different driver mutations had been identified (IOM, 2011). While the development of therapies targeting specific driver mutations is just beginning, genetic classification of diseases holds great promise for tailoring care to patients' genetic variations.

An example of a case in which genetics are beginning to have a substantial impact on care is maturity-onset diabetes of the young (MODY). This rare form of diabetes, generally diagnosed in later adolescence or early adulthood, often is undiagnosed and is easily confused with other forms of diabetes. Treating patients with this condition used to be difficult because different patients would respond very differently to various treatments (O'Rahilly, 2009). With improved genetic understanding, however, MODY was found to be a cluster of diseases, each entailing a specific genetic abnormality. To date, six different varieties of this disease have been identified,

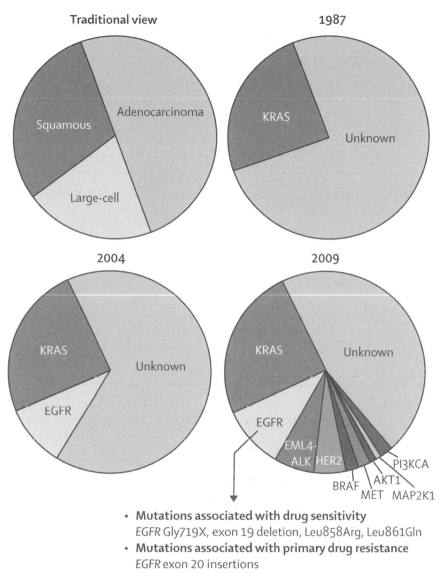

FIGURE 2-6 Evolution in knowledge of the genetic driver mutations associated with non-small-cell lung cancer.
SOURCE: Reprinted from Pao and Girard, 2011. Copyright (2011), with permission from Elsevier.

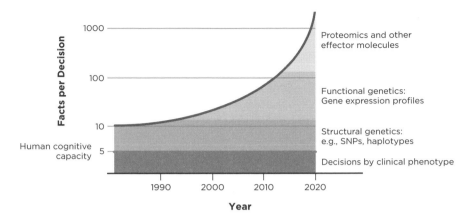

FIGURE 2-7 Schematic describing the sources of complexity in clinical decision making, highlighting their increase over time.
NOTE: SNP = single nucleotide polymorphism.
SOURCE: Adapted with permission from IOM, 2008.

each with a specific genetic component (Chromosome 12, HNF-1α; Chromosome 7, glucokinase; Chromosome 20, HNF-4α; Chromosome 13, insulin promoter factor-1 (IPF-1); Chromosome 17, HNF-1β; Chromosome 2, NeuroD1) (American Diabetes Association, 2011). This progress in genetics has allowed clinicians to personalize treatments based on which form of the disease a patient has. Some patients will respond well to low doses of oral hyperglycemia medications and will not need insulin therapy; others will require insulin injections; and others may have a stable condition and may not need aggressive glucose reduction therapies (Gill-Carey and Hattersley, 2007; Hattersley and Pearson, 2006; O'Rahilly, 2009).

Figure 2-7 illustrates how such advances in genetics and related fields have increased over time, adding to the complexity of clinical decision making. Indeed, as noted earlier, this growth in knowledge may be expanding beyond the limits of what human cognitive capacity can handle.

> *Conclusion 2-1: Diagnostic and treatment options are expanding and changing at an accelerating rate, placing new stresses on clinicians and patients, as well as potentially impacting the effectiveness and efficiency of care delivery.*

Related findings:

- *The volume of clinical studies is increasing rapidly.* On average, approximately 75 clinical trials and a dozen systematic reviews are published daily.

- *New knowledge on the molecular basis of disease is growing exponentially.* In one 3-year period alone, more than 100 genetic variants associated with nearly 40 complex diseases and traits were identified, and in 2008, genetic tests for more than 1,200 clinical conditions became available.
- *Options have changed and increased dramatically for many conditions.* In 1987, for example, only one drug was available to treat HIV; in 2011, 35 different drugs, many of which are used in combination, were available.
- *Clinicians perform more activities per patient and consider more factors in diagnosis and management of disease than ever before.* According to one estimate, more than 21 hours a day of an individual primary care clinician's time would be required to meet all acute and preventive care recommendations for a panel of patients.
- *Given the complexity of information, informed patient preference is an increasingly important consideration.* For the example of localized prostate cancer, it is unknown which treatment works best for a given patient—from watchful waiting, to radical prostatectomy, to radiation and chemotherapy.

Conclusion 2-2: *Chronic diseases and comorbid conditions are increasing, exacerbating the clinical, logistical, decision-making, and economic challenges faced by patients and clinicians.*

Related findings:

- *The prevalence of multiple chronic diseases is increasing.* About 75 million Americans have multiple, concurrent chronic conditions.
- *The population is aging, leading to new health challenges.* The portion of the population over 65 has increased at 1.5 times the rate of the rest of the population in the past decade, with half suffering from a chronic disease.
- *Care of patients with chronic conditions constitutes almost 80 percent of health care costs.* Further, while patients with the highest health care costs represent only 5 percent of the total population, their care consumes 50 percent of total health care resources.

ADMINISTRATIVE COMPLEXITY

Administrative complexity, including complicated workflows and fragmented financing, exacerbate the challenges posed by the clinical complexity described above.

Complicated Workflows

The health care system is characterized by administrative complexity that can waste clinicians' time and interfere with their caring for their patients, as well as increase costs and adversely impact patient outcomes. For example, a study investigating waste in the activities of front-line health care workers found that 35 percent of the workers' time was wasted (Wallace and Savitz, 2008).

Even accomplishing a seemingly straightforward activity such as filling a medication order is marked by unexpected intricacies. As illustrated in Figure 2-8, a medication order at one academic medical center can be filled in 786 different ways, involving a number of different health care professionals and technological channels (Thompson et al., 2003). Another study found that inefficient medication administration practices at one hospital caused nurses to waste 50 minutes per shift looking for the keys to the narcotics cabinet (Spear and Schmidhofer, 2005; Thompson et al., 2003). The results of this administrative complexity and inefficiency are delayed medications, potential errors, waste, and higher costs. Inefficient workflows also restrict the amount of time nurses can spend directly caring for patients; indeed, it has been found that hospital nurses spend only about 30 percent of their time in direct patient care (Hendrich et al., 2008; Hendrickson et al., 1990; Tucker and Spear, 2006).

Studies also have revealed the effects of system complexity on hospital staffing, and in turn on patient outcomes. Despite an average bed occupancy rate of 65 percent, hospitals frequently are overcrowded (Litvak, 2005; Litvak and Bisognano, 2011). Hospital admissions generally come from two sources: emergency departments (EDs), which are unpredictable as a source of admissions, and scheduled elective procedures, which are a seemingly predictable source (Litvak et al., 2005). Because hospitals staff for average occupancy and not for peaks, an unexpected influx of patients creates demands for resources and staff time that are impossible to meet, which can cause problems such as emergency room overcrowding, ICU readmissions, and ICU workload and safety problems (Baker et al., 2009; Carayon and Gurses, 2005; IOM, 2007). Studies have found associations between overcrowding and increased mortality (Needleman et al., 2011), as well as decreased adherence to safety practices, such as reconciling of medications, prevention practices for central-line-associated bloodstream infection, and handwashing (Jayawardhana et al., 2011).

Fragmented Financing

Approximately 60 percent of Americans under age 65 obtain health insurance from more than 1.5 million different employers that purchase

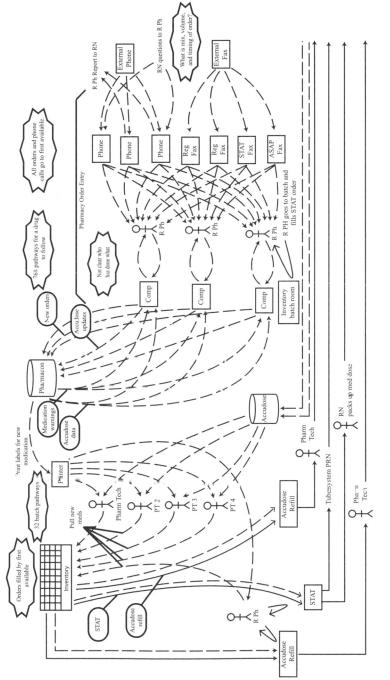

FIGURE 2-8 Diagram of processes for filling a medication order at one academic medical center.
SOURCE: Adapted and reprinted with permission from Thompson et al., 2003.

insurance plans from more than 1,200 insurers (Cebul et al., 2008). In a typical year, moreover, roughly 20 percent of health insurance policy-holders change their plans (Cebul et al., 2008; Cunningham and Kohn, 2000). Switches in health plans can occur because of transitions in job status, changes in eligibility for public programs (such as Medicaid or the Children's Health Insurance Program [CHIP]), or decisions to enroll in another employer-sponsored or individual plan. This frequent turnover in insurance relationships has implications for health care costs and outcomes. While many payers support preventive care and chronic care management, frequent changes in insurance enrollment lessen the incentives for investing in early interventions that can reduce long-term health care costs (Cebul et al., 2008).

Managing the requirements of many different health benefit plans places a heavy administrative burden on clinicians. A recent study found that physicians reported spending an average of 43 minutes a day on inter-actions with health plans—adding up to almost 3 weeks per year on such activities. Nursing staff spent 9 hours per physician per week interacting with health plans, and clerical staff 30 hours per physician per week. In monetary terms, in 2006 practices spent an average of $68,274 per physi-cian per year, the equivalent of roughly $31 billion, interacting with health plans (Casalino et al., 2009).

Continuity of care is compromised as a result of fragmented financing. A study of the overlap among health maintenance organizations (HMOs) in the same cities found that a person switching from one HMO to an-other had a 50 percent chance of having to change his or her primary care physician (Chernew et al., 2004). This finding is significantly problematic, as continuity of care is associated with a reduced likelihood of future hos-pitalizations and emergency visits (Gill and Mainous, 1998; Mainous and Gill, 1998; Menec et al., 2006; van Walraven et al., 2010). A recent study of low-income veterans found that as financing become more fragmented, patients were more likely to be hospitalized; the effect of fragmented financ-ing on hospitalizations was similar to that of being diagnosed with a major chronic disease (Pizer and Gardner, 2011).

Finally, it is important to recognize that health care delivery did not begin this way. Rather, it has evolved into a fragmented, disorganized amalgamation characterized by increasingly unmanageable complexity. Pre-vailing incentives—economic and cultural—allowed for and facilitated this development, and because many health care stakeholders contributed to this evolutionary process, all will need to be engaged in the transition to a continuously learning health care system.

Conclusion 2-3: Care delivery has become increasingly fragmented, leading to coordination and communication challenges for patients and clinicians.

Related findings:

- *Coordinating a patient's care has become more demanding for clinicians.* One study found that in a single year, a typical primary care physician coordinated with an average of 229 other physicians in 117 different practices just for his or her Medicare patient population (see Chapter 3).
- *Patients see a large number and variety of clinicians for their care.* Between 2000 and 2002, fee-for-service Medicare patients saw an average of seven physicians, including five specialists, split among four different practices (see Chapter 3).
- *The involvement of multiple providers tends to blur accountability.* One survey found that 75 percent of hospital patients were unable to identify the clinician in charge of their care (see Chapter 3).

REFERENCES

AHRQ (Agency for Healthcare Research and Quality). 2010. *The CAHPS database: Preliminary comparative data for the CAHPS clinician & group survey (12-month version).* Rockville, MD: AHRQ.

American Diabetes Association. 2011. Diagnosis and classification of diabetes mellitus. *Diabetes Care* 34(Suppl. 1):S62-S69.

Anderson, G. F. 2010. *Chronic care: Making the case for ongoing care.* Princeton, NJ: Robert Wood Johnson Foundation.

Anderson, G. F., and J. Horvath. 2004. The growing burden of chronic disease in America. *Public Health Reports* 119(3):263.

Antman, E. M., J. Lau, B. Kupelnick, F. Mosteller, and T. C. Chalmers. 1992. A comparison of results of meta-analyses of randomized control trials and recommendations of clinical experts. Treatments for myocardial infarction. *Journal of the American Medical Association* 268(2):240-248.

Antman, E. M., D. T. Anbe, P. W. Armstrong, E. R. Bates, L. A. Green, M. Hand, J. S. Hochman, H. M. Krumholz, F. G. Kushner, G. A. Lamas, C. J. Mullany, J. P. Ornato, D. L. Pearle, M. A. Sloan, S. C. Smith, J. S. Alpert, J. L. Anderson, D. P. Faxon, V. Fuster, R. J. Gibbons, G. Gregoratos, J. L. Halperin, L. F. Hiratzka, S. A. Hunt, A. K. Jacobs, American College of Cardiology, American Heart Association Task Force on Practice Guidelines, and Canadian Cardiovascular Society. 2004. ACC/AHA guidelines for the management of patients with ST-elevation myocardial infarction: A report of the American College of Cardiology/American Heart Association Task Force on Practice Guidelines (committee to revise the 1999 guidelines for the management of patients with acute myocardial infarction). *Circulation* 110(9):e82-e292.

Antman, E. M., M. Hand, P. W. Armstrong, E. R. Bates, L. A. Green, L. K. Halasyamani, J. S. Hochman, H. M. Krumholz, G. A. Lamas, C. J. Mullany, D. L. Pearle, M. A. Sloan, S. C. Smith, D. T. Anbe, F. G. Kushner, J. P. Ornato, A. K. Jacobs, C. D. Adams, J. L. Anderson, C. E. Buller, M. A. Creager, S. M. Ettinger, J. L. Halperin, S. A. Hunt, B. W. Lytle, R. Nishimura, R. L. Page, B. Riegel, L. G. Tarkington, C. W. Yancy, Canadian Cardiovascular Society, American Academy of Family Physicians, American College of Cardiology, and American Heart Association. 2008. 2007 focused update of the ACC/AHA 2004 guidelines for the management of patients with ST-elevation myocardial infarction: A report of the American College of Cardiology/American Heart Association Task Force on Practice Guidelines. *Journal of the American College of Cardiology* 51(2):210-247.

Avorn, J. 2010. Transforming trial results into practice change: The final translational hurdle: Comment on "impact of the ALLHAT/JNC7 dissemination project on thiazide-type diuretic use." *Archives of Internal Medicine* 170(10):858-860.

Baker, D. R., P. J. Pronovost, L. L. Morlock, R. G. Geocadin, and C. G. Holzmueller. 2009. Patient flow variability and unplanned readmissions to an intensive care unit. *Critical Care Medicine* 37(11):2882-2887.

Balas, E., and S. Boren. 2000. Managing clinical knowledge for health care improvement. *Yearbook of Medical Informatics* 65-70.

Bastian, H., P. Glasziou, and I. Chalmers. 2010. Seventy-five trials and eleven systematic reviews a day: How will we ever keep up? *PLoS Medicine* 7(9):e1000326.

Bennett, C. L. 2012. A 56-year-old physician who underwent a PSA test. *Archives of Internal Medicine* 172(4):311.

Berner, E. S., and M. L. Graber. 2008. Overconfidence as a cause of diagnostic error in medicine. *American Journal of Medicine* 121(Suppl. 5):S2-S23.

Borden, W. B., R. F. Redberg, A. I. Mushlin, D. Dai, L. A. Kaltenbach, and J. A. Spertus. 2011. Patterns and intensity of medical therapy in patients undergoing percutaneous coronary intervention. *Journal of the American Medical Association* 305(18):1882-1889.

Boyd, C. M., J. Darer, C. Boult, L. P. Fried, L. Boult, and A. W. Wu. 2005. Clinical practice guidelines and quality of care for older patients with multiple comorbid diseases. *Journal of the American Medical Association* 294(6):716.

Braunwald, E., E. M. Antman, J. W. Beasley, R. M. Califf, M. D. Cheitlin, J. S. Hochman, R. H. Jones, D. Kereiakes, J. Kupersmith, T. N. Levin, C. J. Pepine, J. W. Schaeffer, E. E. Smith, D. E. Steward, P. Theroux, J. S. Alpert, K. A. Eagle, D. P. Faxon, V. Fuster, T. J. Gardner, G. Gregoratos, R. O. Russell, and S. C. Smith. 2000. ACC/AHA guidelines for the management of patients with unstable angina and non-ST-segment elevation myocardial infarction. A report of the American College of Cardiology/American Heart Association Task Force on Practice Guidelines (Committee on the Management of Patients with Unstable Angina). *Journal of the American College of Cardiology* 36(3):970-1062.

Braunwald, E., E. M. Antman, J. W. Beasley, R. M. Califf, M. D. Cheitlin, J. S. Hochman, R. H. Jones, D. Kereiakes, J. Kupersmith, T. N. Levin, C. J. Pepine, J. W. Schaeffer, E. E. Smith, D. E. Steward, P. Theroux, R. J. Gibbons, J. S. Alpert, D. P. Faxon, V. Fuster, G. Gregoratos, L. F. Hiratzka, A. K. Jacobs, S. C. Smith, American College of Cardiology, and American Heart Association Committee on the Management of Patients with Unstable Angina. 2002. ACC/AHA 2002 guideline update for the management of patients with unstable angina and non-ST-segment elevation myocardial infarction—summary article: A report of the American College of Cardiology/American Heart Association Task Force on Practice Guidelines (Committee on the Management of Patients with Unstable Angina). *Journal of the American College of Cardiology* 40(7):1366-1374.

Bullen, G., and L. Sacks. 2003. Towards new modes of decision making—complexity and human factors. *Version* 1:1-5.

Burdi, M. D., and L. C. Baker. 1999. Physicians' perceptions of autonomy and satisfaction in California. *Health Affairs* 18(4):134.

Carayon, P., and A. P. Gurses. 2005. A human factors engineering conceptual framework of nursing workload and patient safety in intensive care units. *Intensive & Critical Care Nursing: The Official Journal of the British Association of Critical Care Nurses* 21(5):284-301.

Casalino, L. P., S. Nicholson, D. N. Gans, T. Hammons, D. Morra, T. Karrison, and W. Levinson. 2009. What does it cost physician practices to interact with health insurance plans? *Health Affairs* 28(4):W533-W543.

CDC (Centers for Disease Control and Prevention). 1999. Ten great public health achievements—United States, 1900-1999. *Morbidity and Mortality Weekly Report* 48(12): 241-243.

CDC. 2011a. *National diabetes fact sheet: National estimates and general information on diabetes and prediabetes in the United States, 2011.* Atlanta, GA: U.S. Department of Health and Human Services, CDC.

CDC. 2011b. Ten great public health achievements—United States, 2001-2010. *Morbidity and Mortality Weekly Report* 60(19):619-623.

Cebul, R., J. Rebitzer, L. Taylor, and M. Votruba. 2008. *Organizational fragmentation and care quality in the U.S. health care system.* Cambridge, MA: National Bureau of Economic Research.

Center for Studying Health System Change. 2004-2005. *Physician survey.* http://hscdataonline.s-3.com/psurvey.asp (accessed November 11, 2011).

Certo, C. M. 1985. History of cardiac rehabilitation. *Physical Therapy* 65(12):1793-1795.

Chernew, M. E., W. P. Wodchis, D. P. Scanlon, and C. G. McLaughlin. 2004. Overlap in HMO physician networks. *Health Affairs* 23(2):91.

Cohen, S. B., and W. Yu. 2011. *The concentration and persistence in the level of health expenditures over time: Estimates for the U.S. population, 2008-2009.* Rockville, MD: AHRQ.

Croskerry, P. 2002. Achieving quality in clinical decision making: Cognitive strategies and detection of bias. *Academic Emergency Medicine* 9(11):1184-1204.

Croskerry, P. 2003. The importance of cognitive errors in diagnosis and strategies to minimize them. *Academic Medicine* 78(8):775.

Cunningham, P. J., and L. Kohn. 2000. Health plan switching: Choice or circumstance? *Health Affairs* 19(3):158.

DeVita, V. T., Jr., and E. Chu. 2008. A history of cancer chemotherapy. *Cancer Research* 68(21):8643-8653.

DeVita, V. T., Jr., and S. A. Rosenberg. 2012. Two hundred years of cancer research. *New England Journal of Medicine* 366(23):2207-2214.

Deyell, M. W., C. E. Buller, L. H. Miller, T. Y. Wang, D. Dai, G. A. Lamas, V. S. Srinivas, and J. S. Hochman. 2011. Impact of national clinical guideline recommendations for revascularization of persistently occluded infarct-related arteries on clinical practice in the United States. *Archives of Internal Medicine* 171(18):1636-1643.

Dhar, R. 1997. Consumer preference for a no-choice option. *Journal of Consumer Research* 24(2):215-231.

Donchin, Y., and F. J. Seagull. 2002. The hostile environment of the intensive care unit. *Current Opinion in Critical Care* 8(4):316-320.

Donchin, Y., D. Gopher, M. Olin, Y. Badihi, M. Biesky, C. L. Sprung, R. Pizov, and S. Cotev. 2003. A look into the nature and causes of human errors in the intensive care unit. *Quality & Safety in Health Care* 12(2):143-147.

Fagerlin, A., K. R. Sepucha, M. P. Couper, C. A. Levin, E. Singer, and B. J. Zikmund-Fisher. 2010. Patients' knowledge about 9 common health conditions: The decisions survey. *Medical Decision Making* 30(Suppl 5.):S35-S52.

Fang, J., M. H. Alderman, N. L. Keenan, and C. Ayala. 2010. Acute myocardial infarction hospitalization in the United States, 1979 to 2005. *American Journal of Medicine* 123(3):259-266.

Fauci, A. S. 2003. HIV and AIDS: 20 years of science. *Nature Medicine* 9(7):839-843.

FDA (Food and Drug Administration). 2011a. *Antiretroviral drugs used in the treatment of HIV infection*. http://www.fda.gov/ForConsumers/ByAudience/ForPatientAdvocates/HIVandAIDSActivities/ucm118915.htm (accessed February 1, 2012).

FDA. 2011b. *Timeline/history*. http://www.fda.gov/ForConsumers/ByAudience/ForPatient Advocates/HIVandAIDSActivities/ucm117935.htm (accessed February 2, 2012).

Fischl, M. A., D. D. Richman, M. H. Grieco, M. S. Gottlieb, P. A. Volberding, O. L. Laskin, J. M. Leedom, J. E. Groopman, D. Mildvan, and R. T. Schooley. 1987. The efficacy of azidothymidine (AZT) in the treatment of patients with AIDS and AIDS-related complex. *New England Journal of Medicine* 317(4):185-191.

Floyd, K. C., J. Yarzebski, F. A. Spencer, D. Lessard, J. E. Dalen, J. S. Alpert, J. M. Gore, and R. J. Goldberg. 2009. A 30-year perspective (1975-2005) into the changing landscape of patients hospitalized with initial acute myocardial infarction: Worcester Heart Attack Study. *Circulation. Cardiovascular Quality and Outcomes* 2(2):88-95.

Fraser, A. G., and F. D. Dunstan. 2010. On the impossibility of being expert. *British Medical Journal* 341:c6815.

Gandhi, T. K., A. Kachalia, E. J. Thomas, A. L. Puopolo, C. Yoon, T. A. Brennan, and D. M. Studdert. 2006. Missed and delayed diagnoses in the ambulatory setting: A study of closed malpractice claims. *Annals of Internal Medicine* 145(7):488.

Genetics and Public Policy Center. 2008. *FDA regulation of genetic tests*. http://www.dnapolicy.org/policy.issue.php?action=detail&issuebrief_id=11&print=1 (accessed January 4, 2010).

Gill, J. M., and A. G. Mainous, III. 1998. The role of provider continuity in preventing hospitalizations. *Archives of Family Medicine* 7(4):352.

Gill-Carey, O., and A. T. Hattersley. 2007. Genetics and type 2 diabetes in youth. *Pediatric Diabetes* 8(Suppl. 9):42-47.

Graber, M. L., N. Franklin, and R. Gordon. 2005. Diagnostic error in internal medicine. *Archives of Internal Medicine* 165(13):1493.

Guyer, B., M. A. Freedman, D. M. Strobino, and E. J. Sondik. 2000. Annual summary of vital statistics: Trends in the health of Americans during the 20th century. *Pediatrics* 106(6):1307-1317.

Hattersley, A. T., and E. R. Pearson. 2006. Minireview: Pharmacogenetics and beyond: The interaction of therapeutic response, beta-cell physiology, and genetics in diabetes. *Endocrinology* 147(6):2657-2663.

Hegarty, J., P. V. Beirne, E. Walsh, H. Comber, T. Fitzgerald, and M. Wallace Kazer. 2010. Radical prostatectomy versus watchful waiting for prostate cancer. *Cochrane Database System Reviews* (11):CD006590.

Heidenreich, P. A., and M. McClellan. 2001. Trends in treatment and outcomes for acute myocardial infarction: 1975-1995. *American Journal of Medicine* 110(3):165-174.

Hendrich, A., M. P. Chow, B. A. Skierczynski, and Z. Lu. 2008. A 36-hospital time and motion study: How do medical-surgical nurses spend their time? *Permanente Journal* 12(3):25-34.

Hendrickson, G., T. M. Doddato, and C. T. Kovner. 1990. How do nurses use their time? *Journal of Nursing Administration* 20(3):31-37.

Howden, L. M., and J. A. Meyer. 2011. *Age and sex composition: 2010*. Washington, DC: U.S. Census Bureau, U.S. Department of Commerce.

Howlader, N., A. Noone, M. Krapcho, N. Neyman, R. Aminou, W. Waldron, S. Altekruse, C. Kosary, J. Ruhl, Z. Tatalovich, H. Cho, A. Mariotto, M. Eisner, D. Lewis, H. Chen, E. Feuer, K. Cronin, and B. E. Edwards. 2011. *SEER cancer statistics review, 1975-2008.* http://seer.cancer.gov/statfacts/html/prost.html (accessed December 13, 2011).

Institute for Clinical and Economic Review. 2010. *Management options for low-risk prostate cancer: A report on comparative effectiveness and value.* Boston, MA: Institute for Clinical and Economic Review.

Ioannidis, J. P. A. 2005. Why most published research findings are false. *PLoS Medicine* 2(8):696-701.

IOM (Institute of Medicine). 2007. *Hospital-based emergency care: At the breaking point.* Washington, DC: The National Academies Press.

IOM. 2008. *Evidence-based medicine and the changing nature of health care: 2007 IOM annual meeting summary.* Washington, DC: The National Academies Press.

IOM. 2011. *Toward precision medicine: Building a knowlege network for biomedical research and a new taxonomy of disease.* Washington, DC: The National Academies Press.

Jayawardhana, J., J. M. Welton, and R. Lindrooth. 2011. Adoption of National Quality Forum safe practices by Magnet® hospitals. *Journal of Nursing Administration* 41(9):350-356.

Kampmann, C., and J. D. Sterman. 1998. *Feedback complexity, bounded rationality, and market dynamics.* Cambridge, MA: Massachusetts Institute of Technology.

Litvak, E. 2005. Optimizing patient flow by managing its variability. *Front Office to Front Line: Essential Issues for Health Care Leaders* 91-111.

Litvak, E., and M. Bisognano. 2011. More patients, less payment: Increasing hospital efficiency in the aftermath of health reform. *Health Affairs (Millwood)* 30(1):76-80.

Litvak, E., P. I. Buerhaus, F. Davidoff, M. C. Long, M. L. McManus, and D. M. Berwick. 2005. Managing unnecessary variability in patient demand to reduce nursing stress and improve patient safety. *Joint Commission Journal on Quality and Patient Safety* 31(6):330-338.

Mainous, III, A., and J. Gill. 1998. The importance of continuity of care in the likelihood of future hospitalization: Is site of care equivalent to a primary clinician? *American Journal of Public Health* 88(10):1539.

Makarov, D. V., J. B. Yu, R. A. Desai, D. F. Penson, and C. P. Gross. 2011. The association between diffusion of the surgical robot and radical prostatectomy rates. *Medical Care* 49(4):333-339.

Manolio, T. A. 2010. Emerging genomic information. In *Redesigning the clinical effectiveness research paradigm: Innovation and practice-based approaches: Workshop summary.* Institute of Medicine. Washington, DC: The National Academies Press. Pp. 189-206.

McGlynn, E. A., S. M. Asch, J. Adams, J. Keesey, J. Hicks, A. DeCristofaro, and E. A. Kerr. 2003. The quality of health care delivered to adults in the United States. *New England Journal of Medicine* 348(26):2635-2645.

Mechanic, D., D. D. McAlpine, and M. Rosenthal. 2001. Are patients' office visits with physicians getting shorter? *New England Journal of Medicine* 344(3):198-204.

Menec, V. H., M. Sirski, D. Attawar, and A. Katz. 2006. Does continuity of care with a family physician reduce hospitalizations among older adults? *Journal of Health Services Research & Policy* 11(4):196-201.

Nabel, E. G., and E. Braunwald. 2012. A tale of coronary artery disease and myocardial infarction. *New England Journal of Medicine* 366(1):54-63.

Needleman, J., P. Buerhaus, V. S. Pankratz, C. L. Leibson, S. R. Stevens, and M. Harris. 2011. Nurse staffing and inpatient hospital mortality. *New England Journal of Medicine* 364(11):1037-1045.

O'Rahilly, S. 2009. Human genetics illuminates the paths to metabolic disease. *Nature* 462(7271):307-314.

Panel on Antiretroviral Guidelines for Adults and Adolescents. 2011. *Guidelines for the use of antiretroviral agents in HIV-1-infected adults and adolescents.* Rockville, MD: Department of Health and Human Services.

Pao, W., and N. Girard. 2011. New driver mutations in non-small-cell lung cancer. *Lancet Oncology* 12(2):175-180.

Parekh, A. K., and M. B. Barton. 2010. The challenge of multiple comorbidity for the US health care system. *Journal of the American Medical Association* 303(13):1303-1304.

Payne, J. W., J. R. Bettman, and E. J. Johnson. 1993. *The adaptive decision maker.* Cambridge, United Kingdom: Cambridge University Press.

Pearson, T. A., and T. A. Manolio. 2008. How to interpret a genome-wide association study. *Journal of the American Medical Association* 299(11):1335-1344.

Pizer, S., and J. Gardner. 2011. Is fragmented financing bad for your health? *Inquiry* 48(2):109-122.

Prasad, V., V. Gall, and A. Cifu. 2011. The frequency of medical reversal. *Archives of Internal Medicine* 171(18):1675-1676.

Redberg, R. F. 2011. PCI for late reperfusion after myocardial infarction continues despite negative oat trial: Less is more. *Archives of Internal Medicine* 171(18):1645.

Redelmeier, D. A. 2005. The cognitive psychology of missed diagnoses. *Annals of Internal Medicine* 142(2):115-120.

Rogers, W. J., P. D. Frederick, E. Stoehr, J. G. Canto, J. P. Ornato, C. M. Gibson, C. V. Pollack, J. M. Gore, N. Chandra-Strobos, E. D. Peterson, and W. J. French. 2008. Trends in presenting characteristics and hospital mortality among patients with ST elevation and non-ST elevation myocardial infarction in the National Registry of Myocardial Infarction from 1990 to 2006. *American Heart Journal* 156(6):1026-1034.

Samani, N. J., M. Tomaszewski, and H. Schunkert. 2010. The personal genome—the future of personalised medicine? *Lancet* 375(9725):1497-1498.

Schneider, K. M., B. E. O'Donnell, and D. Dean. 2009. Prevalence of multiple chronic conditions in the United States' Medicare population. *Health and Quality of Life Outcomes* 7:82.

Semel, M. E., A. M. Bader, A. Marston, S. R. Lipsitz, R. E. Marshall, and A. A. Gawande. 2010. Measuring the range of services clinicians are responsible for in ambulatory practice. *Journal of Evaluation in Clinical Practice* 18(2):404-408.

Sepucha, K. R., A. Fagerlin, M. P. Couper, C. A. Levin, E. Singer, and B. J. Zikmund-Fisher. 2010. How does feeling informed relate to being informed? The decisions survey. *Medical Decision Making* 30(Suppl. 5):S77-S84.

Shafir, E., and A. Tversky. 1992. Thinking through uncertainty: Nonconsequential reasoning and choice. *Cognitive Psychology* 24(4):449-474.

Shafir, E., I. Simonson, and A. Tversky. 1993. Reason-based choice. *Cognition* 49(1-2):11-36.

Shrank, W. H., S. M. Asch, J. Adams, C. Setodji, E. A. Kerr, J. Keesey, S. Malik, and E. A. McGlynn. 2006. The quality of pharmacologic care for adults in the United States. *Medical Care* 44(10):936-945.

Simon, H. A. 1979. Rational decision making in business organizations. *American Economic Review* 69(4):493-513.

Simon, H. A. 1990. Invariants of human behavior. *Annual Review of Psychology* 41(1):1-20.

Simon, V., D. D. Ho, and Q. Abdool Karim. 2006. HIV/AIDS epidemiology, pathogenesis, prevention, and treatment. *Lancet* 368(9534):489-504.

Spear, S. J., and M. Schmidhofer. 2005. Ambiguity and workarounds as contributors to medical error. *Annals of Internal Medicine* 142(8):627-630.

Stafford, R. S., L. K. Bartholomew, W. C. Cushman, J. A. Cutler, B. R. Davis, G. Dawson, P. T. Einhorn, C. D. Furberg, L. B. Piller, S. L. Pressel, P. K. Whelton, and ALLHAT Collaborative Research Group. 2010. Impact of the ALLHAT/JNC7 dissemination project on thiazide-type diuretic use. *Archives of Internal Medicine* 170(10):851-858.

Tenopir, C., D. W. King, and A. Bush. 2004. Medical faculty's use of print and electronic journals: Changes over time and in comparison with scientists. *Journal of the Medical Library Association* 92(2):233-241.

Thompson, D. N., G. A. Wolf, and S. J. Spear. 2003. Driving improvement in patient care: Lessons from Toyota. *Journal of Nursing Administration* 33(11):585.

Timmermans, D. 1993. The impact of task complexity on information use in multi-attribute decision making. *Journal of Behavioral Decision Making* 6(2):95-111.

Tinetti, M. E., S. T. Bogardus, and J. V. Agostini. 2004. Potential pitfalls of disease-specific guidelines for patients with multiple conditions. *New England Journal of Medicine* 351(27):2870-2874.

Trude, S. 2003. So much to do, so little time: Physician capacity constraints, 1997-2001. *Tracking Report/Center for Studying Health System Change* (8):1.

Tucker, A. L., and S. J. Spear. 2006. Operational failures and interruptions in hospital nursing. *Health Services Research* 41(3 Pt. 1):643-662.

Tversky, A., and D. Kahneman. 1973. Availability: A heuristic for judging frequency and probability* 1,* 2. *Cognitive Psychology* 5(2):207-232.

Tversky, A., and D. Kahneman. 1974. Judgment under uncertainty: Heuristics and biases. *Science* 185(4157):1124.

van Walraven, C., N. Oake, A. Jennings, and A. J. Forster. 2010. The association between continuity of care and outcomes: A systematic and critical review. *Journal of Evaluation in Clinical Practice* 16(5):947-956.

Wallace, C. J., and L. Savitz. 2008. Estimating waste in frontline health care worker activities. *Journal of Evaluation in Clinical Practice* 14(1):178-180.

Weick, K. E., and K. M. Sutcliffe. 2001. *Managing the unexpected: Assuring high performance in an age of complexity.* San Francisco, CA: Jossey-Bass.

Wilt, T., T. Shamliyan, B. Taylor, R. MacDonald, J. Tacklind, I. Rutks, K. Koeneman, C.-S. Cho, and R. Kane. 2008a. *Comparative effectiveness of therapies for clinically localized prostate cancer. Comparative effectiveness review no. 13.* Rockville, MD: AHRQ.

Wilt, T. J., R. MacDonald, I. Rutks, T. A. Shamliyan, B. C. Taylor, and R. L. Kane. 2008b. Systematic review: Comparative effectiveness and harms of treatments for clinically localized prostate cancer. *Annals of Internal Medicine* 148(6):435-448.

Yarnall, K. S. H., K. Krause, K. Pollak, M. Gradison, and J. Michener. 2009. Family physicians as team leaders: "Time" to share the care. *Preventing Chronic Disease* 6(2):A59.

Zikmund-Fisher, B. J., M. P. Couper, E. Singer, P. A. Ubel, S. Ziniel, F. J. Fowler, Jr., C. A. Levin, and A. Fagerlin. 2010. Deficits and variations in patients' experience with making 9 common medical decisions: The decisions survey. *Medical Decision Making* 30(Suppl. 5):S85-S95.

3

Imperative: Achieving Greater Value in Health Care

Thomas Kundig periodically suffered back pain from an old rock climbing accident. When the pain recurred, he would contact his clinician, only to wait for at least a week to obtain an appointment with a specialist. He would have his back imaged (generally with an x-ray but at least once with magnetic resonance imaging [MRI]) and then receive a prescription for painkillers to get him through the episode. For Thomas, the problem was not just the cost of these therapies, but the hassle and time demands of tests and visits. But Thomas's outlook improved when his health care system changed the way it treated back pain at its spine clinic. Patients now began with physical therapy, with MRIs and intensive imaging being limited to those patients they were most likely to benefit. As a result of this new approach to back pain treatment, when Thomas's back pain returned the next time, the clinic had an appointment available for the next day. Based on an evaluation of his symptoms, a doctor found he did not need an MRI or prescription medications, but instead prescribed physical therapy and an over-the-counter anti-inflammatory drug. After four physical therapy sessions, Thomas's back felt better, and he learned how to continue the exercises on his own, which felt to him like more of a permanent solution to the problem (Fuhrmans, 2007). Nationwide, studies have found that imaging for lower back pain is overused, being prescribed for many patients who will not benefit from these intensive tests (Good Stewardship Working Group, 2011).

As patients and providers struggle with the increased complexity of modern medicine (Chapter 2), the nation struggles with the clear and compelling imperative to improve the value of health care—that is, to achieve better outcomes at lower cost. The challenges of complexity and value are closely linked as the central dilemmas driving the need for attention to opportunities for the continuous learning and improvement that is the focus of this report.

UNACCEPTABLE OUTCOMES

Currently, the U.S. health care system is failing to achieve its potential in either the quality of care or the outcomes of care. These shortfalls can be seen in areas as diverse as patient safety, the evidence basis for care, care coordination, access to care, and health disparities. If the health care system is to realize its potential, a concerted effort to learn and improve on each of these dimensions will be necessary.

Patient Safety

More than a decade ago, the Institute of Medicine (IOM) released *To Err Is Human: Building a Safer Health System,* in which it was estimated that at least 44,000 people, and perhaps as many as 98,000, died in hospitals every year as a result of preventable medical errors (1999). Ten years later, as illustrated in Box 3-1, medical errors still occur routinely (Downey et al., 2012). A study of 10 North Carolina hospitals over a 5-year period, for example, found that approximately 18 percent of patients were harmed by medical care, with 63 percent of those cases being judged as preventable (Landrigan et al., 2010). This finding was reinforced by a nationwide study revealing that one in seven Medicare patients suffered harm from hospital care, with an additional one in seven suffering temporary harm from care-related problems that were detected in time and corrected; 44 percent of these errors were found to be preventable (Levinson, 2010). A third study found that the rate of adverse events in hospitals could be as high as one-third of all admissions (Classen et al., 2011). One of the difficulties of measuring the magnitude of medical errors is that they often are unreported. A recent study found that 86 percent of adverse events were not submitted to existing hospital incident reporting systems, partly because of confusion about what constitutes patient harm (Levinson, 2012). These errors carry substantial financial costs, lengthen patients' hospital stays, and in some cases increase mortality (Zhan and Miller, 2003).

Although infections and complications once were viewed as routine consequences of medical care, it is now recognized that strategies and evidence-based interventions exist that can significantly reduce the incidence

---

BOX 3-1
An Example of Patient Harm

The human impact of medical errors is best appreciated from the lens of the individuals affected. One notable example is that of Ms. Grant, a 68-year-old nondiabetic who underwent cardiac bypass surgery. Two weeks after a series of complications related to her surgery, she was in stable condition in the intensive care unit (ICU). Her doctor noted that she was doing well and appeared to be on the way to a full recovery.

At 6:45 AM, Ms. Grant's arterial line became blocked—a frequent occurrence for this type of case—and her ICU nurse promptly responded with a 1-2 mL heparin flush. Ms. Grant appeared to be recovering from the setback until 8:15 AM, when her ICU nurse heard her coughing and rushed into her room to find her seizing. The nurse gave Ms. Grant labetalol to control her high systolic blood pressure, and the ICU team administered a barrage of diagnostics and therapies.

At 8:45 AM, Ms. Grant's results returned from the laboratory. Her serum glucose level was undetectable. Confused by these results, the ICU team administered two ampules of 50 percent dextrose in water to control Ms. Grant's sudden hypoglycemia, and then began to investigate her rapid deterioration.

At 9:15 AM, the team discovered a near-empty 10 mL vial of insulin on a medicine cart outside Ms. Grant's room, suggesting that earlier that morning, the ICU nurse had inadvertently treated Ms. Grant's arterial line blockage not with heparin but with insulin. Upon further investigation, the ICU team found that multidose vials of both heparin and insulin were on top of the medicine cart outside Ms. Grant's room at the time of the error. The vials looked similar, both held 10 mL of solution, and it was ICU practice to use multidose vials. Even though insulin should have been stored in the refrigerator, it was routinely kept on the medicine cart, and the hospital had no system of double checking or barcode checking high-risk drugs before they were administered.

Ms. Grant spent 7 weeks in a coma, at which point her family withdrew life support and she died (Bates, 2002).

As with many medical errors, the problem was not just the action of the individual clinician but the system that allowed it to happen. This particular error, the incorrect administration of insulin, accounts for 11 percent of serious medication errors, and insulin and heparin are known to be mistaken for one another because they are both administered in similar units and often stored in close proximity. Further, Ms. Grant's case is not unique to the hospital at which she sought care, but involved an error that has been experienced by many patients across the country (Cohen, 1999; Cohen et al., 1998).

---

and severity of such events. For example, there are proven methods for preventing catheter-related bloodstream infections, especially in intensive care unit (ICU) settings (Pronovost et al., 2006). Given that these potentially deadly infections prove fatal 12-25 percent of the time, such interventions can have a substantial impact on mortality (CDC, 2011). Despite progress in reducing the number of these infections with evidence-based interventions, however, 23,000 such infections occurred in inpatient wards in 2009, at an extraordinary cost to the health care system and with an unacceptable risk of serious harm to patients (CDC, 2011). Such evidence-based interventions exist for many aspects of patient safety, yet few are used widely in patient care.

The Evidence Basis for Care

Another area for improvement is ensuring that clinical evidence guides patient care. For example, Americans receive only about half of the preventive, acute, and chronic care recommended by current research and evidence-based guidelines (McGlynn et al., 2003). Patients with diabetes, for instance, receive the recommended preventive care only 21 percent of the time (AHRQ, 2011b).

Estimates vary on the proportion of clinical decisions that are based on evidence, with some studies suggesting only 10-20 percent (Darst et al., 2010; IOM, 1985). The need for evidence also is reflected in clinical guidelines. A study of guidelines for the 10 most common types of cancer found that only 6 percent of the guidelines' recommendations were based on a high level of evidence with uniform consensus (Poonacha and Go, 2011). An examination of 51 guidelines for treating lung cancer, for example, found that less than a third of the recommendations were evidence based (Harpole et al., 2003; IOM, 2009a). Another study found that fewer than half of the guidelines for treatment of infectious diseases are based on clinical trials (Lee and Vielemeyer, 2011).

Even when evidence-based guidelines are available, they are not always followed. For example, a recent analysis of implantable cardioverter-defibrillator (ICD) implants found that 22 percent were implanted in circumstances counter to the recommendations of professional society guidelines (Al-Khatib et al., 2011). While ICDs can be life-saving for many patients, they can be uncomfortable, inconvenient, and even life-threatening when implanted inappropriately.

This failure to deliver evidence-based care to patients results in suboptimal health outcomes. For example, consistently providing preventive services and interventions according to the best clinical evidence could prevent or postpone the majority of deaths from heart disease in the adult population (Kottke et al., 2009). The limited evidence supporting care delivery also contributes to widespread variations in clinical practice. For example, one study found that deliveries of normal-weight babies by caesarean section accounted for 7 percent of all births in some regions and almost 30 percent in others (Baicker et al., 2006).

Care Coordination

The coordination of each patient's care over time is another area for improvement. As patients move among providers and settings, they are subject to treatment errors and duplicative services. A recent survey revealed that patients experience problems with receiving results of medical tests and information about their medical history and that test results frequently are unavailable at the time of doctors' appointments. Almost 20 percent of patients reported that test results or medical records were not transferred from another provider or a laboratory in time for an appointment. Nearly one-quarter of patients said their health care provider had to order a previously performed test to have accurate information for diagnosis (Stremikis et al., 2011). Similarly, care often is not coordinated with the patient. One study found that in 1 of every 14 tests, either the patient was not informed of a clinically significant abnormal test result, or the clinician failed to record reporting the result to the patient (Casalino et al., 2009). In the previously cited study of Stremikis and colleagues (2011), half of survey respondents said they had experienced waste and inefficiency in the health care system, and one-third said the system is poorly organized (Stremikis et al., 2011).

Patients also have reported poor communication between their primary care providers and specialists, and the reported likelihood of these coordination failures increases with the number of physicians seen (Stremikis et al., 2011). This trend is particularly concerning given that, as noted in Chapter 2, Medicare patients see an average of seven physicians, including five specialists, split among four different practices (Pham et al., 2007). The presence of multiple comorbidities only exacerbates this trend. One study found that while the average Medicare patient with type 2 diabetes but no comorbidity saw an average of 5.6 physicians in a year, a patient with 10 comorbidities saw 28.2 physicians (Niefeld et al., 2003). Another study found that in a single year in fee-for-service Medicare, the typical primary care physician had to coordinate with 229 other physicians in 117 different practices (Pham et al., 2009). Further, the rate at which physicians refer patients has doubled over the past decade, and the number of primary care visits resulting in a referral has increased by nearly 160 percent (Barnett et al., 2012). Coordination failures also are likely exacerbated by the wide variety of professionals in health care today (Leape and Berwick, 2005). Modern medicine includes nurses in more than 50 specialties, physicians in more than 50 medical specialties, physician assistants, pharmacists, physical therapists, psychologists, dentists, and many others, all of whom must communicate with each other across specialties and across professional lines to manage a patient's care successfully.[1]

Poor communication and coordination among providers extend to inpatient care. A survey of hospital patients found that 75 percent were unable to identify the clinician in charge of their care (Arora et al., 2009). Moreover, the number of clinicians a patient sees in the hospital is growing; in just the period from 1970 to the late 1990s, the number of clinicians seen by a typical hospital patient increased from 2.5 to more than 15 (Gawande, 2011). A recent study of hospital patients' contact with health care professionals found that during their hospitalization, medical patients saw an average of 18 different doctors, nurses, and other health care workers, while surgical patients saw an average of 27 (Whitt et al., 2007).

Patient handoffs—the transfer of responsibility for a patient from one provider to another—exemplify the care fragmentation experienced by many patients. A study of handoffs from ICUs to inpatient wards found that only 26 percent of receiving physicians communicated verbally with sending physicians during the transfer (Li et al., 2011). Fragmentation among different elements of the health care system continues upon a patient's discharge from the hospital. A study investigating the adequacy of discharge summaries found that they mentioned only 16 percent of tests with pending results and failed to document follow-up providers' information 33 percent of the time (Were et al., 2009). This communication gap makes it difficult for patients' primary care providers and other members of their care team to remain informed of their condition and to guide their care successfully going forward (Leape and Berwick, 2005).

One of the most dramatic results of this lack of care coordination is the number of patients who must reenter the hospital soon after discharge. One study found that almost one-fifth of Medicare patients were rehospitalized within 30 days (Jencks et al., 2009). These rehospitalizations were responsible for $15 billion in Medicare spending in 2005 alone (Medicare Payment Advisory Commission, 2008). While a patient may have to be rehospitalized for many reasons, one of the most prominent is a lack of effective transition between hospital care and care delivered in community settings. Indeed, half of patients who were quickly rehospitalized were not seen by a health care provider before being readmitted (Jencks et al., 2009), suggesting that no provider was responsible for transitioning the patient back into the community. Figure 3-1 shows a representative timeline of

---

[1]The number of specialties was calculated based on specialty and subspecialty certificates provided by American Board of Medical Specialties member boards, American Osteopathic Association specialty certifying boards, and American Board of Nursing Specialties approved certification programs.

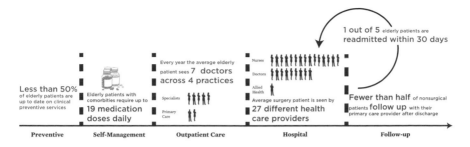

FIGURE 3-1 Representative timeline of a patient's experiences in the U.S. health care system.
SOURCE: Data derived from Boyd et al., 2005; Jencks et al., 2009; Pham et al., 2007; Shenson et al., 2007; Whitt et al., 2007.

the preventive, self-management, outpatient, hospital, and follow-up care patients experience in the U.S. health care system.

Multiple evidence-based interventions exist to improve care coordination. These range from the transitional care model (Naylor et al., 1994, 1999, 2004) to guided care (Boult et al., 2008, 2011; Boyd et al., 2010), to many varieties of medical homes (Rosenthal, 2008). Many care coordination problems thus could be resolved if the knowledge that currently exists were applied.

Access to Care

A lack of timely access to care is another concerning impact of complexity on the quality of health care. Many studies have explored the number of Americans who lack insurance coverage and the deleterious impact on their health (IOM, 2002, 2003a,b, 2004, 2009b). Other obstacles to accessing care exist as well. In one survey, 29 percent of patients reported having difficulty obtaining an appointment with their health care provider when sick, while almost 60 percent noted problems with obtaining care outside of traditional business hours (nights, weekends, holidays) without going to the emergency room (Stremikis et al., 2011).

As a result of these access issues, many Americans are forced to visit the emergency room—one of the most costly settings for care—for treatment of chronic illnesses that could be managed in an outpatient setting. For example, asthma can be properly managed entirely through outpatient care. However, many patients fail to receive high-quality asthma management, which results in 1.75 million visits to the emergency room and almost 0.5 million hospitalizations each year (Akinbami et al., 2011). As a result, the United States has a higher rate of hospital admissions for asthma than other developed nations (Squires, 2011).

Health Disparities

The complexity of modern health care often has impeded efforts to close unacceptable gaps in quality of care and health outcomes based on race, ethnicity, and income. As noted in previous IOM studies, the use of evidence-based treatments and the quality of care vary by race and ethnicity (IOM, 2003c). These disparities continue to be reported; for example, one recent study noted three-fold differences among different ethnic groups in the use of intravenous tissue plasminogen activator (tPA) for eliminating cerebral blood clots in stroke patients (Hsia et al., 2011). Moreover, an evaluation by the Agency for Healthcare Research and Quality (AHRQ) found that individuals with lower incomes received lower-quality care on 80 percent of the AHRQ core quality measures (AHRQ, 2011a). These disparities in care, along with social determinants, contribute to disparities in overall health (Woolf and Braveman, 2011). For example, life expectancy at birth is 4-6 years less for African Americans than for Caucasians, and the mortality rate for African American infants is double the national average (National Center for Health Statistics, 2011).

Overall Impact

The above shortfalls in the generation, diffusion, and application of knowledge on effective clinical care have a measurable impact on Americans' health. One way to measure this impact is through mortality amenable to health care, defined as the number of deaths that should not occur in the presence of timely and effective health care. Examples of amenable mortality include childhood infections, surgical complications, and diabetes. The level of amenable mortality varies almost threefold among states, ranging from 64 to 158 deaths per 100,000 population (McCarthy et al., 2009; Schoenbaum et al., 2011). If all states had provided care of the quality delivered by the highest-performing state, 75,000 fewer deaths would have occurred across the country in 2005.

It is important to stress that there are multiple areas of excellence in the U.S. health care system in which technically advanced, compassionate care improves the health of patients and extends their lives. One such area is cancer care. The outcomes for cancer patients in the United States tend to be better than those in other countries (Coleman et al., 2008; Gatta et al., 2000). For breast, colorectal, and cervical cancers, 5-year survival rates are high compared with rates in other developed nations, while overall mortality is comparatively low (Squires, 2011). The positive outcomes for cancer care underscore the potential for the health care system to improve in overall quality and address the areas for improvement discussed above.

Conclusion 3-1: Health care safety, quality, and outcomes for Americans fall substantially short of their potential and vary significantly for different populations of Americans.

Related findings:

- *Medical care is guided insufficiently by evidence.* Americans receive only about half of the preventive, acute, and chronic care recommended by current research and guidelines.
- *Preventable medical harm is pervasive, despite proven methods for its reduction.* One study found that nearly one in five hospital patients are harmed during their stay, and nearly two-thirds of that harm is preventable.
- *The nature and quality of health care vary considerably among states, with serious health and economic consequences.* If all states could provide care of the quality provided by the highest-performing state, an estimated 75,000 fewer deaths would have occurred across the country in 2005.
- *Poor continuity of care is both harmful and costly.* In 2004, one-fifth of Medicare patients were rehospitalized within 30 days, and Medicare rehospitalizations were responsible for $15 billion of Medicare spending in 2005 alone.

UNSUSTAINABLE COSTS

In addition to quality shortfalls, the value of health care is compromised by excess costs and waste (Brook, 2010). In 2012, the United States will spend $2.8 trillion, about 18 percent of the nation's gross domestic product, on the health care system (Keehan et al., 2011). The high cost of health care by itself might not be a reason for concern. Patients, consumers, and the public might simply be choosing to invest more of their resources in health care because this investment is improving their health (Baicker and Chandra, 2011; Cutler et al., 2006). What is concerning, however, is the unsustainable rate of growth in health care costs. For 31 of the past 40 years, health care costs have increased at a greater rate than the economy as a whole, and health care spending is expected to continue increasing more rapidly than the total economy, growing 4 to 8 percent per year through 2020 (CMS, 2012; Keehan et al., 2011). To put these cost increases into perspective, if the cost of other goods had risen as quickly as health care costs in the post–World War II period, a dozen eggs now would cost $55,

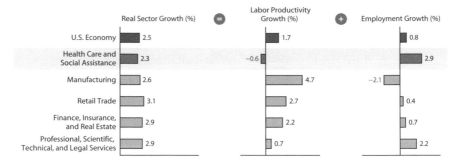

FIGURE 3-2 Real sector growth, broken into labor productivity and employment growth, for health care and other sectors of the U.S. economy.
SOURCE: Kocher and Sahni, 2011. Copyright © (2011) Massachusetts Medical Society. Reprinted with permission from Massachusetts Medical Society.

a gallon of milk would cost $48, and a dozen oranges would cost $134.[2,3] Notably, moreover, growth in health care costs has not been accompanied by a commensurate growth in the productivity of the health care labor force similar to the gains seen in other industries (see Figure 3-2) (Kocher and Sahni, 2011).

In considering the growth in health care costs, it is important to consider the specific impact of this growth on different stakeholders. For governments, health care expenditures are quickly consuming larger and larger fractions of the overall budget. Health care costs for the Department of Defense alone now top $50 billion a year, almost a tenth of its budget (Government Accountability Office, 2011). Likewise, Medicaid expenditures now consume almost 20 percent of state budgets, crowding out other priorities, such as education (National Association of State Budget Officers, 2011). State funding for higher education has seen decreases of up to 20 percent as a result of increasing Medicaid costs (Kane and Orszag, 2003). These decreases in spending for education and other national priorities can be expected to continue unless the rate of health care spending is slowed.

For the public, the cost of health care is consuming more of every paycheck and rising higher than any increases in pay. In the past decade, the average income for a family of four with health insurance rose by 30 percent, while the family's health care costs (including health insurance premiums

---

[2]All monetary estimates were converted to 2009 dollars using the Consumer Price Index inflation estimates unless otherwise noted (U.S. Bureau of Labor Statistics, 2011b).

[3]For the estimate of the cost of various food products assuming health care inflation rates, food prices from 1945 were calculated from the 1945 U.S. Statistical Abstract, with health care prices being drawn from national health expenditure accounts (Hansen, 1945; Keehan et al., 2011; Rice and Cooper, 1971).

and out-of-pocket costs) increased by 76 percent, effectively eliminating any wage increases (Auerbach and Kellermann, 2011). In 2012, almost 4 in 10 Americans with a serious illness, medical condition, injury, or disability reported that medical costs were a serious financial problem for them or their families (NPR et al., 2012). As a result of these rising costs, many families must forgo care; the percentage of the public unable to receive needed care in the past year because of its cost rose from 9 percent in 1999 to 15 percent in 2009. That figure for 2009 was fully 37 percent for those who were uninsured (National Center for Health Statistics, 2011). These high costs have strained families' budgets and put coverage out of reach for many, contributing to the 50 million Americans without health insurance coverage (DeNavas-Walt et al., 2011).

In addition to unsustainable cost growth, there is evidence that a substantial proportion of health care expenditures is wasted, leading to little improvement in health or in the quality of care. Estimates vary on waste and excess health care costs, but they are large. The IOM work shop summary *The Healthcare Imperative: Lowering Costs and Improving Outcomes* assesses waste by evaluating excess costs in six domains: unnecessary services, services inefficiently delivered, prices that are too high,[4] excess administrative costs, missed prevention opportunities, and medical fraud (IOM, 2010). These estimates, presented by workshop speakers with respect to their areas of expertise and based on assumptions from limited observations, suggest the substantial contribution of each domain to excess health care costs (see Table 3-1). Although these estimates have unknown overlap, their sum—$765 billion—indicates the significant scale of waste in the system.

Two other independent and differing analytic approaches—considering regional variation in costs and comparing costs across countries—produce similar estimates, with total excess costs approaching $750-$760 billion in 2009 (Farrell et al., 2008; IOM, 2010; Wennberg et al., 2002). One approach entailed analyzing health care spending in the United States versus that in peer countries of the Organisation for Economic Co-operation and Development (OECD) after adjusting for wealth. Based on 2006 data, excess U.S. health expenditures compared with those of OECD countries were estimated to constitute almost one-third of overall spending. After adjusting to 2009 health care expenditures, this estimate would be approximately $750 billion (Farrell et al., 2008). The second analysis examined variations

---

[4]In this report, *price* refers to the amount charged for a given health care service or product. It is important to note that there are frequently multiple prices for the same service or product, depending on the patient's insurance status and payer, as well as other factors. *Cost* is the total sum of money spent at a given level (episodes, patients, organizations, state, national), or price multiplied by the volume of services or products used.

TABLE 3-1 Sources of Estimated Excess Costs in Health Care (2009)

Category	Sources	Estimate of Excess Costs
Unnecessary Services	• Overuse—beyond evidence-established levels • Discretionary use beyond benchmarks • Unnecessary choice of higher-cost services	$210 billion
Inefficiently Delivered Services	• Mistakes—errors, preventable complications • Care fragmentation • Unnecessary use of higher-cost providers • Operational inefficiencies at care delivery sites	$130 billion
Excess Administrative Costs	• Insurance paperwork costs beyond benchmarks • Insurers' administrative inefficiencies • Inefficiencies due to care documentation requirements	$190 billion
Prices That Are Too High	• Service prices beyond competitive benchmarks • Product prices beyond competitive benchmarks	$105 billion
Missed Prevention Opportunities	• Primary prevention • Secondary prevention • Tertiary prevention	$55 billion
Fraud	• All sources—payers, clinicians, patients	$75 billion

SOURCE: Adapted with permission from IOM, 2010.

in Medicare spending across the country. It found that if Medicare spending were at the same level as the lowest decile, after adjusting for age, sex, and race, almost 30 percent of Medicare spending could be saved (Wennberg et al., 2002). Extrapolating this result to national health care spending in 2009 would lead to an estimated $750 billion in excess costs. While there are methodological issues with each approach to estimating excess costs, the consistently large figures resulting from each approach signal the potential for reducing health care costs while improving quality and health outcomes.

To highlight one factor in Table 3-1, higher prices are a major contributor to higher health care spending in the United States. A 2012 review found that the average commercial price in the United States was higher than that in the country with the next-highest price by 150 percent for a daily stay in a hospital, by 120 percent for an appendectomy, and by 50 percent for a hip replacement (International Federation of Health Plans, 2012). While prices do not fully explain the differences in costs among different countries, they are one major factor (Anderson et al., 2003).

To understand the scale of this waste, it is useful to compare it against other national expenses. For example, the estimated unnecessary costs and waste in health care outstrip the Fiscal Year 2009 outlays for the Department of Defense by more than $100 billion (OMB, 2010). Similarly, it is more than 1.5 times the nation's total infrastructure investment in 2004, including roads, railroads, aviation, drinking water, telecommunications, and other structures, counting both public and private funding.[5]

This represents a tremendous opportunity cost, because this money could be directed toward higher-value health care uses. For instance, one-quarter of the amount could provide all recommended childhood and adolescent vaccinations to 152 million children (nearly the number of children born in the 40 years between 1968 and 2008).[6] If this health care waste were eliminated, the redirected funds could provide health insurance coverage for more than 150 million workers (including both employer and employee contributions), equal to the entirety of the civilian labor force.[7] And just a fraction of the unnecessary expenditures in health care could fund the $24 billion investment in public health needed to enable the delivery of a minimum level of public health services to every community in the United States (IOM, 2012).

Such waste also has opportunity costs for society more broadly. If only half of these excess expenditures were applied to other functions, it would be enough to buy groceries for every household in America for an entire

---

[5]Comparisons of health care waste with the national infrastructure investment were drawn from a Congressional Budget Office analysis (Congressional Budget Office, 2008), while the Department of Defense budget was calculated from the Fiscal Year 2009 outlays listed in the Fiscal Year 2011 U.S. Government Budget (OMB, 2010).

[6]The cost of childhood and adolescent vaccinations was drawn from a paper by Lindley et al. (2009), while the number of children born between 1968 and 2008 came from Centers for Disease Control and Prevention (CDC) data (Martin et al., 2010).

[7]The average premiums for a single worker were calculated using the Kaiser Family Foundation's 2009 Employer Health Benefits survey, with the size of the 2009 civilian labor force being derived from Bureau of Labor Statistics estimates (Kaiser Family Foundation and Health Research & Educational Trust, 2009; U.S. Bureau of Labor Statistics, 2012).

year.[8] If the waste in health care were redirected, it could provide every young person in America aged 18-24 the average annual tuition and fees of a 4-year institution of higher learning for 2 years.[9] Or the total could pay the salaries of all of the nation's first response personnel, including fire-fighters, police officers, and emergency medical technicians, for 12 years.[10]

> **Conclusion 3-2: The growth rate of health care expenditures is unsustainable, with waste that diverts major resources from necessary care and other priorities at every level—individual, family, community, state, and national.**

Related findings:

- *Health care costs in the United States far outpace the growth rate of costs in the rest of the economy.* For 31 of the past 40 years, health care costs have increased at a greater rate than the economy as a whole, and now constitute 18 percent of national gross domestic product.
- *The growth in health care costs has contributed to stagnation in real income gains for American families.* Although income for families with health insurance has increased by 30 percent over the past decade, these gains have effectively been eliminated by a 76 percent increase in health care costs.
- *A substantial portion of health care spending is wasteful.* The total amount of unnecessary health care costs and waste in 2009 was an estimated $750-$765 billion, more than a third of total health care expenditures.
- *Wasteful health expenditures directly stifle progress on other priorities.* State Medicaid expenditures have displaced education investments, for example. If the waste in health care were redirected, it

---

[8]The cost of groceries was estimated from household expenditures on food for home use as listed in the Consumer Expenditure Survey, while the number of households was obtained from census estimates (U.S. Bureau of Labor Statistics, 2011a; U.S. Census Bureau, 2010).

[9]To calculate the years of tuition that could be available for young adults, the average cost of a 4-year institution of higher learning was obtained from U.S. Department of Education statistics, while the number of young adults aged 18 to 24 came from 2010 census estimates (Aud et al., 2011; U.S. Census Bureau, 2011).

[10]The comparison with expenditures on first responders was calculated from the annual salary data for firefighters, police officers, and emergency medical technicians provided in the 2009 National Compensation Survey, while the total number of individuals in those occupations was drawn from the 2009 Occupational Employment Statistics (U.S. Bureau of Labor Statistics, 2010a,b).

could provide every young person in America 2 years of education at a 4-year institution of higher learning.

CONSEQUENCES OF INACTION

The examples discussed in this chapter highlight areas in which the health care system is failing to achieve its potential. They demonstrate the unevenness of the system's performance, with many organizations and clinicians providing good care while others struggle in an increasingly complex and chaotic environment. Overcoming these problems will require transforming how the health care enterprise generates, processes, and applies information to improve the care of patients.

The stakes are high, with measurable impacts on care effectiveness, the economy, and overall health. If the nation's care reached the quality of the highest-performing state, an estimated 75,000 fewer deaths would have occurred nationwide in 2005 (McCarthy et al., 2009; Schoenbaum et al., 2011). And several estimates suggest that up to $750 billion is lost annually as a result of care delivered inefficiently and ineffectively (IOM, 2010). If the necessary transformation does not occur, the health care system will continue on its current path, and each of these shortfalls will persist or worsen. While some patients will continue to receive world-class, excellent care, too many others will experience unnecessary harm and poor-quality care. Stress on clinicians will grow as they try to coordinate increasingly complex care with an increasing number of other health care providers. Costs and waste will continue to grow as well, squeezing out other important priorities. This future does not have to occur. The problems of shortfalls in outcomes and cost excesses can be addressed through the application of tools and strategies that enable continuous learning and improvement in care delivery, the subject of the next chapter.

REFERENCES

AHRQ (Agency for Healthcare Research and Quality). 2011a. *2010 national healthcare disparities report*. Rockville, MD: U.S. Department of Health and Human Services.

AHRQ. 2011b. *National healthcare quality report, 2011*. Rockville, MD: U.S. Department of Health and Human Services, AHRQ.

Akinbami, L. J., J. E. Moorman, and X. Liu. 2011. Asthma prevalence, health care use, and mortality: United States, 2005-2009. *National Health Statistics Report* (32):1-14.

Al-Khatib, S. M., A. Hellkamp, J. Curtis, D. Mark, E. Peterson, G. D. Sanders, P. A. Heidenreich, A. F. Hernandez, L. H. Curtis, and S. Hammill. 2011. Non-evidence-based ICD implantations in the United States. *Journal of the American Medical Association* 305(1):43-49.

Anderson, G. F., U. E. Reinhardt, P. S. Hussey, and V. Petrosyan. 2003. It's the prices, stupid: Why the United States is so different from other countries. *Health Affairs (Millwood)* 22(3):89-105.

Arora, V., S. Gangireddy, A. Mehrotra, R. Ginde, M. Tormey, and D. Meltzer. 2009. Ability of hospitalized patients to identify their in-hospital physicians. *Archives of Internal Medicine* 169(2):199-201.

Aud, S., W. Hussar, G. Kena, K. Bianco, L. Frohlich, J. Kemp, and K. Tahan. 2011. *The condition of education 2011.* Washington, DC: U.S. Department of Education, National Center for Education Statistics.

Auerbach, D. I., and A. L. Kellermann. 2011. A decade of health care cost growth has wiped out real income gains for an average US family. *Health Affairs* 30(9):1630-1636.

Baicker, K., and A. Chandra. 2011 (unpublished). *Aspirin, angioplasty, and proton beam therapy: The economics of smarter health care spending.* Cambridge, MA: Harvard University.

Baicker, K., K. S. Buckles, and A. Chandra. 2006. Geographic variation in the appropriate use of cesarean delivery. *Health Affairs (Millwood)* 25(5):w355-w367.

Barnett, M. L., Z. Song, and B. E. Landon. 2012. Trends in physician referrals in the United States, 1999-2009. *Archives of Internal Medicine* 172(2):163-170.

Bates, D. W. 2002. Unexpected hypoglycemia in a critically ill patient. *Annals of Internal Medicine* 137(2):110-116.

Boult, C., L. Reider, K. Frey, B. Leff, C. M. Boyd, J. L. Wolff, S. Wegener, J. Marsteller, L. Karm, and D. Scharfstein. 2008. Early effects of "guided care" on the quality of health care for multimorbid older persons: A cluster-randomized controlled trial. *The Journals of Gerontology. Series A, Biological Sciences and Medical Sciences* 63(3):321-327.

Boult, C., L. Reider, B. Leff, K. D. Frick, C. M. Boyd, J. L. Wolff, K. Frey, L. Karm, S. T. Wegener, T. Mroz, and D. O. Scharfstein. 2011. The effect of guided care teams on the use of health services: Results from a cluster-randomized controlled trial. *Archives of Internal Medicine* 171(5):460-466.

Boyd, C. M., J. Darer, C. Boult, L. P. Fried, L. Boult, and A. W. Wu. 2005. Clinical practice guidelines and quality of care for older patients with multiple comorbid diseases: Implications for pay for performance. *Journal of the American Medical Association* 294(6):716-724.

Boyd, C. M., L. Reider, K. Frey, D. Scharfstein, B. Leff, J. Wolff, C. Groves, L. Karm, S. Wegener, J. Marsteller, and C. Boult. 2010. The effects of guided care on the perceived quality of health care for multi-morbid older persons: 18-month outcomes from a cluster-randomized controlled trial. *Journal of General Internal Medicine* 25(3):235-242.

Brook, R. H. 2010. The end of the quality improvement movement: Long live improving value. *Journal of the American Medical Association* 304(16):1831-1832.

Casalino, L. P., D. Dunham, M. H. Chin, R. Bielang, E. O. Kistner, T. G. Karrison, M. K. Ong, U. Sarkar, M. A. McLaughlin, and D. O. Meltzer. 2009. Frequency of failure to inform patients of clinically significant outpatient test results. *Archives of Internal Medicine* 169(12):1123-1129.

CDC (Centers for Disease Control and Prevention). 2011. Vital signs: Central line-associated blood stream infections—United States, 2001, 2008, and 2009. *Morbidity and Mortality Weekly Report* 60(8):243-248.

Classen, D. C., R. Resar, F. Griffin, F. Federico, T. Frankel, N. Kimmel, J. C. Whittington, A. Frankel, A. Seger, and B. C. James. 2011. 'Global trigger tool' shows that adverse events in hospitals may be ten times greater than previously measured. *Health Affairs (Millwood)* 30(4):581-589.

CMS (Centers for Medicare & Medicaid Services). 2012. *National health expenditures summary and GDP: Calendar years 1960-2010.* http://www.cms.gov/Research-Statistics-Data-and-Systems/Statistics-Trends-and-Reports/NationalHealthExpendData/downloads/tables.pdf (accessed August 31, 2012).

Cohen, M. R. 1999. *Medication errors.* Washington, DC: American Pharmaceutical Association Publications.

Cohen, M. R., S. M. Proulx, and S. Y. Crawford. 1998. Survey of hospital systems and common serious medication errors. *Journal of Healthcare Risk Management* 18(1):16-27.

Coleman, M. P., M. Quaresma, F. Berrino, J. M. Lutz, R. De Angelis, R. Capocaccia, P. Baili, B. Rachet, G. Gatta, T. Hakulinen, A. Micheli, M. Sant, H. K. Weir, J. M. Elwood, H. Tsukuma, S. Koifman, G. A. E Silva, S. Francisci, M. Santaquilani, A. Verdecchia, H. H. Storm, J. L. Young, and CONCORD Working Group. 2008. Cancer survival in five continents: A worldwide population-based study (CONCORD). *Lancet Oncology* 9(8):730-756.

Congressional Budget Office. 2008. *Issues and options in infrastructure investment.* Washington, DC: Congressional Budget Office.

Cutler, D. M., A. B. Rosen, and S. Vijan. 2006. The value of medical spending in the United States, 1960-2000. *New England Journal of Medicine* 355(9):920-927.

Darst, J. R., J. W. Newburger, S. Resch, R. H. Rathod, and J. E. Lock. 2010. Deciding without data. *Congenital Heart Disease* 5(4):339-342.

DeNavas-Walt, C., B. D. Proctor, and J. C. Smith. 2011. *Income, poverty, and health insurance coverage in the United States: 2010.* Washington, DC: U.S. Census Bureau.

Downey, J. R., T. Hernandez-Boussard, G. Banka, and J. M. Morton. 2012. Is patient safety improving? National trends in patient safety indicators: 1998-2007. *Health Services Research* 47(1 Pt. 2):414-430.

Farrell, D., E. Jensen, B. Kocher, N. Lovegrove, F. Melhem, L. Mendonca, and B. Parish. 2008. *Accounting for the cost of US health care: A new look at why Americans spend more.* Washingtion, DC: McKinsey Global Institute.

Fuhrmans, V. 2007. A novel plan helps hospital wean itself off pricey tests. *Wall Street Journal,* January 12.

Gatta, G., R. Capocaccia, M. P. Coleman, L. A. Gloeckler Ries, T. Hakulinen, A. Micheli, M. Sant, A. Verdecchia, and F. Berrino. 2000. Toward a comparison of survival in American and European cancer patients. *Cancer* 89(4):893-900.

Gawande, A. 2011. Cowboys and pit crews. *New Yorker,* May 26.

Good Stewardship Working Group. 2011. The "top 5" lists in primary care: Meeting the responsibility of professionalism. *Archives of Internal Medicine* 171(15):1385-1390.

Government Accountability Office. 2011. *DoD health care: Prohibition on financial incentives that may influence health insurance choices for retirees and their dependents under age 65.* Washington, DC: Government Accountability Office.

Hansen, M. H. 1945. *Statistical abstract of the United States: 1944-45.* Washington, DC: U.S. Department of Commerce, Bureau of the Census.

Harpole, L. H., M. J. Kelley, G. Schreiber, E. M. Toloza, J. Kolimaga, and D. C. McCrory. 2003. Assessment of the scope and quality of clinical practice guidelines in lung cancer. *Chest* 123(Suppl. 1):S7-S20.

Hsia, A. W., D. F. Edwards, L. B. Morgenstern, J. J. Wing, N. C. Brown, R. Coles, S. Loftin, A. Wein, S. S. Koslosky, S. Fatima, B. N. Sánchez, A. Fokar, M. C. Gibbons, N. Shara, A. Jayam-Trouth, and C. S. Kidwell. 2011. Racial disparities in tissue plasminogen activator treatment rate for stroke: A population-based study. *Stroke* 42(8):2217-2221.

International Federation of Health Plans. 2012. *IFHIP 2011 comparative price report.* London, UK: International Federation of Health Plans.

IOM (Institute of Medicine). 1985. *Assessing medical technologies.* Washington, DC: National Academy Press.

IOM. 1999. *To err is human: Building a safer health system.* Washington, DC: National Academy Press.

IOM. 2002. *Care without coverage: Too little, too late.* Washington, DC: National Academy Press.

IOM. 2003a. *A shared destiny: Community effects of uninsurance.* Washington, DC: The National Academies Press.

IOM. 2003b. *Hidden costs, value lost: Uninsurance in America.* Washington, DC: The National Academies Press.

IOM. 2003c. *Unequal treatment: Confronting racial and ethnic disparities in health care.* Washington, DC: The National Academies Press.

IOM. 2004. *Insuring America's health: Principles and recommendations.* Washington, DC: The National Academies Press.

IOM. 2009a. *America's uninsured crisis: Consequences for health and health care.* Washington, DC: The National Academies Press.

IOM. 2009b. *Initial national priorities for comparative effectiveness research.* Washington, DC: The National Academies Press.

IOM. 2010. *The healthcare imperative: Lowering costs and improving outcomes: Workshop series summary.* Washington, DC: The National Academies Press.

IOM. 2012. *For the public's health: Investing in a healthier future.* Washington, DC: The National Academies Press.

Jencks, S. F., M. V. Williams, and E. A. Coleman. 2009. Rehospitalizations among patients in the Medicare fee-for-service program. *New England Journal of Medicine* 360(14):1418-1428.

Kaiser Family Foundation and Health Research & Educational Trust. 2009. *Employer health benefits: 2009 annual survey.* Menlo Park, CA: Henry J. Kaiser Family Foundation.

Kane, T. J., and P. R. Orszag. 2003. *Funding restrictions at public universities: Effects and policy implications.* Washington, DC: Brookings Institution.

Keehan, S. P., A. M. Sisko, C. J. Truffer, J. A. Poisal, G. A. Cuckler, A. J. Madison, J. M. Lizonitz, and S. D. Smith. 2011. National health spending projections through 2020: Economic recovery and reform drive faster spending growth. *Health Affairs (Millwood)* 30(8):1594-1605.

Kocher, R., and N. R. Sahni. 2011. Rethinking health care labor. *New England Journal of Medicine* 365(15):1370-1372.

Kottke, T. E., D. A. Faith, C. O. Jordan, N. P. Pronk, R. J. Thomas, and S. Capewell. 2009. The comparative effectiveness of heart disease prevention and treatment strategies. *American Journal of Preventive Medicine* 36(1):82-88.

Landrigan, C. P., G. J. Parry, C. B. Bones, A. D. Hackbarth, D. A. Goldmann, and P. J. Sharek. 2010. Temporal trends in rates of patient harm resulting from medical care. *New England Journal of Medicine* 363(22):2124-2134.

Leape, L. L., and D. M. Berwick. 2005. Five years after to err is human: What have we learned? *Journal of the American Medical Association* 293(19):2384-2390.

Lee, D. H., and O. Vielemeyer. 2011. Analysis of overall level of evidence behind infectious diseases society of America practice guidelines. *Archives of Internal Medicine* 171(1):18.

Levinson, D. R. 2010. *Adverse events in hospitals: National incidence among Medicare beneficiaries.* Washington, DC: U.S. Department of Health and Human Services, Office of Inspector General.

Levinson, D. R. 2012. *Hospital incident reporting systems do not capture most patient harm.* Washington, DC: U.S. Department of Health and Human Services, Office of Inspector General.

Li, P., H. T. Stelfox, and W. A. Ghali. 2011. A prospective observational study of physician handoff for intensive-care-unit-to-ward patient transfers. *American Journal of Medicine* 124(9):860-867.

Lindley, M. C., A. K. Shen, W. A. Orenstein, L. E. Rodewald, and G. S. Birkhead. 2009. Financing the delivery of vaccines to children and adolescents: Challenges to the current system. *Pediatrics* 124(Suppl. 5):S548-S557.

Martin, J. A., B. E. Hamilton, P. D. Sutton, S. J. Ventura, T. J. Mathews, and M. J. K. Osterman. 2010. *Births: Final data for 2008*. Hyattsville, MD: National Center for Health Statistics.

McCarthy, D., S. How, C. Schoen, J. Cantor, and D. Belloff. 2009. *Aiming higher: Results from a state scorecard on health system performance*. New York: Commonwealth Fund Commission on a High Performance Health System.

McGlynn, E. A., S. M. Asch, J. Adams, J. Keesey, J. Hicks, A. DeCristofaro, and E. A. Kerr. 2003. The quality of health care delivered to adults in the United States. *New England Journal of Medicine* 348(26):2635-2645.

Medicare Payment Advisory Commission. 2008. *Reforming the delivery system*. Washington, DC: Medicare Payment Advisory Commission.

National Association of State Budget Officers. 2011. *State expenditure report 2010: Examining fiscal 2009-2011 state spending*. Washington, DC: National Association of State Budget Officers.

National Center for Health Statistics. 2011. *Health, United States, 2010: With special feature on death and dying*. Hyattsville, MD: U.S. Department of Health and Human Services, CDC.

Naylor, M., D. Brooten, R. Jones, R. Lavizzo-Mourey, M. Mezey, and M. Pauly. 1994. Comprehensive discharge planning for the hospitalized elderly. A randomized clinical trial. *Annals of Internal Medicine* 120(12):999-1006.

Naylor, M. D., D. Brooten, R. Campbell, B. S. Jacobsen, M. D. Mezey, M. V. Pauly, and J. S. Schwartz. 1999. Comprehensive discharge planning and home follow-up of hospitalized elders: A randomized clinical trial. *Journal of the American Medical Association* 281(7):613-620.

Naylor, M. D., D. A. Brooten, R. L. Campbell, G. Maislin, K. M. McCauley, and J. S. Schwartz. 2004. Transitional care of older adults hospitalized with heart failure: A randomized, controlled trial. *Journal of the American Geriatrics Society* 52(5):675-684.

Niefeld, M. R., J. B. Braunstein, A. W. Wu, C. D. Saudek, W. E. Weller, and G. F. Anderson. 2003. Preventable hospitalization among elderly Medicare beneficiaries with type 2 diabetes. *Diabetes Care* 26(5):1344-1349.

NPR, Robert Wood Johnson Foundation, and Harvard School of Public Health. 2012. *Poll: Sick in America (summary)*. http://www.npr.org/documents/2012/may/poll/summary.pdf (accessed May 21, 2012).

OMB (Office of Management and Budget). 2010. *Fiscal year 2011 budget of the U.S. government*. Washington, DC: OMB.

Pham, H. H., D. Schrag, A. S. O'Malley, B. Wu, and P. B. Bach. 2007. Care patterns in Medicare and their implications for pay for performance. *New England Journal of Medicine* 356(11):1130-1139.

Pham, H. H., A. S. O'Malley, P. B. Bach, C. Saiontz-Martinez, and D. Schrag. 2009. Primary care physicians' links to other physicians through Medicare patients: The scope of care coordination. *Annals of Internal Medicine* 150(4):236-242.

Poonacha, T. K., and R. S. Go. 2011. Level of scientific evidence underlying recommendations arising from the national comprehensive cancer network clinical practice guidelines. *Journal of Clinical Oncology* 29(2):186-191.

Pronovost, P., D. Needham, S. Berenholtz, D. Sinopoli, H. Chu, S. Cosgrove, B. Sexton, R. Hyzy, R. Welsh, G. Roth, J. Bander, J. Kepros, and C. Goeschel. 2006. An intervention to decrease catheter-related bloodstream infections in the ICU. *New England Journal of Medicine* 355(26):2725-2732.

Rice, D. P., and B. S. Cooper. 1971. National health expenditures, 1929-70. *Social Security Bulletin* 34(1):3-18.

Rosenthal, T. C. 2008. The medical home: Growing evidence to support a new approach to primary care. *Journal of the American Board of Family Medicine* 21(5):427-440.

Schoenbaum, S. C., C. Schoen, J. L. Nicholson, and J. C. Cantor. 2011. Mortality amenable to health care in the United States: The roles of demographics and health systems performance. *Journal of Public Health Policy* 32(4):407-529.

Shenson, D., J. Bolen, and M. Adams. 2007. Receipt of preventive services by elders based on composite measures, 1997-2004. *American Journal of Preventive Medicine* 32(1):11-18.

Squires, D. 2011. *The U.S. health system in perspective: A comparison of twelve industrialized nations.* New York: Commonwealth Fund.

Stremikis, K., C. Schoen, and A.K. Fryer. 2011. *A call for change: The 2011 Commonwealth Fund survey of public views of the U.S. health system.* New York: Commonwealth Fund.

U.S. Bureau of Labor Statistics. 2010a. *May 2009 national occupational employment and wage estimates.* http://www.bls.gov/oes/2009/may/oes_nat.htm (accessed May 22, 2012).

U.S. Bureau of Labor Statistics. 2010b. *National compensation survey: Occupational earnings in the United States, 2009.* http://www.bls.gov/ncs/ocs/sp/nctb1346.pdf (accessed May 22, 2012).

U.S. Bureau of Labor Statistics. 2011a. *Average annual expenditures and characteristics of all consumer units, consumer expenditure survey, 2006-2010.* http://www.bls.gov/cex/2010/standard/multiyr.pdf (accessed August 31, 2012).

U.S. Bureau of Labor Statistics. 2011b. *Consumer Price Index (CPI).* http://www.bls.gov/cpi/ (accessed September 25, 2011).

U.S. Bureau of Labor Statistics. 2012. *Labor force statistics from the current population survey.* http://data.bls.gov/pdq/SurveyOutputServlet?request_action=wh&graph_name=LN_cpsbref1 (accessed May 23, 2012).

U.S. Census Bureau. 2010. *Households and families: 2010.* http://www.census.gov/prod/cen2010/briefs/c2010br-14.pdf (accessed September 25, 2011).

U.S. Census Bureau. 2011. *Age and sex composition: 2010.* http://www.census.gov/prod/cen2010/briefs/c2010br-03.pdf (accessed May 22, 2012).

Wennberg, J. E., E. S. Fisher, and J. S. Skinner. 2002. Geography and the debate over Medicare reform. *Health Affairs (Millwood)* (Suppl. Web Exclusives):W96-W114.

Were, M., X. Li, J. Kesterson, J. Cadwallader, C. Asirwa, B. Khan, and M. Rosenman. 2009. Adequacy of hospital discharge summaries in documenting tests with pending results and outpatient follow-up providers. *Journal of General Internal Medicine* 24(9):1002-1006.

Whitt, N., R. Harvey, G. McLeod, and S. Child. 2007. How many health professionals does a patient see during an average hospital stay? *New Zealand Medical Journal* 120(1253):U2517.

Woolf, S. H., and P. Braveman. 2011. Where health disparities begin: The role of social and economic determinants—and why current policies may make matters worse. *Health Affairs (Millwood)* 30(10):1852-1859.

Zhan, C., and M. R. Miller. 2003. Excess length of stay, charges, and mortality attributable to medical injuries during hospitalization. *Journal of the American Medical Association* 290(14):1868-1874.

4

Imperative: Capturing Opportunities from Technology, Industry, and Policy

Carolyn Thornton was at home baking on Thanksgiving day when her heart palpitations, which she had been experiencing for some time, suddenly got worse. A visit to her doctor confirmed that Carolyn had myocarditis and congestive heart failure. But Carolyn's treatment would be different from that of other patients with her condition. After being discharged from the hospital, Carolyn was enrolled in Partners HealthCare's Connected Cardiac Care program, a home monitoring and education program for patients at risk for hospitalization. Each morning, patients in the program use home telemonitoring technology to take their own weight, blood pressure, pulse, and oxygen levels and answer questions about their symptoms. The data from these tests are sent to a telemonitoring nurse, who reviews patients' vitals and takes appropriate follow-up steps for out-of-parameter readings, including calling the patient or coordinating care with the patient's care team (Partners Health-Care Center for Connected Health, 2012). These prompt interventions can often help avoid unplanned hospital admissions—to date, the Connected Cardiac Care program has achieved a 51 percent reduction in heart failure readmissions (Cosgrove et al., 2012). Telemonitoring nurses also guide patients through structured heart failure education sessions to help make them aware of the impact of their daily behaviors on their condition and to help them develop new self-management skills (Partners HealthCare Center for Connected Health, 2012). The program illustrates how

new remote monitoring and connectivity capabilities can help pa-
tients like Carolyn and others monitor and manage complex health
conditions.

Although the challenges of complexity and value confronting U.S. health care today are formidable, opportunities exist to mold the system into one characterized by continuous learning and improvement. Advances have made vast computational power affordable and widely available, while improvements in connectivity have allowed information to be accessible in real time virtually anywhere. Progress in these areas has the potential to improve health care by increasing the reach of research knowledge, providing access to clinical records when and where needed, and assisting patients and providers in managing chronic diseases. Another area of opportunity lies with the human and organizational capabilities developed by diverse industries to improve safety, quality, reliability, and value; many of these capabilities can be adapted to health care settings to improve performance. Finally, recent changes in health policies present opportunities that can be leveraged to promote the growth of a learning health care system. Together, these opportunities can operate synergistically to enable more transformative change than can be accomplished with any of them individually. The path toward a more effective and efficient health care system will not be an easy one, but recent advances demonstrate the real potential for the necessary transformation.

THE DIGITAL INFRASTRUCTURE: COMPUTING, THE INTERNET, AND MOBILE TECHNOLOGIES

The past several decades have seen remarkable advances in technology, from personal computers, to cellular phones, to portable music players. The first mainframe computer offering a magnetic hard drive, the IBM RAMAC 305, was introduced in 1956, weighed a full ton, cost $250,000-$300,000 a year to lease in today's dollars, and stored less than 5 megabytes (Lesser and Haanstra, 1957; Levy, 2006). The price and capacity of computer storage have changed dramatically since then: in 2011, one could purchase a 32 gigabyte microSD card for $40,[1] which could store almost 7,000 times more information than the IBM RAMAC 305 at almost a thousandth of the price. One could also buy a disk drive capable of storing all of the world's music for only $600 (Manyika et al., 2011). And computer processing speed has grown by an average rate of 60 percent per year over the past several decades (Hilbert and López, 2011).

---

[1] Based on searches of major vendors.

Advanced technologies that rely on this computing power have become widespread. In the United States, 85 percent of adults own a cellphone, almost half own a digital music player, and 76 percent own a laptop or desktop computer (Zickuhr, 2011). The ability to generate, communicate, share, and access information has also been revolutionized by the rapid growth of digital networks. The Internet pervades modern life, allowing for quick access to multiple sources of information and rapid communication. The number of Americans with access to the Internet grew from 14 percent in 1995 to almost 80 percent in 2011 (Pew Internet & American Life Project, 2011). The Internet has given rise to new ways to connect with others, such as through social networking sites. These sites are now pervasive, being used by 65 percent of Internet users as of 2011 (Purcell, 2011).

In recent years, connectivity has become mobile and ubiquitous. Since the turn of the century, the capacity to share information across telecommunications networks has grown by an average of 30 percent per year (Hilbert and López, 2011). With the rise of tablets and smartphones that offer Internet connectivity and additional applications, mobile devices have become more sophisticated and have gained greater functionality. It is estimated that by 2020, 10 billion such mobile Internet-connected devices will be in use (Huberty et al., 2011).

These advances have dramatically changed numerous sectors of the U.S. economy, and even society more broadly. Companies have developed new ways to streamline their work processes, share information within their organizations, and analyze trends and knowledge (see Box 4-1 for an example). Individuals now have a wealth of information at their fingertips, with the ability to learn about almost any new topic in seconds.

While technologies and communications have led to widespread societal changes, these capacities are still relatively early in their development in the health care arena, and there is substantial room for progress and improvements as technologies are implemented in the field. One way digital connectivity can lead to better performance in health care is by ensuring that clinical information for a given patient is available when and where it is needed. The infrastructure for this type of connectivity, however, is largely lacking. As of 2011, only 34 percent of office-based physicians used a basic electronic health record system (although projections are for 90 percent to have access by 2019) (Congressional Budget Office, 2009; Hsiao et al., 2011), and only 18 percent of hospitals had a basic system (DesRoches et al., 2012). Thus, substantial opportunities exist to improve the safety and efficiency of medical care by promoting greater use of digital records. Once in place, these systems create the potential for advanced uses of clinical data to improve outcomes (see Box 4-2 for an example). For instance, they allow providers to analyze their patient populations and identify those who may benefit from preventive care or other proactive clinical services.

BOX 4-1
Using Data to Transform Business Practices

The explosion of data, along with new mechanisms for mining the data for insights, has transformed many businesses. One business that has made extensive use of this new opportunity is Ceasars Entertainment, which has focused on using data to improve its customer retention. These data originate from the company's loyalty program, Total Rewards, which has generated a customer information database that grew to more than 40 million members in 2010. The data, tracked by each customer's Total Rewards card, range from the total number of visits customers have made to a particular casino, to their buffet activity, to the amount of money they win or lose on an average visit. When it appears that customers may be frustrated in their experience, the company's analysis allows the Total Rewards staff to make data-supported decisions on the timing, type, and magnitude of promotional offers that have the highest likelihood of bringing those customers back. By tracking these offers and customers' subsequent visits, the company is able to monitor the success of the predictions. Through the use of evidence to predict the most effective offer for each customer, the company can ensure that a high proportion of customers will be enticed to return, which translates to guaranteed revenue for the business.

SOURCES: Greenfeld, 2010; National Public Radio, 2011.

Several early results have been promising, with digital records encouraging greater adherence to national best practices and leading to improvements in health outcomes (Cebul et al., 2011; Friedberg et al., 2009).

Increasing the diffusion of a digital infrastructure that supports health care processes and access to information provides the necessary foundation for a continuously improving, learning health care system (President's Information Technology Advisory Committee, 2001, 2004). Using this infrastructure, the system can capture and use knowledge from clinical care in real time. However, the sheer scale and complexity of the digital health infrastructure, including legacy systems, new electronic health record systems, financial data systems, and other data sources, necessitate conceptualizing this infrastructure in a new way. As noted in the Institute of Medicine (IOM) publication *Digital Infrastructure for the Learning Health System*, managing this complex technological resource effectively will require allowing local users of the data maximum flexibility, minimizing the number of standards necessary, and promoting adaptability and incremental innovation. Achieving this vision will require addressing a number of challenges, including the need for interoperability (see Chapter 6), supportive care processes (see Chapter 9), governance, the building of trust among clinicians and patients, and patient and public engagement (see Chapter 7) (IOM, 2011).

Improved connectivity increases patients' access to clinical knowledge—from guidelines, to clinical research results, to peer support—and may improve their engagement in their care. The fact that 80 percent of Internet users now look for health information online, making this the third most popular Internet activity, demonstrates that individuals are interested in obtaining more health care information (Fox, 2011a,b). Patients also are increasingly interested in finding information that is customized to their particular circumstances and that relates to the experiences of similar patients (Fox, 2011b).

Likewise, these technologies can help clinicians access clinical evidence, as well as additional information about their patients. Several examples exist of initiatives, such as the National Library of Medicine's MedlinePlus Connect and Kaiser Permanente's Clinical Library, aimed at seamlessly integrating clinical information with an electronic medical record. Evidence indicates that clinicians already have started to take advantage of these

---

BOX 4-2
Gleaning Real-Time Insights from Clinical Data

Although there has been an increase in the clinical knowledge being produced (see Chapter 2), the necessary evidence is lacking in many areas. However, the increased use of electronic medical records provides an opportunity to expand the evidence base on which clinicians can draw, especially in the absence of published data. For example, a group of pediatricians was treating a 13-year-old girl with systemic lupus erythematosus (SLE). Her autoimmune disease was complicated by conditions that put her at risk for blood clots, and her physicians considered the administration of an anticoagulant as a preventive measure. However, the physicians could not find any evidence (either peer-reviewed literature or expert opinion) pertaining to the patient's situation. Given the need to make a decision quickly, they reviewed the medical records from their institution, collating the records of 98 other pediatric SLE cases handled by their division in the past 5 years. Based on these data, they conducted a cohort review and ascertained that children with similar complicating conditions had been more likely to develop blood clots. They then recommended anticoagulant use within 24 hours of the patient's admission. The patient did not develop blood clots or experience any anticoagulant-related complications. Although this form of data review does not eliminate more extensive clinical research protocols, the data in the electronic medical records allowed a real-time clinical decision to be made based on the best available data, an approach that holds promise for larger-scale use.

SOURCE: Frankovich et al., 2011.

types of resources. In a 2010 survey, 86 percent of physicians reported using the Internet to gather health, medical, or prescription drug information (Dolan, 2010). Moreover, new digital data systems can automatically apply clinical knowledge to patient situations and flag potential problems. For example, computerized physician order entry (CPOE) systems can highlight patients' allergies to medications or potential interactions between different prescriptions, as well as ensure that medications are delivered more reliably. Although there are benefits and drawbacks to any technology, studies have found that using such electronic systems can potentially improve safety. One study found a 41 percent reduction in potential adverse drug events following the implementation of a CPOE system, while another found that overall medication error rates dropped by 81 percent (Bates et al., 1998, 1999; Potts et al., 2004). Further improvements may be seen with the use of new computational designs, such as the IBM Watson system, which can review large numbers of journal articles, clinical trials, guidelines, and medical records to apply the best evidence to a specific patient care situation.

Digital technologies also provide a paradigm for managing chronic diseases. Remote monitoring, such as devices that monitor heart conditions and blood sugar levels, can feed data in near real time to electronic health record systems (Manyika et al., 2011). With these technologies, for example, diabetics could monitor changes in their blood sugar after eating different foods and after different levels of exercise, giving them greater control over their condition. Additionally, at each consecutive appointment their provider could see blood sugar data for every day since their previous appointment, giving the provider greater ability to spot trends and precisely fine-tune medications.

On another front, increases in computing power allow for the use of advanced statistical analysis, simulation, and modeling. These new statistical techniques can help segment results for different populations, as well as highlight the impact of different interventions on population health (Berry et al., 2006). Advanced analysis, simulation, and modeling techniques may also allow for more sophisticated population-level planning and policy development. In addition, the growth in computational power makes possible simulation models that can replicate physiological pathways and disease states (Eddy and Schlessinger, 2003; Stern et al., 2008). These models can then be used to simulate clinical trials and tailor clinical guidelines to a patient's particular situation and biology (Eddy et al., 2011). As computational power increases, the potential applications of these simulation and modeling tools will continue to advance.

Conclusion 4-1: Advances in computing, information science, and connectivity can improve patient-clinician communication, point-of-care guidance, the capture of experience, population surveillance, planning and evaluation, and the generation of real-time knowledge—features of a continuously learning health care system.

Related findings:

- *Computing capacity is improving rapidly, enabling large-scale data analysis and improved care.* Over the past three decades, computer processing speed has grown by an average rate of 60 percent per year, and the capacity to share information across telecommunications networks has grown by an average of 30 percent per year.
- *The digital infrastructure for routine health care is developing rapidly.* Projections are for 90 percent of physicians to have access to fully operational electronic health records by 2019, up from 34-35 percent in 2011.
- *Digital capacity to provide electronic decision support prompts at the point of choice holds promise for transforming the safety and effectiveness of care.* One study found that implementation of a computerized physician order entry (CPOE) system reduced potential adverse drug events by 41 percent.
- *Developing digital communication capacity opens up the possibility of rapidly and seamlessly connecting researchers, patients, and providers.* The number of Americans with access to the Internet grew from 14 percent in 1995 to almost 80 percent in 2011, and by 2020 there will be 10 billion mobile Internet-connected devices in use.
- *Web-based health information holds considerable promise for informing patient decisions.* Fully 80 percent of Internet users now look for health information online, making this the third most popular Internet activity.

LESSONS IN CONTINUOUS IMPROVEMENT FROM OTHER INDUSTRIES

Over the past several decades, many industries have developed new methods to improve safety, reliability, quality, and value. Several organizations have learned how to manage and analyze large volumes of information; how to coordinate their workers (numbering in the hundreds or thousands) to create products or services with consistent quality; and how to ensure reliable performance, even under conditions of high risk. Several of these methods could be adapted to health care to improve the system's performance. In such adaptation, it is important to consider unique aspects of health care, such as patient diversity and the technical complexity of modern medicine, that may limit the methods' applicability, as well as the many factors that could affect their implementation. A discussion of the factors that influence the diffusion of innovation, including characteristics of the discovery, characteristics of the potential adopter, and environmental factors, can be found in Chapter 6.

Lessons for Enhancing Safety

The IOM publication *To Err Is Human: Building a Safer Health System* highlights several practices from other industries that health care practitioners could adopt to improve the safety of care (IOM, 1999). In particular, the health care system has opportunities to leverage the knowledge gained by industries that also confront high risk and complexity. Several of these industries have developed methods for substantially reducing the number of accidents and effectively mitigating human error.

One high-risk industry that has made substantial progress in safety is aviation. Improving mechanical components and ensuring that redundancies exist resulted in a sharp decline in aviation accidents. Even after these improvements, however, a residual level of accidents remained. Further improvement in the accident rate required addressing human factors. The industry adopted advanced safety measures centered on the assumptions that human error is inevitable and that systems must be designed to correct for individual mistakes (Nance, 2011; Wiegmann and Shappell, 2001). As a result, the safety of commuter air travel has improved dramatically. Domestic commercial commuter airlines reported 2.1 fatalities per 100,000 aircraft departures in 1980 and zero fatalities from 2007 to 2010 (Bureau of Transportation Statistics, 2011).

Industries that manage complex risks, such as aviation and nuclear power, operate on the assumption that accidents can be prevented through good organizational design and management. These industries are characterized by a commitment to safety, standard work processes, and a strong organizational culture for continuous learning (IOM, 1999). For example, the culture of these organizations encourages workers to search routinely for environmental factors or processes that could cause failure. Uncovering these safety concerns as a matter of common practice can allow the organization to address problems at a stage when they are easily fixed and before they have led to an accident (Chassin and Loeb, 2011).

Efforts to introduce safety practices from other high-risk industries into health care have yielded positive results for patient safety. One initiative, for example, introduced several methods drawn from aviation, such as checklists and a focus on teamwork and communication, to address catheter-related bloodstream infections. These methods eliminated such infections in the intensive care units of most hospitals and resulted in an 80 percent decrease in infections per catheter-day (Pronovost et al., 2006, 2009). The checklist concept has been diffused through the World Health Organization's Surgical Safety Checklist. Implementing this checklist has reduced fatalities and surgical complications by approximately one-third globally (Haynes et al., 2009). In another example, Great Ormond Street Hospital for Children drew on the pit stop techniques of the Ferrari Formula One race car team to redesign several aspects of its process for handoff from cardiac surgery to intensive care unit, yielding a 50 percent reduction in error rates (Catchpole et al., 2007). While not all industry safety methods will be effective in a health care setting, these examples illustrate the potential for practices pioneered in other industries to improve patient safety when adapted to a health care environment (Lewis et al., 2011). Chapter 9 explores additional lessons for managing errors in terms of reporting, organizational culture, and mitigation of impacts.

Lessons for Improving Quality and Value

Other potential lessons for health care come from commercial strategies for managing and improving the quality and value of goods and services (Hammer, 2004; Kenney, 2008). These strategies, including lean, Six Sigma, and others, introduce methods for coordinating complex work across diverse organizations, identifying existing and potential problems, and addressing those problems systematically (Chassin and Loeb, 2011; Kaplan et al., 2010). All of these strategies imply that the goal should not be to make the system work perfectly immediately, but to establish a process of gradual improvement (Young et al., 2004).

One notable strategy for improvement is the Toyota production system (Bohmer, 2010; Kenney, 2011). Under this system and related strategies, work is viewed as a series of ongoing experiments that immediately reveal problems. First, each worker's tasks are broken down into highly regimented sequences of steps. These steps make clear when workers are deviating from specifications and help both workers and their supervisors monitor adherence to the work process. Second, connections and communications among workers and between workers and outside suppliers and customers are standardized. Each communication unambiguously states the expected result of the request, the person or people responsible, and the time within which the request will be met. The third step of Toyota's production system is to create simple, defined workflows for the products, services, and help requests that make up the company's production lines. These workflows deliberately and systematically link sets of tasks and communications together, thereby reducing ambiguities. When ambiguities do arise, the fourth and final step of Toyota's production system is to teach workers how to address them, requiring that changes to workflows be in accordance with the scientific method, guided by a teacher, and made at the lowest possible level of the organization. To meet this requirement, Toyota trains its workers to frame problems and to formulate and test solutions. In this way, the organization fosters a learning environment in which workers at all levels are invested in identifying the root cause of problems and developing practical, implementable solutions (Spear and Bowen, 1999).

Additional methods that have shown success in improving quality come from the fields of systems engineering, industrial engineering, and operations research. Major corporations, from Wal-Mart to Boeing, could not operate their complex organizations without extensive use of engineering tools for the design, analysis, and control of complex production and distribution systems. These tools help companies coordinate deliveries from suppliers and manage complex production across multiple sites, and allow production to improve continuously. Several of these tools, including statistical process controls, supply chain management, modeling, and simulation, could be applied to improve health care processes (Agwunobi and London, 2009; IOM, 2005; IOM and NAE, 2011).

Initial results from the application of these methods to health care settings have been positive. For example, one hospital that applied the lessons of queuing theory and variability methodology was able to smooth the flow of patients, thereby increasing its surgical volume by 7 percent annually for 2 years without increasing staff or adding beds, while simultaneously improving the quality of care (Litvak and Bisognano, 2011). Similarly, a pharmacy unit at a large hospital applied production system methods to streamline its work. By undertaking systematic problem solving, the unit not only reduced the time spent searching for medications by 60 percent and the number of times medications were out of stock by 85 percent, but also substantially decreased the amount of medication that was spoiled or wasted (Spear, 2005).

Conclusion 4-2: Systematic, evidence-based process improvement methods applied in various sectors to achieve often striking results in safety, quality, reliability, and value can be similarly transformative for health care.

Related findings:

- *Industries that regularly confront high risk and complexity have successfully transformed performance.* For example, domestic commercial commuter airlines reported 2.1 fatalities per 100,000 aircraft departures in 1980 and zero fatalities from 2007 to 2010.

- *The introduction of safety practices from high-risk industries into health care has already improved patient safety.* In one study, the use of checklists inspired by the aviation industry eliminated catheter-related bloodstream infections in the intensive care units of most hospitals in the study and resulted in an 80 percent decrease in infections per catheter-day.
- *Commercial strategies for improving the reliability of the delivery of goods and services have potential applicability to health care.* A pharmacy unit, for example, undertook systematic problem solving and reduced the time spent searching for medications by 60 percent and the frequency of out-of-stock medications by 85 percent.

OPPORTUNITIES FROM A CHANGING HEALTH POLICY LANDSCAPE

Across the United States, there is growing momentum to implement novel partnerships and collaborations that test delivery system innovations aimed at high-value, high-quality health care. In many settings, federal, state, and local governments; public and private insurers; health care delivery organizations; employers; patients and consumers; and others are working together to pursue shared interests of controlling health care costs and improving health care quality. The convergence of these novel partnerships, a changing health care landscape, and investments in needed knowledge infrastructure establishes a potentially unique opportunity in the nation's history to achieve a learning health care system.

Many states have been at the forefront of initiatives to expand health insurance coverage, improve care quality and value, and advance the overall health of their residents. Massachusetts, the first state to enact a plan to achieve universal health insurance coverage for its residents, achieved a 98 percent coverage rate for its population following the passage of its 2006 health care reform law (Raymond, 2011). To extend coverage to previously uninsured state residents, the state established the Commonwealth Care Health Insurance Program (CommCare), a publicly funded health insurance program for low-income adults; Commonwealth Choice (CommChoice), a program that assists those individuals who are ineligible for CommCare but do not have access to employer-sponsored insurance; and the Connector, which provides an exchange that residents can use to purchase insurance plans. The Quality and Cost Council, established as a provision of the health care reform law, was charged with developing and coordinating quality improvement goals, with the objectives of lowering costs and improving care quality, and further legislative action on these goals is likely (McDonough et al., 2008; Raymond, 2011; Song and Landon, 2012). At the same time, private initiatives are being established to focus on health care payment and value.

Utah is another state that has established a health insurance exchange, which was created by legislation in 2009. The exchange supplies a technological foundation for providing information on health insurance and comparing different plans, as well as a standardized electronic application and enrollment system for purchasing insurance. One question that states consider when establishing exchanges is the extent to which they prefer to engage actively in the market, such as by setting minimum quality standards for plans, limiting variations in plan offerings, or including a bidding process. Some states have taken a more active role, while others have preferred to take a more market-oriented position (Corlette et al., 2011).

Vermont also has initiated a number of health care reforms, simultaneously establishing its own Vermont Health Benefit Exchange and beginning the transition to a single-payer system (State of Vermont, 2011). These reforms build on Vermont's 2006 health care reform legislation, which established the Catamount Health Plan to provide an insurance option for uninsured individuals with incomes below 300 percent of the poverty level, and developed initiatives to create a statewide, integrated electronic health information infrastructure (Kaiser Family Foundation, 2007). In parallel with coverage- and insurance-oriented reforms, Vermont passed legislation to implement delivery system reforms, including patient-centered medical homes, community-based support teams, coordinated transitions with medical and nonmedical services, multi-insurer payment reforms that align incentives with health care goals, a statewide health information network, and the data systems necessary to support knowledge generation and a learning health care system (Bielaszka-DuVernay, 2011).

Potential opportunities also lie in leveraging changes in recent national health care legislation. Recent legislation includes initiatives related to three objectives of particular relevance for a learning health care system: expanding clinical research knowledge, increasing digital capacity, and improving the value achieved from health care. While this legislation provides one potential path for advancing these three objectives, several other paths are possible. Regardless of the path followed, however, each of these objectives is critical for advancing a learning system.

Seeking to increase the level of clinical effectiveness research, the Patient Protection and Affordable Care Act (ACA) of 2010 established the Patient-Centered Outcomes Research Institute (PCORI), an independent, not-for-profit, private research organization. To accomplish its mission, the organization will support patient-centered outcomes research that compares the benefits and risks of different interventions, therapies, or delivery system initiatives. In support of these priorities, funding of $210 million has been provided for the first 3 years, rising to $500 million annually from

2014 to 2019 (Washington and Lipstein, 2011). While it is premature to judge PCORI's work, increasing the level of knowledge about comparative effectiveness is critical to building a learning system.

To promote the adoption of health information technologies, the Health Information Technology for Economic and Clinical Health (HITECH) Act, part of the American Recovery and Reinvestment Act, formalized the Office of the National Coordinator for Health Information Technology in the Department of Health and Human Services and provided substantial financial incentives for health care providers and hospitals to adopt and use electronic health records. Resources devoted to those programs include $2 billion for programs by the National Coordinator, as well as almost $30 billion in Medicare and Medicaid incentive payments to physicians and hospitals (Blumenthal, 2009; Buntin et al., 2010). Notably, the act encourages not only the adoption but also the meaningful use of such record systems, which is projected to yield savings of $93 billion between 2011 and 2019 (Congressional Budget Office, 2009).

A considerable portion of the ACA is focused on value initiatives. The law established pilot programs to test bundled payments, created value-based purchasing for several common conditions, and reduced Medicare payments to hospitals with high rates of avoidable readmissions and health care–acquired conditions (see Appendix C). One prominent program designed to improve value is the development of accountable care organizations (ACOs). ACOs are voluntary groups of physicians, hospitals, and other health care providers that assume responsibility for specified patient populations. As noted in the final October 20, 2011, regulation for the Medicare Shared Savings Plan, ACOs are responsible for delivering high-quality care as defined by specified quality measures, and share with Medicare any savings that result from better care coordination (Berwick, 2011). These programs are intended to spread the concept of coordinated care beyond Medicare to all payer arrangements.

Another ACA provision focused on value is the creation of the Center for Medicare & Medicaid Innovation. The Center is charged with testing and evaluating innovative payment and delivery system models that could improve care quality while slowing cost growth in Medicare, Medicaid, and the Children's Health Insurance Program (CHIP). While the ACA outlines approximately 20 areas the Center could consider at the outset, it gives the Center substantial flexibility to explore different models. Successful models may be extended to a larger patient population with approval by the Secretary of Health and Human Services. The Center's ultimate goal is to promote the rapid development and diffusion of innovative payment and delivery models that can improve quality and value (Guterman et al., 2010). In its first year, the Center introduced 16 initiatives and stimulated numerous other activities (Center for Medicare & Medicaid Innovation, 2012).

Passage of legislation alone will not lead to fundamental change in the health care enterprise. The legislation will have to be carefully implemented to better orient health care toward science and value. These reforms are an ongoing process and will evolve over time in response to changing national conditions.

Federal and state government actions are complemented by multiple initiatives on the part of employers, specialty societies, patient and consumer groups, health care delivery organizations, health plans, and others seeking to improve the health care system:

- In 2012, the American Board of Internal Medicine (ABIM), along with nine other specialty societies, released its Choosing Wisely campaign, focused on reducing overuse of specific medical tests or procedures in different health care specialties (Cassel and Guest, 2012). The first stage of the campaign, piloted by the National Physicians Alliance, developed a list for use by primary care practitioners to promote the more effective use of health care resources (Good Stewardship Working Group, 2011); current initiatives are working to expand this list to additional medical specialties.

- Drawing on their experiences in improving outcomes and lowering costs through initiatives in their own institutions, a group of health care delivery leaders has developed "A CEO Checklist for High-Value Health Care," which describes system-change approaches that can be adopted in most health care settings to improve outcomes and reduce costs of care (Cosgrove et al., 2012) (Appendix B).

- The Patient-Centered Primary Care Collaborative is an initiative that seeks to spread patient-centered medical homes.

- Other innovative approaches are being explored by partnerships among health systems, employers, payers, and other key stakeholders. In 2004, for example, Virginia Mason negotiated an arrangement with Aetna by which Virginia Mason production system's lean methods would be used to provide care more efficiently in exchange for Aetna's providing analyses of claims data to support the endeavor. Four major employers in the Seattle market—Costco, Starbucks, King Country, and Nordstrom—also participated, each choosing a condition prevalent among their workforces on which Virginia Mason should concentrate its efforts to deliver high-value care (Ginsburg et al., 2007; Pham et al., 2007).

- In Wisconsin, two multistakeholder groups—the Wisconsin Collaborative for Healthcare Quality and the Wisconsin Health Information Organization—work to collect, measure, and report health

care quality and efficiency data with the aim of encouraging value-based payment (Toussaint et al., 2011).
- All-payer databases are being established in various states around the country.
- Community-based initiatives include the Aligning Forces for Quality program and the Chartered Value Exchange project.

As these examples illustrate, sustained transformation will require initiatives and partnerships that nurture continuous learning and promote improvement and innovation.

Conclusion 4-3: Innovative public- and private-sector health system improvement initiatives, if adopted broadly, could support many elements of the transformation necessary to achieve a continuously learning health care system.

Related findings:

- *Many states have undertaken productive health system improvement initiatives.* States ranging from Massachusetts to Utah to Vermont have introduced initiatives aimed at expanding health insurance coverage, improving care quality and value, and advancing the overall health of their residents.
- *Incentives for the adoption of health information technology may promote learning and yield substantial savings.* The Health Information Technology for Economic and Clinical Health (HITECH) Act provides $30 billion in Medicare and Medicaid incentive payments for the meaningful use of health information technology by clinicians and hospitals, which has been estimated to yield savings of $93 billion between 2011 and 2019.
- *Efforts to encourage innovative payment and delivery models may help steward the transition to a continuously learning system.* The Center for Medicare & Medicaid Innovation, created to promote the rapid development and diffusion of innovation that could improve the effectiveness and efficiency of care, has stimulated activities beyond the 16 initiatives introduced in its first year.
- *Increased comparative effectiveness research may yield insights that can help clinicians and patients make better-informed health care decisions.* The Patient-Centered Outcomes Research Institute (PCORI), created to increase the quality and quantity of information about what works best for whom, will receive annual funding of $500 million from 2014 through 2019.

- *Partnerships and collaborations are increasingly identifying and testing opportunities for improving care delivery.* Multiple initiatives by employers, specialty societies, patient and consumer groups, health care delivery organizations, health plans, and others are aimed at improving the health care system. These initiatives include the American Board of Internal Medicine (ABIM) Choosing Wisely campaign, the Good Stewardship project, the Patient-Centered Primary Care Collaborative, and others.

REFERENCES

Agwunobi, J., and P. A. London. 2009. Removing costs from the health care supply chain: Lessons from mass retail. *Health Affairs (Millwood)* 28(5):1336-1342.

Bates, D. W., L. L. Leape, D. J. Cullen, N. Laird, L. A. Petersen, J. M. Teich, E. Burdick, M. Hickey, S. Kleefield, B. Shea, M. Vander Vliet, and D. L. Seger. 1998. Effect of computerized physician order entry and a team intervention on prevention of serious medication errors. *Journal of the American Medical Association* 280(15):1311-1316.

Bates, D. W., J. M. Teich, J. Lee, D. Seger, G. J. Kuperman, N. Ma'Luf, D. Boyle, and L. Leape. 1999. The impact of computerized physician order entry on medication error prevention. *Journal of the American Medical Informatics Association* 6(4):313-321.

Berry, D. A., L. Inoue, Y. Shen, J. Venier, D. Cohen, M. Bondy, R. Theriault, and M. F. Munsell. 2006. Modeling the impact of treatment and screening on U.S. breast cancer mortality: A Bayesian approach. *Journal of the National Cancer Institute Monographs* (36):30-36.

Berwick, D. M. 2011. Making good on ACOs' promise—the final rule for the Medicare shared savings program. *New England Journal of Medicine* 65(19):1753-1756.

Bielaszka-DuVernay, C. 2011. Vermont's blueprint for medical homes, community health teams, and better health at lower cost. *Health Affairs (Millwood)* 30(3):383-386.

Blumenthal, D. 2009. Stimulating the adoption of health information technology. *New England Journal of Medicine* 360(15):1477-1479.

Bohmer, R. 2010. *Virginia Mason Medical Center (abridged).* Cambridge, MA: Harvard Business School.

Buntin, M. B., S. H. Jain, and D. Blumenthal. 2010. Health information technology: Laying the infrastructure for national health reform. *Health Affairs (Millwood)* 29(6):1214-1219.

Bureau of Transportation Statistics. 2011. *National transportation statistics.* Washington, DC: Research and Innovation Technology Administration, U.S. Department of Transportation.

Cassel, C. K., and J. A. Guest. 2012. Choosing wisely: Helping physicians and patients make smart decisions about their care. *Journal of the American Medical Association* 307(17):1801-1802.

Catchpole, K. R., M. R. De Leval, A. Mcewan, N. Pigott, M. J. Elliott, A. Mcquillan, C. Macdonald, and A. J. Goldman. 2007. Patient handover from surgery to intensive care: Using formula 1 pit stop and aviation models to improve safety and quality. *Pediatric Anesthesia* 17(5):470-478.

Cebul, R. D., T. E. Love, A. K. Jain, and C. J. Hebert. 2011. Electronic health records and quality of diabetes care. *New England Journal of Medicine* 365(9):825-833.

Center for Medicare & Medicaid Innovation. 2012. *One year of innovation: Taking action to improve care and reduce costs.* http://www.innovations.cms.gov/Files/reports/Innovation-Center-Year-One-Summary-document.pdf (accessed March 27, 2012).

Chassin, M. R., and J. M. Loeb. 2011. The ongoing quality improvement journey: Next stop, high reliability. *Health Affairs (Millwood)* 30(4):559-568.

Congressional Budget Office. 2009. *Health Information Technology for Economic and Clinical Health Act*. Washington, DC: Congressional Budget Office.

Corlette, S., J. Alker, J. Touschner, and J. Volk. 2011. *The Massachusetts and Utah health insurance exchanges: Lessons learned*. Washington, DC: Georgetown University Health Policy Institute.

Cosgrove, D., M. Fisher, P. Gabow, G. Gottlieb, G. C. Halvorson, B. James, G. Kaplan, J. Perlin, R. Petzel, G. Steele, and J. Toussaint. 2012. *A CEO checklist for high-value health care*. Discussion Paper, Institute of Medicine, Washington, DC. http://www.iom.edu/CEOChecklist (accessed August 31, 2012).

DesRoches, C. M., C. Worzala, M. S. Joshi, P. D. Kralovec, and A. K. Jha. 2012. Small, non-teaching, and rural hospitals continue to be slow in adopting electronic health record systems. *Health Affairs* 31(5):1092-1099.

Dolan, P. L. 2010. 86% of physicians use Internet to access health information. *American Medical News*, January 11.

Eddy, D. M., and L. Schlessinger. 2003. Archimedes: A trial-validated model of diabetes. *Diabetes Care* 26(11):3093-3101.

Eddy, D. M., J. Adler, B. Patterson, D. Lucas, K. A. Smith, and M. Morris. 2011. Individualized guidelines: The potential for increasing quality and reducing costs. *Annals of Internal Medicine* 154(9):627-634.

Fox, S. 2011a. *Health topics: 80% of Internet users look for health information online*. Washington, DC: Pew Research Center.

Fox, S. 2011b. *The social life of health information, 2011*. Washington, DC: Pew Research Center.

Frankovich, J., C. A. Longhurst, and S. M. Sutherland. 2011. Evidence-based medicine in the EMR era. *New England Journal of Medicine* 365(19):1758-1759.

Friedberg, M. W., K. L. Coltin, D. G. Safran, M. Dresser, A. M. Zaslavsky, and E. C. Schneider. 2009. Associations between structural capabilities of primary care practices and performance on selected quality measures. *Annals of Internal Medicine* 151(7):456-463.

Ginsburg, P. B., H. H. Pham, K. McKenzie, and A. Milstein. 2007. Distorted payment system undermines business case for health quality and efficiency gains. *Spine* 400(415):15.

Good Stewardship Working Group. 2011. The "top 5" lists in primary care: Meeting the responsibility of professionalism. *Archives of Internal Medicine* 171(15):1385-1390.

Greenfeld, K. 2010. How to survive in vegas. *Bloomberg Businessweek*, August 5. http://www.businessweek.com/magazine/content/10_33/b4191070705858.htm (accessed December 12, 2011).

Guterman, S., K. Davis, K. Stremikis, and H. Drake. 2010. Innovation in Medicare and Medicaid will be central to health reform's success. *Health Affairs (Millwood)* 29(6):1188-1193.

Hammer, M. 2004. Deep change. How operational innovation can transform your company. *Harvard Business Review* 82(4):84-93, 141.

Haynes, A. B., T. G. Weiser, W. R. Berry, S. R. Lipsitz, A. H. Breizat, E. P. Dellinger, T. Herbosa, S. Joseph, P. L. Kibatala, M. C. Lapitan, A. F. Merry, K. Moorthy, R. K. Reznick, B. Taylor, A. A. Gawande, and Safe Surgery Saves Lives Study Group. 2009. A surgical safety checklist to reduce morbidity and mortality in a global population. *New England Journal of Medicine* 360(5):491-499.

Hilbert, M., and P. López. 2011. The world's technological capacity to store, communicate, and compute information. *Science* 332(6025):60-65.

Hsiao, C.-J., E. Hing, T. C. Socey, and B. Cai. 2011. *Electronic health record systems and intent to apply for meaningful use incentives among office-based physician practices: United States, 2001-2011*. Hyattsville, MD: National Center for Health Statistics.

Huberty, K., M. Lipacis, A. Holt, E. Gelblum, S. Devitt, B. Swinburne, F. Meunier, K. Han, F. A. Y. Wang, J. Lu, G. Chen, B. Lu, M. Ono, M. Nagasaka, K. Yoshikawa, and M. Schneider. 2011. *Tablet demand and disruption.* New York: Morgan Stanley.

IOM (Institute of Medicine). 1999. *To err is human: Building a safer health system.* Washington, DC: National Academy Press.

IOM. 2005. *Building a better delivery system: A new engineering/health care partnership.* Washington, DC: The National Academies Press.

IOM. 2011. *Digital infrastructure for the learning health system: The foundation for continuous improvement in health and health care: A workshop summary.* Washington, DC: The National Academies Press.

IOM and NAE (National Academy of Engineering). 2011. *Engineering a learning healthcare system: A look at the future: Workshop summary.* Washington, DC: The National Academies Press.

Kaiser Family Foundation. 2007. *Vermont health care reform plan.* http://www.kff.org/uninsured/upload/7723.pdf (accessed December 20, 2011).

Kaplan, H. C., P. W. Brady, M. C. Dritz, D. K. Hooper, W. M. Linam, C. M. Froehle, and P. Margolis. 2010. The influence of context on quality improvement success in health care: A systematic review of the literature. *Milbank Quarterly* 88(4):500-559.

Kenney, C. 2008. *The best practice: How the new quality movement is transforming medicine.* 1st ed. New York: Public Affairs.

Kenney, C. 2011. *Transforming health care: Virginia Mason Medical Center's pursuit of the perfect patient experience.* Boca Raton, FL: CRC Press.

Lesser, M. L., and J. W. Haanstra. 1957. The random-access memory accounting machine, 1. System organizations of the IBM-305. *IBM Journal of Research and Development* 1(1):62-71.

Levy, S. 2006. The hard disk that changed the world. *Newsweek,* August 6.

Lewis, G. H., R. Vaithianathan, P. M. Hockey, G. Hirst, and J. P. Bagian. 2011. Counterheroism, common knowledge, and ergonomics: Concepts from aviation that could improve patient safety. *Milbank Quarterly* 89(1):4-38.

Litvak, E., and M. Bisognano. 2011. More patients, less payment: Increasing hospital efficiency in the aftermath of health reform. *Health Affairs (Millwood)* 30(1):76-80.

Manyika, J., M. Chui, B. Brown, J. Bughin, R. Dobbs, C. Roxburgh, and A. H. Byers. 2011. *Big data: The next frontier for innovation, competition, and productivity.* Washington, DC: McKinsey Global Institute.

McDonough, J. E., B. Rosman, M. Butt, L. Tucker, and L. K. Howe. 2008. Massachusetts health reform implementation: Major progress and future challenges. *Health Affairs (Millwood)* 27(4):w285-w297.

Nance, J. J. 2011. Airline safety. In *Engineering a learning healthcare system: A look at the future: Workshop summary.* Institute of Medicine. Washington, DC: The National Academies Press.

National Public Radio. 2011. From Harvard economist to casino CEO. *Planet Money,* November 15.

Partners HealthCare Center for Connected Health. 2012. *Connected cardiac care.* http://www.connected-health.org/programs/cardiac-care/center-for-connected-health-initiatives/connected-cardiac-care.aspx (accessed April 13, 2012).

Pew Internet & American Life Project. 2011. *Internet adoption, 1995-2011.* http://www.pewinternet.org/Trend-Data/Internet-Adoption.aspx (accessed October 27, 2011).

Pham, H. H., P. B. Ginsburg, K. McKenzie, and A. Milstein. 2007. Redesigning care delivery in response to a high-performance network: The Virginia Mason Medical Center. *Health Affairs* 26(4):w532-w544.

Potts, A. L., F. E. Barr, D. F. Gregory, L. Wright, and N. R. Patel. 2004. Computerized physician order entry and medication errors in a pediatric critical care unit. *Pediatrics* 113(1 Pt. 1):59-63.

President's Information Technology Advisory Committee. 2001. *Transforming health care through information technology.* http://www.nitrd.gov/Pubs/pitac/pitac-hc-9feb01.pdf (accessed August 31, 2012).

President's Information Technology Advisory Committee. 2004. *Revolutionizing health care through information technology.* http://www.itrd.gov/pitac/meetings/2004/20040617/20040615_hit.pdf (accessed August 31, 2012).

Pronovost, P., D. Needham, S. Berenholtz, D. Sinopoli, H. T. Chu, S. Cosgrove, B. Sexton, R. Hyzy, R. Welsh, G. Roth, J. Bander, J. Kepros, and C. Goeschel. 2006. An intervention to decrease catheter-related bloodstream infections in the ICU. *New England Journal of Medicine* 355(26):2725-2732.

Pronovost, P. J., C. A. Goeschel, K. L. Olsen, J. C. Pham, M. R. Miller, S. M. Berenholtz, J. B. Sexton, J. A. Marsteller, L. L. Morlock, A. W. Wu, J. M. Loeb, and C. M. Clancy. 2009. Reducing health care hazards: Lessons from the commercial aviation safety team. *Health Affairs (Millwood)* 28(3):w479-w489.

Purcell, K. 2011. *Search and email still top the list of most popular online activities.* Washington, DC: Pew Research Center.

Raymond, A. G. 2011. *Massachusetts health reform: A five-year progress report.* http://bluecrossfoundation.org/Health-Reform/~/media/0FF9BF33E14E4E089335AD12E8DEB77E.pdf (accessed December 20, 2011).

Song, Z., and B. E. Landon. 2012. Controlling health care spending—the Massachusetts experiment. *New England Journal of Medicine* 366(17):1560-1561.

Spear, S. J. 2005. Fixing health care from the inside, today. *Harvard Business Review* 83(9):78.

Spear, S. J., and H. K. Bowen. 1999. Decoding the DNA of the Toyota production system. *Harvard Business Review.* http://twi-institute.com/pdfs/article_DecodingToyotaProductionSystem.pdf (accessed August 31, 2012).

State of Vermont. 2011. *Brief summary of Act 48 Vermont Health Reform Law of 2011.* http://hcr.vermont.gov/health-care-reform-initiatives/2011 (accessed December 20, 2011).

Stern, M., K. Williams, D. Eddy, and R. Kahn. 2008. Validation of prediction of diabetes by the Archimedes model and comparison with other predicting models. *Diabetes Care* 31(8):1670-1671.

Toussaint, J. S., C. Queram, and J. W. Musser. 2011. Connecting statewide health information technology strategy to payment reform. *American Journal of Managed Care* 17(3):e80-e88.

Washington, A. E., and S. H. Lipstein. 2011. The Patient-Centered Outcomes Research Institute—promoting better information, decisions, and health. *New England Journal of Medicine* 365(15):e31.

Wiegmann, D., and S. Shappell. 2001. Human error analysis of commercial aviation accidents: Application of the Human Factors Analysis and Classification System (HFACS). *Aviation Space and Environmental Medicine* 72(11):1006-1016.

Young, T., S. Brailsford, C. Connell, R. Davies, P. Harper, and J. H. Klein. 2004. Using industrial processes to improve patient care. *British Medical Journal* 328(7432):162-164.

Zickuhr, K. 2011. *Generations and their gadgets.* Washington, DC: Pew Research Center.

Part II

The Vision

5

A Continuously Learning
Health Care System

In 1982, results of the Beta-Blocker Heart Attack Trial were pub-
lished, showing that the use of beta-blockers after a heart attack re-
duced mortality by at least 25 percent (Beta-Blocker Heart Attack
Trial Research Group, 1982). Further studies validated these re-
sults (Yusuf et al., 1985). Yet, by the mid-1990s, beta-blockers were
being prescribed after a heart attack only 30 to 50 percent of the
time (Brand et al., 1995; Burwen et al., 2003; Gottlieb et al., 1998;
Krumholz et al., 1998). Even as utilization remained low, trials in
the 1990s showed that the mortality reduction from beta-blocker
use was as high as 40 percent and that more patients benefited from
the treatment than had originally been estimated (Gottlieb et al.,
1998). The use of this treatment was encouraged in the 1990s by
its inclusion in professional guidelines and by efforts to measure
the extent of its use. The American College of Cardiology and the
American Heart Association recommended beta-blocker treatment
after heart attack in their guidelines (Ryan et al., 1996, 1999).
On the measurement front, the Joint Commission established a
performance measurement program for hospitals, including in its
measures the level of prescribing of beta-blockers after heart at-
tack hospitalizations; the Health Care Financing Administration
(now the Centers for Medicare & Medicaid Services) began col-
lecting similar data for Medicare patients (Krumholz et al., 1998;
Marciniak et al., 1998), and the National Committee for Quality
Assurance (NCQA) included beta-blocker usage in its Healthcare
Effectiveness Data and Information Set (HEDIS) measures (Health

Plan Employer Data and Information Set) (Bradley et al., 2001; Lee, 2007). Beyond guidelines and measures, some health plans offered financial incentives under pay-for-performance contracts to increase the rates at which beta-blocker therapy was delivered (Lee, 2007). In addition to developing guidelines, the American College of Cardiology and American Heart Association both created programs to encourage clinicians to implement these guidelines in their practices. And the Institute for Healthcare Improvement included beta-blocker use as one component of its 100,000 Lives Campaign (Gosfield and Reinertsen, 2005). After this considerable amount of effort, on May 8, 2007, NCQA retired the use of a beta-blocker measure. The measure finally was no longer necessary because most patients under most health plans were now receiving this therapy for heart attack care (Lee, 2007).

Advances in science and technology have allowed health care to make great strides in treating diseases. Some diseases considered fatal just a generation ago are now routinely managed. Despite this progress, however, health care today displays notable shortcomings on each of the six aims for high-quality care identified in the Institute of Medicine (IOM) report *Crossing the Quality Chasm*: safety, effectiveness, efficiency, equity, timeliness, and patient-centeredness (2001). Care varies significantly from one part of the country to another and even from one town to another, with some areas offering high-quality, high-value care and others falling short of their potential. Substantial variations exist as well in the dissemination and adoption of new innovations. Some interventions and treatments with little evidence for superior outcomes spread rapidly, while others with a strong evidence base languish in obscurity. The shortfalls of the current health care system are captured by this simple fact: fully 160 years after Semmelweis discovered the importance of hand hygiene, many American health care institutions are finding it necessary to mount campaigns to encourage providers to wash their hands (Chassin and Loeb, 2011).

The health care environment itself places unnecessary burdens on health care professionals, siloing care activities, insufficiently meeting patient needs, and failing to disseminate knowledge broadly. The "system" has few elements that are systematic. Patients often report their frustration with a health care delivery enterprise that is fragmented, uncoordinated, and diffusely organized. As a result, they often are lost in the gaps and frustrated in trying to access the care they need.

Further, as discussed in Part I of this report, evidence on what is effective for a given patient under specific clinical circumstances often is lacking, poorly disseminated, or inconsistently implemented. The sheer volume of new clinical trials, journal articles, clinical guidelines, and other medical information far exceeds individual human cognitive capacity—no clinician can read, process, and apply all of this constantly emerging information to regular patient care. Future developments in genomics, proteomics, informatics, and technology will only exacerbate these challenges.

Asking, urging, or demanding that clinicians keep pace with new clinical knowledge will not improve the quality of care. Such an approach would only impose unnecessary and demoralizing stress on these health care providers and associated professionals. Indeed, the problems described here persist even as individual physicians, nurses, technicians, pharmacists, and others involved in patient care work diligently at performing difficult health care tasks and at providing high-quality, compassionate care to their patients. Yet, they work within a system that lags far behind other industries in the ability to assimilate and disseminate information in real time and useful form—a system impaired by the weight of its own complexity. The path to improvement, then, is to transform the current environment into a coordinated system of care. This new environment would provide tools and resources, actionable real-time information, and appropriate incentives to help providers successfully manage the increasing complexity of medical care. In short, by making the right thing easy to do, systemwide change can be achieved.

The example at the beginning of this chapter of the diffusion of the use of beta-blockers after heart attack is a success story in many ways: high-quality evidence was produced; it was incorporated into clinical care guidelines, quality improvement initiatives, and quality-of-care measures; and several health plans offered financial incentives for its uptake. Yet even with this level of effort, it took 25 years from the time the initial results were published until the time the treatment saw general use in clinical practice. This example speaks to the need to create infrastructure that makes the process of learning and improvement easier, so that the next discovery does not require 25 years of sustained effort before it is widely used to help patients.

Improving quality and controlling costs requires moving from this unsustainable and flawed organizational arrangement to a system that gains knowledge from every care delivery experience and is engineered to promote continuous improvement. In short, the nation needs a health care system that learns, and the committee believes a learning health care system is both possible and necessary for the nation today. This chapter outlines the vision for such a system, highlighting specific characteristics and aims for improvement.

DEFINITION

A Learning Health Care System

A learning health care system is one in which science, informatics, incentives, and culture are aligned for continuous improvement and innovation, with best practices seamlessly embedded in the care process, patients and families active participants in all elements, and new knowledge captured as an integral by-product of the care experience. (Roundtable on Value & Science-Driven Health Care, 2012)

As noted in Part I of this report, the supply of knowledge currently available to health care providers and patients has several deficiencies. Providers and patients often lack reliable evidence on the effectiveness of different treatment options, interventions, and technologies and on how the effectiveness of treatments varies for different patients. Moreover, the quality of care depends not only on the effectiveness of a given treatment but also on the way that treatment is delivered. Thus it is necessary to build knowledge about different methods of delivering care and provide clinicians and health care organizations with tools to improve care processes.

Learning processes must also be tailored to the circumstances and needs of the various stakeholders in the health care system. Each stakeholder has a different role in the generation and dissemination of knowledge, so each will need different tools to support continuous learning and improvement. Furthermore, organizations and individuals are at different stages in their learning journey; some have developed advanced systems for continuously improving care (see Chapter 9 for examples), while others are just starting out. New opportunities, such as digital technologies with which to share information and measure progress, can increase the learning potential of every stakeholder. Figure 5-1 illustrates the committee's vision of how systematically capturing and translating information generated from clinical research and from care delivery can close now open-ended learning loops.

CHARACTERISTICS

To foster transition to a health care system characterized by continuous learning and improvement, public and private purchasers, health care organizations, clinicians, patients, and other stakeholders should focus their efforts on the foundational elements of a learning health care system, as detailed below and summarized in Table 5-1.

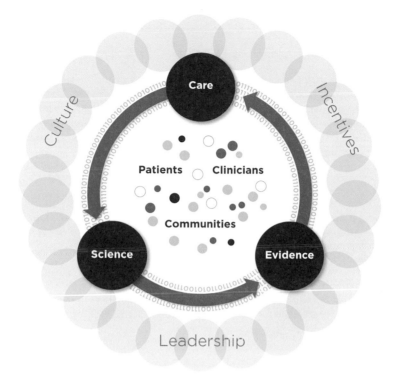

FIGURE 5-1 Schematic of a learning health care system.

Engaged, empowered public and patients. The people served by the health care system—patients, caregivers, and the public—must serve as both the system's unwavering focus and its fully engaged agents for change. This implies that patient perspectives and needs should be fundamental in the design of health care delivery and in its daily operations. Further, patients and the public should be active contributors, supporters, and actors in the learning process. Yet, currently, the notion of patient-centeredness feels unfamiliar, even disruptive, and the health care culture is not conducive to patient involvement in care—this despite the evidence for positive benefits of such involvement (Berwick, 2009). As noted in prior IOM publications, patients often are limited in their ability to participate as full partners in their health care (IOM, 2001, 2011). Few patients receive clear information on the benefits and potential adverse effects of screenings, tests, treatments, and interventions under consideration for their condition.

TABLE 5-1 Characteristics of a Continuously Learning Health Care
System

Science and Informatics

> *Real-time access to knowledge*—A learning health care system continuously and reliably captures, curates, and delivers the best available evidence to guide, support, tailor, and improve clinical decision making and care safety and quality.
>
> *Digital capture of the care experience*—A learning health care system captures the care experience on digital platforms for real-time generation and application of knowledge for care improvement.

Patient-Clinician Partnerships

> *Engaged, empowered patients*—A learning health care system is anchored on patient needs and perspectives and promotes the inclusion of patients, families, and other caregivers as vital members of the continuously learning care team.

Incentives

> *Incentives aligned for value*—A learning health care system has incentives actively aligned to encourage continuous improvement, identify and reduce waste, and reward high-value care.
>
> *Full transparency*—A learning health care system systematically monitors the safety, quality, processes, prices, costs, and outcomes of care, and makes information available for care improvement and informed choices and decision making by clinicians, patients, and their families.

Continuous Learning Culture

> *Leadership-instilled culture of learning*—A learning health care system is stewarded by leadership committed to a culture of teamwork, collaboration, and adaptability in support of continuous learning as a core aim.
>
> *Supportive system competencies*—A learning health care system constantly refines complex care operations and processes through ongoing team training and skill building, systems analysis and information development, and creation of the feedback loops for continuous learning and system improvement.

In contrast, the central focus of a learning health care system is those it serves—patients, their families and caregivers, and the broader public. In a learning health care system, patient needs and perspectives are factored into the design of health care processes, the creation and use of technologies, and the training of clinicians.

To increase the engagement of patients and consumers in health care, it will be necessary to develop new communication strategies that provide understandable evidence on care options and account for individual patient needs, preferences, and capabilities. In addition, tools that allow the patient to be a partner in clinical decisions need to be diffused widely. One way to disseminate these communication strategies and tools is through changes in clinician education and training. In addition, several new initiatives, such as those centered on participatory medicine, shift the model of health care to one in which patients are key actors in their health and full partners with clinicians in their care. The vision for engaging and empowering patients and the public in a learning health care system is discussed in detail in Chapter 7.

Data infrastructure. The current methods for generating clinical knowledge, while effective in many ways, are slow, cumbersome, and expensive. Yet, the need for knowledge to guide clinical and policy decisions has never been greater. The increasing rate at which new interventions and medical technologies are developed, along with new data on individual variations in conditions and their optimum treatment, requires the development of a new engine for generating clinical knowledge.

An array of clinical effectiveness research strategies, ranging from controlled clinical trials to research drawn from clinical practice, can provide the evidence needed to guide high-quality patient care. Today, more evidence exists about the effectiveness of different treatments and interventions than at any other time in history. But clinical trials often are not structured in a way that delivers the most meaningful results for general clinical use. Despite being expensive and lengthy, large experimental trials frequently generate evidence that may not be applicable to all practice circumstances or patient populations. Trials routinely focus on younger and healthier patients, which introduces uncertainty when the results are extrapolated to real-world patient populations.

In a learning health care system, nimble and efficient approaches, including emerging statistical techniques, research designs, and analytic models that can be applied across all population groups, drive the creation of clinical knowledge. As clinical datasets expand and become more numerous, the potential for generating new insights on the effectiveness of interventions through data mining approaches becomes greater (IOM, 2010). Further, in a true learning system, information is developed as a natural by-product of the care process; knowledge on effectiveness, quality, and value is gained from each patient experience. Increased use of data collected and measured at the point of care, of clinical datasets, and of emerging research techniques in conjunction with traditional research methods can help ensure that research informs the real-world settings of clinical practice. The vision of a robust data infrastructure in a learning health care system is discussed in detail in Chapter 6.

Real-time access to knowledge. Information has transformed modern life. Most individuals are bombarded with information throughout the day, every day. The increasing availability of information has led to widespread societal changes, altered the way governments interact with their citizens, and resulted in extraordinary changes in the way most industries do business. Many industries have used this access to information to increase their productivity and develop new ways of delivering services.

In the health care sector, a dynamic biomedical research enterprise produces some of the world's most advanced and innovative clinical discoveries. Unfortunately, important knowledge produced by this research often is not applied to clinical decision making. Recommended practices are delivered only approximately half of the time (McGlynn et al., 2003). One of the major barriers to the consistent application of evidence is the overwhelming quantity of knowledge that is produced every year. The volume and complexity of medical evidence are beyond the capabilities of any individual to aggregate, synthesize, and interpret for clinical practice. The result is uneven quality of care and patient health outcomes.

In a learning health care system, the data, information, and knowledge produced from both biomedical research and clinical encounters is captured, stored, exchanged, and managed using tools that are reliable and secure, and that support continuous quality improvement and health management for a population of patients. New technological tools are used to translate evidence and guidelines into a format that is usable by clinicians and integrated seamlessly at the point of care, such as through clinical decision support software. Finally, patients and their caregivers are engaged in knowledge generation and dissemination through privacy and security policies that build and maintain public trust while incorporating patient-generated data and improving patients' access to their health information. The vision for increasing clinicians' and patients' real-time access to data, information, and knowledge in a learning health care system is discussed in detail in Chapter 6.

Leadership-instilled culture of learning. Strong, visible leadership will be necessary from all sectors of the health care system if the vision of a learning health care system is to be realized (NRC, 2011). For individual health care organizations, leadership has a special significance because it establishes the organization's vision, communicates its core values, and makes learning and improvement a priority. In addition, health care system leaders help guide the culture of their organization, which has a substantial impact on health outcomes, patient experience, and the satisfaction of employees. A poor culture can present barriers to learning, while a strong culture can drive change (IOM, 2001; Schein, 2004). In promoting safety, for example, the culture must encourage coordination and teamwork among clinicians, as well as promote a nonpunitive environment in which health care professionals feel free to report potential problems. In contrast, the current health care culture is centered on the autonomy of the individual health professional. Clinician expertise is crucial, but this type of culture often leads to a system in which each individual pursues his or her own judgment instead of collaborating to provide the best care for the patient.

The culture of a learning health care system emphasizes teamwork, adaptability, and coordination and strives for continuous learning and improvement. To promote such an environment, health care leaders must know how to influence, support, and measure their organization's culture. Further, leadership must require visible accountability for improved performance in such areas as quality and safety. This does not mean that leaders must personally spearhead improvement initiatives, but that they must be responsible for devoting resources to such initiatives and supporting the individuals involved. These leadership qualities are not innate to every health care leader and worker; they must be actively taught and reinforced if strong leadership is to become widely available throughout the system.

This is not to say that all elements of the current culture must be reworked. Most physicians, nurses, and other health care professionals are passionate about their work. Every day, in every hospital or clinic across the country, individuals go above and beyond to care for patients, regardless of the system's limitations. However, changes are necessary to support and augment that passion and dedication. The vision of a leadership-instilled culture of learning in a learning health care system is discussed in detail in Chapter 9.

Competencies that promote continuous improvement. Given the complexity of the health care system and the limits of human capacity, human errors are inevitable. Yet many health care systems are designed and operated under the mistaken assumption that their workers will never err. Adverse events result in part from the variability in the flow of patients through the health care delivery system. And the siloed nature of health care, which boasts hundreds of specialties and often is marked by a lack of communication within and among providers and health care organizations, leads to quality lapses during transitions in patient care.

In a learning health care system, health care organizations design care delivery with an understanding of these limitations. System analysis tools such as root cause analyses and standard protocols for clinical processes are used to identify and overcome human error and support consistent performance. Teamwork and coordination among professionals help integrate care and reduce adverse events at the interfaces between different care processes. Variations in care quality are reduced through the use of variability methodologies and operations management. This type of deliberate system design allows health care providers to harness their strengths—compassion and an emphasis on meeting individual patient needs—more effectively instead of focusing on factors beyond their control. The vision of continuous improvement in a learning health care system is discussed in detail in Chapter 9.

Alignment of incentives. The current health care system fails to support high-value care, and the result has been serious long-term fiscal challenges for the nation. Health care costs consistently outpace inflation rates; squeeze the budgets of states, employers, and individuals; and reduce individual and family income—all without commensurate health improvements. Medical practice varies significantly from state to state, hospital to hospital, and clinician to clinician, degrading patient care and resulting in uneven quality and safety. Counteracting these trends will require a stronger focus on ways to enhance both health and economic returns from health care investments.

In a learning health care system, the best practices, drawn from research and experience, are the starting point for care. Reliably employing established best practices and building them into routine care leads to system excellence. New technologies provide new opportunities for reducing variations in care, such as through decision support tools. Incentives also are powerful agents for change. To support the transition to a learning health care system, payment incentives must be directly aligned with the goals of a high-quality health care system; promote a focus on the needs of patients and families; and provide the resources and time necessary to support a culture of continuous improvement in the effectiveness, efficiency, and safety of care. Further, a learning health care system fosters value by advancing the science of value incentives so the effects of different payment and incentive models can be better understood. The vision of alignment of incentives in a learning health care system is discussed in detail in Chapter 8.

Transparency. While many definitions of transparency exist, in its basic sense transparency means ensuring that complete, timely, and understandable information is available to support wise decisions. Such information often is missing in the modern health care environment. Yet transparency can be a powerful motivator for change, encouraging providers and organizations to reassess their own practices in order to improve. Most clinicians lack critical data on their own performance and how it relates to that of their peers. Transparency in this regard empowers providers to improve their performance and helps organizations eliminate waste and improve care processes.

Further, patients and consumers lack the information they need to make health care decisions, from which course of medical treatment to pursue to the selection of health care providers. While there are unanswered questions about the best way to present this information to a public audience, the current opacity of the health care system prevents people from discovering basic information, from the cost of a proposed treatment to the average outcomes for a particular intervention. Without meaningful and trustworthy sources of information on costs and outcomes of care, patients and consumers cannot make fully informed decisions. The vision of increased transparency in a learning health care system is discussed in detail in Chapter 8.

THE PATH TO A CONTINUOUSLY
LEARNING HEALTH CARE SYSTEM

On each of the dimensions discussed above, the current health care system falls short of its potential. Achieving the core aims of the health care system—better patient health, enhanced experience of care, and improved value from care—will require a fundamental transformation on all these fronts. As outlined in Part I, the imperatives are clear. Too much is spent on health care without concomitant benefits. Equally clear is the path to improvement. Even as the health care system struggles in the face of increasing complexity and costs, it can achieve its potential by transforming into a system that continuously learns and improves. The goal of such a system is to draw on the best evidence in providing care, emphasize prevention and health promotion, continuously improve in value and care quality, and foster advances in the nation's health.

Yet there are challenges to implementing this vision in real-world clinical environments. Clinicians routinely report moderate or high levels of stress, feel there is not enough time to meet their patients' needs, and find their work environment chaotic (Burdi and Baker, 1999; Linzer et al., 2009; Trude, 2003). As described in Chapter 2, clinicians struggle to deliver care while confronting inefficient workflows, administrative burdens, and uncoordinated systems. These time pressures, stresses, and inefficiencies limit clinicians from focusing on additional tasks and initiatives, even those that have important goals for improving care. Similarly, professionals working in health care organizations are overwhelmed by the sheer volume of initiatives currently under way to improve various aspects of the care process, initiatives that appear to be unconnected with the organization's priorities. Often, these initiatives may be successful in one setting yet may not translate to other parts of the same organization.

Given such real-world impediments, initiatives that focus merely on incremental improvements and add to a clinician's daily workload are unlikely to succeed. Just as the quantity of clinical information now available exceeds the capacity of any individual to absorb and apply it, the number of tasks needed for regular care outstrips the capabilities of any individual. Rather, significant improvements can occur only if the environment, context, and systems in which these professionals practice are reconfigured. Strategies for building this type of system that supports clinicians' efforts focus on three major areas: providing the foundations for learning, establishing a suitable environment for improvement, and ensuring that learning focuses on the right targets. Essential as well are expanding the evidence base to ensure that clinicians have the information they need, expanding the capacity to capture patient data in digital records, and developing metrics for assessing different aspects of learning and improvement. In creating a supportive environment, the levers for change include developing incentives that promote improvement, ensuring that payment and contracting policies support learning, promoting transparency that helps clinicians and patients make informed decisions, and building cultures that encourage improvement. Finally, focusing learning on the right targets requires approaches for engaging patients to ensure that care addresses their needs, goals, and circumstances. Part III of this report explores each of these strategies in more detail.

REFERENCES

Berwick, D. M. 2009. What "patient-centered" should mean: Confessions of an extremist. *Health Affairs (Millwood)* 28(4):w555-w565.

Beta-Blocker Heart Attack Trial Research Group. 1982. A randomized trial of propranolol in patients with acute myocardial infarction. I. Mortality results. *Journal of the American Medical Association* 247(12):1707-1714.

Bradley, E. H., E. S. Holmboe, J. A. Mattera, S. A. Roumanis, M. J. Radford, and H. M. Krumholz. 2001. A qualitative study of increasing beta-blocker use after myocardial infarction: Why do some hospitals succeed? *Journal of the American Medical Association* 285(20):2604-2611.

Brand, D. A., L. N. Newcomer, A. Freiburger, and H. Tian. 1995. Cardiologists' practices compared with practice guidelines: Use of beta-blockade after acute myocardial infarction. *Journal of the American College of Cardiology* 26(6):1432-1436.

Burdi, M. D., and L. C. Baker. 1999. Physicians' perceptions of autonomy and satisfaction in California. *Health Affairs* 18(4):134.

Burwen, D. R., D. H. Galusha, J. M. Lewis, M. R. Bedinger, M. J. Radford, H. M. Krumholz, and J. M. Foody. 2003. National and state trends in quality of care for acute myocardial infarction between 1994-1995 and 1998-1999: The Medicare health care quality improvement program. *Archives of Internal Medicine* 163(12):1430-1439.

Chassin, M. R., and J. M. Loeb. 2011. The ongoing quality improvement journey: Next stop, high reliability. *Health Affairs (Millwood)* 30(4):559-568.

Gosfield, A. G., and J. L. Reinertsen. 2005. The 100,000 lives campaign: Crystallizing standards of care for hospitals. *Health Affairs (Millwood)* 24(6):1560-1570.

Gottlieb, S. S., R. J. McCarter, and R. A. Vogel. 1998. Effect of beta-blockade on mortality among high-risk and low-risk patients after myocardial infarction. *New England Journal of Medicine* 339(8):489-497.

IOM (Institute of Medicine). 2001. *Crossing the quality chasm: A new health system for the 21st century*. Washington, DC: National Academy Press.

IOM. 2010. *Redesigning the clinical effectiveness research paradigm: Innovation and practice-based approaches: Workshop summary*. Washington, DC: The National Academies Press.

IOM. 2011. *Patients charting the course: Citizen engagement in the learning health system: Workshop summary*. Washington, DC: The National Academies Press.

Krumholz, H. M., M. J. Radford, Y. Wang, J. Chen, A. Heiat, and T. A. Marciniak. 1998. National use and effectiveness of beta-blockers for the treatment of elderly patients after acute myocardial infarction: National cooperative cardiovascular project. *Journal of the American Medical Association* 280(7):623-629.

Lee, T. H. 2007. Eulogy for a quality measure. *New England Journal of Medicine* 357(12):1175-1177.

Linzer, M., L. B. Manwell, E. S. Williams, J. A. Bobula, R. L. Brown, A. B. Varkey, B. Man, J. E. McMurray, A. Maguire, B. Horner-Ibler, M. D. Schwartz, and MEMO (Minimizing Error, Maximizing Outcome) Investigators. 2009. Working conditions in primary care: Physician reactions and care quality. *Annals of Internal Medicine* 151(1):28-36, W26-W29.

Marciniak, T. A., E. F. Ellerbeck, M. J. Radford, T. F. Kresowik, J. A. Gold, H. M. Krumholz, C. I. Kiefe, R. M. Allman, R. A. Vogel, and S. F. Jencks. 1998. Improving the quality of care for medicare patients with acute myocardial infarction: Results from the cooperative cardiovascular project. *Journal of the American Medical Association* 279(17):1351-1357.

McGlynn, E. A., S. M. Asch, J. Adams, J. Keesey, J. Hicks, A. DeCristofaro, and E. A. Kerr. 2003. The quality of health care delivered to adults in the United States. *New England Journal of Medicine* 348(26):2635-2645.

NRC (National Research Council). 2011. *Strategies and priorities for information technology at the Centers for Medicare & Medicaid Services.* Washington, DC: The National Academies Press.

Roundtable on Value & Science-Driven Health Care. 2012. *The Roundtable.* Washington, DC: Institute of Medicine.

Ryan, T. J., J. L. Anderson, E. M. Antman, B. A. Braniff, N. H. Brooks, R. M. Califf, L. D. Hillis, L. F. Hiratzka, E. Rapaport, B. J. Riegel, R. O. Russell, E. E. Smith Iii, W. D. Weaver, J. L. Ritchie, M. D. Cheitlin, K. A. Eagle, T. J. Gardner, J. A. Garson, R. J. Gibbons, R. P. Lewis, and R. A. O'Rourke. 1996. ACC/AHA guidelines for the management of patients with acute myocardial infarction: A report of the American College of Cardiology/American Heart Association task force on practice guidelines (committee on management of acute myocardial infarction). *Journal of the American College of Cardiology* 28(5):1328-1419.

Ryan, T. J., E. M. Antman, N. H. Brooks, R. M. Califf, L. D. Hillis, L. F. Hiratzka, E. Rapaport, B. Riegel, R. O. Russell, E. E. Smith, W. D. Weaver, R. J. Gibbons, J. S. Alpert, K. A. Eagle, T. J. Gardner, A. Garson, G. Gregoratos, and S. C. Smith. 1999. 1999 update: ACC/AHA guidelines for the management of patients with acute myocardial infarction: Executive summary and recommendations: A report of the American College of Cardiology/American Heart Association Task Force on Practice Guidelines (Committee on Management of Acute Myocardial Infarction). *Circulation* 100(9):1016-1030.

Schein, E. H. 2004. *Organizational culture and leadership.* San Francisco, CA: Jossey-Bass.

Trude, S. 2003. So much to do, so little time: Physician capacity constraints, 1997-2001. *Tracking Report/Center for Studying Health System Change* (8):1.

Yusuf, S., R. Peto, J. Lewis, R. Collins, and P. Sleight. 1985. Beta blockade during and after myocardial infarction: An overview of the randomized trials. *Progress in Cardiovascular Diseases* 27(3):335-371.

Part III

The Path

6

Generating and Applying
Knowledge in Real Time

*In 2008, Ann Morrison received two all-metal hip replacements at
the age of 50. Soon after the procedure, she experienced intense
rashes, pain, and inflammation at the sites of her surgery. The inju-
rious devices were replaced in 2010, just 2 years after she received
her initial hip replacements; hip replacements typically last 15 years
or more. Today, as a result of extensive tissue damage caused by
metal debris shed from the original replacements, Ann requires a
brace to walk, and she still has not been able to return to her work
as a physical therapist. With the proper digital infrastructure—
electronic health records, the use of clinical data to compare the
effectiveness and efficiency of different interventions, and registries
to track side effects and safety—Ann's experience could have been
avoided. Instead, the U.S. health care system currently lacks the
data, monitoring, and analysis capabilities necessary to effectively
evaluate, disseminate, and implement the ever-increasing amount
of health information and technologies (Meier and Roberts, 2011).*

Although an unprecedented amount of information is available in journals, guidelines, and other sources, patients and clinicians often lack access
to information they can feel confident is relevant, timely, and useful for
the circumstances at hand. Moreover, the current system for disseminating
knowledge is strained by the quantity of information now available, which
means that new evidence often is not applied to care. After explaining the
need for a new approach to generating clinical and biomedical knowledge,

149

this chapter describes emerging capacities, methods, and approaches that hold promise for helping to meet this need. It then examines what is necessary to create the data utility that will be essential to a continuously learning and improving health care system. Next, the critical issue of building a learning bridge from knowledge to practice is explored. This is followed by a discussion of the crucial role of people, patients, and consumers as active stakeholders in the learning enterprise. The chapter concludes with recommendations for achieving the vision of a health care system that generates and applies knowledge in real time.

NEED FOR A NEW APPROACH TO KNOWLEDGE GENERATION

The current approach to generating new medical knowledge falls short in delivering the evidence needed to support the delivery of quality care. The evidence base is inadequate, and methods for generating medical knowledge have notable limitations.

Inadequacy of the Evidence Base

Clinical and biomedical research emerges at a remarkable rate, with almost 2,100 scientific publications, 75 clinical trials, and 11 systematic reviews being produced every day (Bastian et al., 2010).[1] Although clinicians need not review every study to provide high-quality care, the ever-increasing volume of evidence makes it difficult to maintain a working knowledge of new clinical information.

Even so, however, the availability of such high-quality evidence is not keeping pace with the ever-increasing demand for clinical information that can help guide decisions on different diagnostics, interventions and therapies, and care delivery approaches (see Box 6-1 for an example of this information paradox). Rather, the gap between the evidence possible and the evidence produced continues to grow, and studies indicate that the number of guideline statements backed by evidence is not at the level that should be expected. In some cases, 40 to 50 percent of the recommendations made in guidelines are based on expert opinion, case studies, or standards of care rather than on multiple clinical trials or meta-analyses (Chauhan et al., 2006; IOM, 2008, 2011b; Tricoci et al., 2009). A study of the strength of the current recommendations of the Infectious Diseases Society of America, for example, found that only 14 percent were based on more than one randomized controlled trial, and more than half were based

---

[1]The number of journal publications was determined from searches on PubMed for 2010 (National Library of Medicine: http://www.ncbi.nlm.nih.gov/pubmed/) using the methodology described in Chapter 2.

BOX 6-1
The Information Paradox

The treatment of breast cancer is one example of the information paradox in clinical medicine. Relative to years past, a vast array of information about breast cancer is available. Five decades ago, breast cancer was detected from a physical exam, no biopsy was performed, and mastectomy was the recommended treatment for all detected breast cancers (Harrison, 1962). Today, multiple imaging technologies exist for the detection and diagnosis of the disease, including standard x-ray mammography, computed tomography (CT), ultrasound, positron emission tomography (PET), and magnetic resonance imaging (MRI) (IOM, 2001b, 2005). Similarly, traditional biopsies required surgical excision of the area of interest, whereas new methods allow for a less invasive evaluation, such as fine needle aspiration biopsy and core needle biopsy, and may be performed under imaging guidance (Bevers et al., 2009). Once diagnosed, the cancer can be further characterized by genetic characteristics (such as BRCA1, BRCA2, HER-2, and now multigene tests), in addition to its estrogen and progesterone receptor status. Treatments have developed at a similarly fast pace, with a number of surgical, radiological, chemotherapy, and endocrine therapies now being available, along with targeted therapies such as monoclonal antibodies (Kasper and Harrison, 2005; National Comprehensive Cancer Network, 2012). While progress in breast cancer diagnosis and treatment has been swift, however, the comparative efficacy and safety of these diagnostic technologies and treatments have not been evaluated; these innovations are administered without an adequate evidence basis. Likewise, the efficacy of many treatments or the accuracy of many diagnostic technologies is unknown for a given patient with a given condition (IOM, 2008). The results include widespread variation in patient care, confusion among patients and providers on the best methods for treating a specific disease or condition, and waste due to delivering services that are ineffective or even harmful for the patient.

---

on expert opinion alone (Lee and Vielemeyer, 2011). Another study, examining the joint cardiovascular clinical practice guidelines of the American College of Cardiology and the American Heart Association, found that the current guidelines were based largely on lower levels of evidence or expert opinion (Tricoci et al., 2009).

The inadequacy of the evidence base for clinical guidelines has consequences for the evidence base for care delivered. Estimates vary on the proportion of clinical decisions in the United States that are adequately informed by formal evidence gained from clinical research, with some studies suggesting a figure of just 10-20 percent (Darst et al., 2010; IOM, 1985). These results suggest that there are substantial opportunities for improvement in ensuring that the knowledge generated by the clinical research enterprise meets the demands of evidence-based care.

Even after identifying relevant information for a given condition, clinicians still must ensure that the information is of high quality—that the risk of contradiction by later studies is minimal, that the information is uncolored by bias or conflicts of interest, and that it applies to a particular patient's clinical circumstances. Several recent publications have observed that the rate of medical reversals is significant, with one recent paper finding that 13 percent of articles about medical practice in a high-profile journal contradicted the evidence for existing practices (Ioannidis, 2005b; Prasad et al., 2011). Another concern is managing conflicts of interest—which can occur in the research, education, and practice domains. As noted in the 2009 Institute of Medicine (IOM) report *Conflict of Interest in Medical Research, Education, and Practice*, patients can benefit when clinicians and researchers collaborate with the life science industry to develop new products, yet there are concerns that financial ties could unduly influence professional judgments. These tensions must be balanced to ensure that conflicts of interest do not negatively impact the integrity of the scientific research process, the objectivity of health professionals' training and education, or the public's trust in health care. There are approaches to managing conflicts of interest, especially financial relationships, without stifling important collaborations and innovations (IOM, 2009b).

Concerns exist as well about whether the current evidence base applies to the circumstances of particular patients. A study of clinical practice guidelines for nine of the most common chronic conditions, for example, found that fewer than half included guidance for the treatment of older patients with multiple comorbid conditions (Boyd et al., 2005). For patients and their health care providers, this lack of knowledge limits the ability to choose the most effective treatment for a condition. Furthermore, health care payers may not have the evidence they need to make coverage decisions for the patients enrolled in their plans. One analysis of Medicare payment policies for cardiovascular devices, for example, found that participants in the trials that provided evidence for coverage decisions differed from the Medicare population. Participants in the trials often were younger and healthier and had a different prevalence of comorbid conditions (Dhruva and Redberg, 2008).

Further, without greater capacity, the challenges to evidence production will only continue to grow. This is particularly true given the projected proliferation of new medical technologies; the increased complexity of managing chronic diseases; and the growing use of genomics, proteomics, and other biological factors to personalize treatments and diagnostics (Califf, 2004). As noted in Chapter 2, in one 3-year period, genome-wide scans were able to identify more than 100 genetic variants associated with nearly 40 diseases and traits; this growth in genetic understanding led to the availability in 2008 of more than 1,200 genetic tests for clinical conditions

(Genetics and Public Policy Center, 2008; Manolio, 2010; Pearson and Manolio, 2008).

Even as clinical research strains to keep pace with the rapid evolution of medical interventions and care delivery methods, improving and increasing the supply of knowledge with which to answer health care questions is a core aim of a learning health care system. The current research knowledge base provides limited support for answering important types of clinical questions, including those related to comparative effectiveness and long-term patient outcomes (*British Medical Journal*, 2011; Gill et al., 1996; IOM, 1985; Lee et al., 2005a; Tunis et al., 2003). This lack of knowledge is demonstrated by the fact that many technologies are not adequately evaluated before they see widespread clinical use. For example, cardiac computed tomography angiography (CTA) has been adopted widely throughout the medical community despite limited data on its effectiveness compared with alternative interventions, the risks of its use, and its substantial cost (Redberg, 2007). New opportunities in technology and research design can mitigate these limitations and offer a dynamic view of evidence and outcomes; leveraging these opportunities can bridge the gap between research and practice to accelerate the use of research in routine care.

Limitations of Current Methods

At present, support for clinical research often focuses on the randomized controlled trial as the gold standard for testing the effectiveness of diagnostics and therapeutics. The randomized controlled trial has gained this status because of its ability to control for many confounding factors and to provide direct evidence on the efficacy of different treatments, interventions, and care delivery methods (Hennekens et al., 1987). Yet, while the randomized controlled trial has a highly successful track record in generating new clinical knowledge, it has, like most research methods available today, several limitations: such trials are not practical or feasible in all situations, are expensive and time-consuming, address only the questions they were designed to answer, and cannot answer every type of research question.

A study of head-to-head randomized controlled trials for comparative effectiveness research purposes found that their costs ranged from $400,000 to $125 million, with the average costs for larger studies averaging $15-$20 million (Holve and Pittman, 2009, 2011). Randomized controlled trials also are slow to address the research questions they set out to answer. Half of all trials are delayed, 80 to 90 percent of these because of a shortage of willing trial participants (Grove, 2011). As currently designed and operated, moreover, randomized controlled trials do not address all clinically relevant populations, which may limit a trial's generalizability to regular clinical practice and many patient populations (Frangakis, 2009; Greenhouse et al., 2008; Stewart et al., 2007; Weisberg et al., 2009). At a time when many patients have multiple chronic conditions (Alecxih et al., 2010; Tinetti and Studenski, 2011), for example, patients with comorbidities are routinely excluded from most randomized controlled trials (Dhruva and Redberg, 2008; Van Spall et al., 2007). In addition, many current trials collect data only for a limited period of time, which means they may not capture long-term effects or low-probability side effects and may not reflect the practice conditions of many health care providers.

Other research methods have limitations as well. For instance, the strength of observational studies is that they capture health practices in real-world situations, which aids in generalizing their results to more medical practices. This research design can provide data throughout a product's life cycle and allow for natural experiments provided by variations in care. However, observational studies are challenged to minimize bias and ensure that their results were due to the intervention under consideration. For this reason, as demonstrated by the use of hormone replacement therapy (see Box 6-2) and Vitamin E for the treatment of coronary disease, results of observational trials do not always accord with those of randomized

---

BOX 6-2
Considerations for Producing Evidence:
The Story of Hormone Replacement Therapy Trials

Research on the impact of hormone replacement therapy on coronary heart disease provides a cautionary note for less traditional research methods (Manson, 2010). Initial observational studies of women taking hormone replacement therapy suggested a reduction in the risk of heart disease in the range of 30 to 50 percent (Grady et al., 1992; Grodstein et al., 2000). However, later randomized trials, especially the Women's Health Initiative, found no effect or even an elevated risk (Ioannidis, 2005a; Manson et al., 2003). Several factors may have led to these divergent results, including traditional confounding elements, the fact that these studies were limited in their ability to assess short-term or acute outcomes, and the predominance of follow-up data among long-term hormone therapy users. This example demonstrates that observational studies need to be careful to capture both short- and long-term outcomes (Grodstein et al., 2003). In addition, these types of studies need to consider the differential effects on clinically relevant subgroups; in this case, hormone therapy may have different impacts depending on whether it is started before or after the onset of menopause (Grodstein et al., 2006; IOM, 2008). The experience of hormone replacement therapy research highlights several areas for improvement in observational research design.

TABLE 6-1 Examples of Research Methods and Questions Addressed by Each

Research Design	Questions Addressed
Traditional randomized controlled trial	Efficacy, therapeutic efficacy
Active comparator randomized controlled trials, matched-pair studies	Comparative effectiveness
Surveillance studies	Safety, side effects, indications
Cohort studies, retrospective audit studies, prospective case series	Effectiveness (generalizability to regular clinical practice and larger patient populations)

SOURCE: Data derived from Walach et al., 2006.

controlled trials (Lee et al., 2005b; Rossouw et al., 2002), although some studies have shown concordance between the results derived from the two methods (Concato et al., 2000).

The challenge, therefore, is not determining which research method is the best for a particular condition but rather which provides the information most appropriate to a particular clinical need. Table 6-1 summarizes different research designs and the questions most appropriately addressed by each. In the case of examining biomedical treatments and diagnostic technologies, different types of studies will be more appropriate for different stages of a product's life cycle. Early studies will need to focus on safety and efficacy, which will require randomized controlled trials, while later studies will need to focus on comparative effectiveness and surveillance of unexpected effects, requiring a mix of observational studies and randomized controlled trials. (See Figure 6-1 for a depiction of the change in appropriate research methods over time.) As this report was being written, the methodology committee of the Patient-Centered Outcomes Research Institute (PCORI) had developed a translation table to aid in determining the research methods most appropriate for addressing certain comparative clinical effectiveness research questions (PCORI, 2012). Each study must be tailored to provide useful, practical, and reliable results for the condition at hand.

Conclusion 6-1: Despite the accelerating pace of scientific discovery, the current clinical research enterprise does not sufficiently address pressing clinical questions. The result is decisions by both patients and clinicians that are inadequately informed by evidence.

Related findings:

- *Clinical and biomedical research studies are being produced at an increasing rate.* As noted in the findings supporting Conclusion 2-1, on average approximately 75 clinical trials and a dozen systematic reviews are published daily (see Chapter 2).
- *The evidence basis for clinical guidelines and recommendations needs to be strengthened.* In some cases, 40 to 50 percent of the recommendations made in guidelines are based on expert opinion, case studies, or standards of care rather than on multiple clinical trials or meta-analyses.
- *Even at the current pace of production, the knowledge base provides limited support for answering many of the most important types of clinical questions.* A study of clinical practice guidelines for nine of the most common chronic conditions found that fewer than half included guidance for the treatment of patients with multiple comorbid conditions.
- *New methods are needed to address current limitations in clinical research.* The cost of current methods for clinical research averages $15-$20 million for larger studies—and much more for some—yet the studies do not reflect the practice conditions of many health care providers.

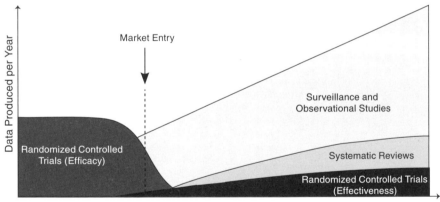

FIGURE 6-1 Different types of research are needed at different stages of a medical product's life cycle. Early trials will need to focus on therapeutic efficacy, while later research will need to focus on comparative effectiveness and surveillance.
SOURCE: Adapted from IOM, 2010a.

EMERGING CAPACITIES, METHODS, AND APPROACHES

As discussed above, there is a clear need for new approaches to knowledge generation, management, and application to guide clinical care, quality improvement, and delivery system organization. The current clinical research enterprise requires substantial resources and takes significant time to address individual research questions. Moreover, the results provided by these studies do not always generate the information needed by patients and their clinicians and may not always be generalizable to a larger population. New research methods are needed that address these serious limitations. Developments in information technology and research infrastructure have the potential to expand the ability of the research system to meet this need. For example, the anticipated growth in the adoption of digital records presents an unprecedented opportunity to expand the supply of data available for learning, generating insights from the regular delivery of care (see the discussion of the data utility in the next section for further detail on these opportunities). These new developments can increase the output derived from the substantial clinical research investments of agencies and foundations, including the Agency for Healthcare Research and Quality (AHRQ), the National Institutes of Health (NIH), and PCORI.

New tools are extending research methods and overcoming many of the limitations highlighted in the previous section (IOM, 2010a). The scientific community has recognized the need for change. High-profile efforts—including NIH's Clinical and Translational Science Awards and the U.S. Food and Drug Administration's Clinical Trials Transformation Initiative—have been undertaken to improve the quality, efficiency, and applicability of clinical trials, and new translational research paradigms have been developed (Lauer and Skarlatos, 2010; Luce et al., 2009; Woolf, 2008; Zerhouni, 2005). Based on these efforts and the work of academic research leaders, new forms of experimental designs have been developed, including pragmatic clinical trials, delayed design trials, and cluster randomized controlled trials[2] (Campbell et al., 2007; Eldridge et al., 2008; Tunis et al., 2003, 2010). Other new methods have been devised to develop knowledge from data produced during the regular course of care. Initial results derived with these new methods have shown promise (see Box 6-3 for a description of one new method). Advanced statistical methods, including Bayesian analysis, allow for adaptive research designs that can learn as a study advances, making studies more flexible (Chow and Chang, 2008). Taken together,

---

[2]In pragmatic clinical trials, the questions faced by decision makers dictate the study design (Tunis et al., 2003b). In delayed design trials, participants are randomized to either receive the intervention or have it withheld for a period of time, with both groups receiving the intervention by the end of the study (Tunis et al., 2010). In cluster randomized controlled trials, groups of subjects, rather than individual subjects, are randomized (Campbell et al., 2007).

BOX 6-3
New Methods for Randomized Clinical Trials:
Point-of-Care Clinical Trial

One new method for conducting experimental research is the point-of-care clinical trial. These trials currently are being conducted at the Boston Veterans Affairs Health Care System, with similar trials being proposed or conducted at other locations (Vickers and Scardino, 2009). The method entails using an electronic health records system to conduct randomized controlled trials by automatically flagging patients who have a choice between competing treatments. If patients do not express a preference, they are asked whether they would be willing to participate in a trial and if so, are randomly assigned to a treatment protocol. The electronic health record system records outcome data and automatically calculates the effectiveness of the treatment protocols. Disadvantages of such trials are that they do not allow for a control group and can be used only for treatments that are already approved for standard care. This type of trial has started being applied to consideration of competing methods for insulin administration (a sliding scale versus a weight-based regimen) for blood sugar control (Fiore et al., 2011).

---

these new methods are designed to reduce the expense and effort of conducting research, improve the applicability of the results to clinical decisions, improve the ability to identify smaller effects, and be applied when traditional methods cannot be used.

In addition to new research methods, advances in statistical analysis, simulation, and modeling have supplemented traditional methods for conducting trials. Given that even the most tightly controlled trials show a distribution in patient responses to a given treatment or intervention, new statistical techniques can help segment results for different populations. Further, new Bayesian techniques for data analysis can separate out the effects of different clinical interventions on overall population health (Berry et al., 2006). With the growth in computational power, new models have been developed that can replicate physiological pathways and disease states (Eddy and Schlessinger, 2003; Stern et al., 2008). These models can then be used to simulate clinical trials and individualize clinical guidelines to a patient's particular situation and biology; this approach thus holds promise for improving health status while reducing costs (Eddy et al., 2011). As computational power grows, the potential applications of these simulation and modeling tools will continue to increase. Despite the opportunities afforded by new research methods, several challenges must be addressed as these methods are improved. One such challenge for the clinical research enterprise is keeping pace with the introduction of new procedures, treatments, diagnostic technologies, and care delivery models. As currently structured, clinical trials often are not comparable, so that a new trial must be conducted to compare the effectiveness of new treatments, diagnostics, or care delivery models with that of existing ones. One solution to this problem is to create standard comparators for a given disease or clinical condition, which would allow new innovations to be compared easily using existing data for current treatments or diagnostic technologies. Additionally, as the research enterprise is expanded, additional emphasis may be required in fields that are underserved by the current clinical research paradigm, such as pediatrics (Cohen et al., 2007; IOM, 2009c; Simpson et al., 2010). One exception to this observation is pediatric cancer care. Virtually all of the treatment provided in pediatric oncology is recorded and applied to registries or active clinical trials, which then inform future care for children undergoing treatment (IOM, 2010b; Pawlson, 2010).

CREATION OF THE DATA UTILITY

In considering how to take advantage of opportunities to create a more nimble, timely, and targeted clinical research enterprise, three basic questions should be considered: (1) What does the system need to know? (2) How will the information be captured and used? and (3) How will the resulting knowledge be organized and shared? These questions have important ramifications for the design and operation of the overall data system.

With respect to the first question, stakeholders in the health care system are interested in comparing the effectiveness of different treatments and interventions, monitoring the current safety of medical products through surveillance, undertaking quality improvement activities, and understanding the quality and performance of different providers and health care organizations. Achieving these goals will require capturing data on the care that is delivered to patients, such as processes and structures of care delivery, and the outcomes of that care, such as longitudinal health outcomes and other outcomes important to patients. With respect to how these data will be used to generate new health care knowledge, uses will include comparing the effects of different treatments, interventions, or care protocols; establishing guidelines and best practices; and searching for unexpected effects of treatments or interventions. Finally, the new knowledge generated will have little impact if not shared broadly with all involved in delivering care for a given patient or, for research cases, all those involved in research. Each of these three questions is explored in further detail below.

What Does the System Need to Know?

Data on how patients respond to diagnostic technologies, treatments, interventions, or care delivery methods are the raw material for generating new clinical knowledge. However, gathering this raw material currently requires significant effort through specialized research protocols. Substantial quantities of clinical data are generated every day in the regular process of care. Unfortunately, most of this information remains locked inside paper records, which are difficult to access, transfer, and query. As of 2011, only about 34-35 percent of office-based physicians were using a basic electronic health record (EHR) system (Decker et al., 2012; Hsiao et al., 2011), while only 18 percent of hospitals had a basic system (DesRoches et al., 2012).

The anticipated growth in the adoption of digital records presents an unprecedented opportunity to improve the supply of data available for learning, particularly as data sources are designed to capture information generated during the delivery of care. Examples of such sources include larger clinical and administrative databases, clinical registries, personal electronic devices (such as smartphones and mobile sensors), clinical trials for regulatory purposes (such as new drug applications), and advanced EHR systems. New sources for data capture are fueled in part by the infusion of capital provided by the Health Information Technology for Economic and Clinical Health (HITECH) Act,[3] which included financial incentives for the meaningful use of EHR systems. Just as the information revolution has transformed many other fields, growing stores of data hold the same promise for improving clinical research, clinical practice, and clinical decision making.

Health care providers play a critical role in supplying clinical data for research and ensuring the quality of the data. To achieve strong provider participation in the learning enterprise, data capture must be seamlessly integrated into providers' daily workflow and must not disrupt the clinical routine. In addition, professional and specialty societies might be engaged to increase the number of providers willing to participate in the clinical research enterprise. Finally, aligning financial incentives and reimbursement can encourage providers and health care organizations to gather, store, and manage clinical data. Currently, many individuals and organizations donate their time when collecting data for research, which limits the amount of effort they can expend on these initiatives. Specific incentives for generating clinical data could increase the supply of data available for research and the quality of the overall enterprise.

---

[3]Included in the American Recovery and Reinvestment Act, Public Law 111-5, 111th Congress (February 17, 2009).

How Will the Information Be Captured and Used?

New sources of health care data, combined with existing resources, offer unprecedented opportunities to learn from health care delivery and patient care. These sources include, for example, EHR systems; registries on diseases, treatments, or specific populations; claims databases from insurers and payers; and mobile devices and sensors that capture local data. In addition to the capacity these sources bring to the collection of clinical data, they also support clinical effectiveness research; surveillance for safety, public health, and other purposes; quality improvement initiatives; population health management; cost and quality reporting; and tools for patient education.

As noted above, EHR systems provide a substantial opportunity for learning by unlocking information currently stored in paper medical records. For example, one study found that real-time analysis of clinical data from EHRs could have identified the increased risk of heart attack associated with rosiglitazone, a diabetes drug, within 18 months of its introduction, as opposed to the 7-8 years between the medication's introduction and when concerns were raised publicly (Brownstein et al., 2010). In considering how to maximize the clinical knowledge gained from EHR systems, a tension exists between the data needs of research studies and the resources required to collect and store clinical data on care processes and patient outcomes. Given the range of health care research studies, it is likely to be infeasible for every system to capture the full amount of data needed to fulfill all potential research needs. A compromise solution to this tension is to identify those core pieces of information that are needed for many research questions and ensure that this limited set of information is captured faithfully by most digital health record systems. This method of identifying a core dataset that satisfies both research and clinical care needs has been used by several organizations. For example, the National Quality Forum's (NQF's) Quality Data Model defines a set of standardized clinical and administrative data that are needed to calculate quality measures using information from EHRs (National Quality Forum, 2010), while the HMO Research Network's Virtual Data Warehouse (discussed further on page 165) maps data from the EHRs and medical claims of multiple health maintenance organization (HMO) plans into a standardized dataset. Other efforts focus on population health; for example, popHealth software integrates with providers' EHRs to automate and simplify the reporting and exchange of quality data on the providers' patient populations, and the Query Health project is setting data standards to enable research on population health (Fridsma, 2011; popHealth, 2012). In addition to the research benefits, routine adoption of core datasets in EHRs can enhance the capacity for exchange of consistent health information across systems and organizations, thereby supporting improved coordination of health services.

As EHR systems become more widespread, it will be necessary to provide flexibility to address new and unforeseen research questions. The sheer scale and complexity of the digital utility, its use by a variety of individuals with conflicting needs, and its constant evolution will require new ways to set standards, develop applications, and interact with the users of clinical data. One technological solution is to ensure that these digital systems are designed in the modular fashion popular in other industries, as with smartphone applications and computer software. This modular approach could also provide additional capacity for meeting new research needs without necessitating an overhaul of the central structure of the digital system.

Registries, which are distinguished by their focus on a specific disease, procedure, treatment, intervention, or resource use, are another important tool for developing new knowledge (Robert Wood Johnson Foundation, 2010) (see Box 6-4). A registry collects uniform clinical data using observational methods to evaluate specified outcomes for a specific population and for a specific purpose (AHRQ, 2010). By collecting detailed data not contained in other sources, registries have been able to determine the clinical effectiveness of a variety of health care interventions and treatments (Akhter et al., 2009; Grover et al., 2001; Meadows et al., 2009; Savage et al., 2003). Further, the clinical and financial payoffs of this method of aggregating and generating knowledge can be substantial.

In addition to EHRs and registries, mobile technologies for providers and patients will play an increasingly important role in capturing and storing health care data. These technologies include a wide range of patient-focused devices that monitor patient health, with the potential to support improved diagnosis or treatment. Provider-focused tools include applications that are built into existing personal digital assistants, smartphones, and tablet computers to store patient health information or access clinical databases. According to industry reports, global sales of these portable devices for health care uses reached $8.2 billion in 2009, and growth of up to 7 percent per year is projected for the next 5 years (Kalorama Information, 2010).

Conclusion 6-2: Growing computational capabilities to generate, communicate, and apply new knowledge create the potential to build a clinical data infrastructure to support continuous learning and improvement in health care.

Related findings:

- *The application of computing capacity and new analytic approaches enables the development of real-time research insights from existing patient populations.* One study found that real-time analysis of clinical data from electronic health records could have identified the increased risk of heart attack associated with rosiglitazone, a diabetes drug, within 18 months of its introduction.
- *Computational capabilities offer the prospect of speeding the delivery of important new insights from the care experience.* For example, a comprehensive disease registry in Sweden has helped facilitate a 65 percent reduction in 30-day mortality and a 49 percent decrease in 1-year mortality for heart attack patients.
- *Computational capabilities present promising, as yet unrealized, opportunities for care improvement.* For example, mining data

---

BOX 6-4
Registries: An Important Source for Developing Knowledge

Registries that are well designed and well managed can promote continuous learning and improvement. One leader in the development and implementation of disease registries is Sweden, which has nearly 90 government supported registries and where almost 25 percent of the nation's medical expenses are covered and monitored by disease-specific registries. In the case of acute myocardial infarction (AMI), the *Register of Information and Knowledge about Swedish Heart Intensive-Care Admissions*, first established in 1991, collects data from all 74 of the nation's major hospitals and covers approximately 80 percent of patients in Sweden who suffer an AMI. In 2005, the *Register* created a publicly reported quality index that ranked hospitals on their adherence to clinical guidelines, and by 2009, the average hospital quality index score was growing at an annual rate of 22 percent, with the lowest-performing hospitals improving at a rate of 40 percent per year. By 2009, the *Register* had helped facilitate a 65 percent reduction in the average 30-day mortality rate for patients who had suffered an acute heart attack, as well as a 49 percent decrease in the 1-year mortality rate from heart attacks.

A recent study estimated the savings that could occur if the United States had a registry for hip replacement surgery comparable to Sweden's. Such a registry could yield savings amounting to $2 billion by 2015 by decreasing the number of surgeries needed to replace or repair failing hip prostheses. Absent such a registry, the total costs for these surgeries are expected to amount to $24 billion by that time.

SOURCE: Larsson et al., 2011.

on patient outcomes and care processes at Intermountain's LDS Hospital allows for continuous improvement of clinical practice guidelines. Implementation of an improved guideline for acute respiratory distress syndrome increased patient survival from 9.5 percent to 44 percent (see Chapter 9).

How Will Knowledge Be Organized and Shared?

Although each individual data source presents an opportunity for learning, the capacity for learning increases exponentially when the system can draw knowledge from multiple sources. Expanding the ability to share data requires developing technological solutions, building a data sharing culture, and addressing privacy and security concerns. Nevertheless, several organizations have successfully overcome these hurdles and implemented large-scale data sharing. Examples include large health care delivery organizations with extensive EHR capabilities, such as Kaiser Permanente and the Veterans Health Administration, and major initiatives in data sharing between different organizations, such as the Nationwide Health Information Network, the Care Connectivity Consortium, the Shared Health Research Information Network, and Informatics for Integrating Biology and the Bedside (i2b2) (Kuperman, 2011; Lohr, 2011; Murphy et al., 2010; Weber et al., 2009).

The technological aspects of sharing depend on the sources of the data. For EHR systems, sharing is complicated by the fact that there is a variety of EHR systems, each of which stores data using different methods and in different formats (Detmer, 2003). An additional complication is the inevitability of systems of different ages being in use, some that incorporate newer technologies and others that are legacy systems. Overcoming these barriers will require several technological solutions, such as interoperability strategies; methods for highlighting the quality of the data; and ways to identify the source, context, and provenance of the data (IOM, 2011c). The challenge to sharing between registries and EHRs is that many registries were developed before EHRs existed, so that in most cases, the two are not interoperable (Physician Consortium for Performance Improvement, 2011). However, improved sharing of data from EHRs may provide a new means of populating registries. One additional technological and policy hurdle is the difficulty of linking records for the same patient across multiple data sources, as different methods (from statistical linkages to unique patient identifiers) strike different balances between the desire for research accuracy and concerns about the privacy of health information (Detmer, 2003).

One method for sharing data securely and efficiently is through distributed data networks. In this design, each organization in the network stores its information locally, often in a common format. When a researcher seeks to answer a specific research question, the organizations execute identical computer programs that analyze the organizations' own data, create a summary of the results for each site, and share those summaries with the entire network. The advantage of this approach is that the institutions share only deidentified summary data instead of patient records. (See Box 6-5 for a description of one distributed data network, the Virtual Data Warehouse of the HMO Research Network, alluded to earlier.) Other models that could be used to share data include centralized databases, whereby data are submitted to and accessed at one central source, and alternative distributed designs, whereby clinical data are shared directly between different institutions (Brown et al., 2010).

BOX 6-5
An Example of a Distributed Data Network

One example of a distributed data network is the Virtual Data Warehouse of the HMO Research Network, formed in 1993, which links 16 integrated delivery systems. The participating health maintenance organizations (HMOs) collaborate to develop and implement common study designs and share standardized data (Vogt et al., 2004). Data from electronic health records (EHRs) and claims are mapped to a standardized set of definitions, names, and codes. The data for each local system are in a database format, structured so that the same computer program can be used at all sites for data analysis (Bocchino, 2011; Larson, 2007). Each site receives direction from the Virtual Data Warehouse Operational Committee, which provides implementation guidance, documentation, and quality control evaluation, and also manages the activities of cross-disciplinary workgroups on different data domains. The HMO Research Network has generated several collaborative projects, including the Cancer Research Network and Cardiovascular Research Network (Go et al., 2008; Hornbrook et al., 2005; Wagner et al., 2005). Types of questions that have been considered by this distributed network include changes in women's use of hormone replacement therapy after the Women's Health Initiative (Wei et al., 2005), the risks of birth defects for cases in which a mother took two common heart medications (beta-blockers or calcium channel blockers) during pregnancy (Davis et al., 2011), and the frequency of potentially inappropriate prescriptions for elderly patients (Simon et al., 2005).

Other examples of this approach include the National Bioterrorism Syndromic Surveillance Demonstration Program, which uses this distributed approach for surveillance of potential bioterrorism events and clusters of naturally occurring illness (Lazarus et al., 2006; Platt, 2010; Yih et al., 2004); the Shared Health Research Information Network, a federated query tool for three clinical data repositories created using the i2b2 open source software platform (Murphy et al., 2010; Weber et al., 2009); the Food and Drug Administration's Mini-Sentinel network (Behrman et al., 2011; Lee et al., 2005a); and the Pediatric EHR Data Sharing Network (PedsNET).

While the above technical considerations are important, problems associated with data ownership may pose a greater challenge to the sharing and exchange of information (Blumenthal, 2006; Let data speak to data, 2005; Piwowar et al., 2008). Researchers have invested significant energy and resources in collecting data and thus may be hesitant to share the data freely with others. Clinical data may be viewed as a proprietary good that belongs to its owner, rather than a societal good that can benefit the population at large. Overcoming this barrier will require a shift toward research and organizational cultures that value open sharing of data. This culture change will in turn require efforts on the part of organizational and national leadership, recognition and rewards for data sharing, and education of researchers in the potential benefits of data sharing (Piwowar et al., 2008).

Significant testimony as to the importance of patient and public engagement, support, and demand for the use of clinical data to produce new knowledge is offered by the misinterpretation of the privacy rule of the Health Insurance Portability and Accountability Act (HIPAA), which led to restricted use of data for new insights. Privacy is a highly important societal and personal value, but the current formulation and interpretation of this rule not only offer limited protection to patients, but also may impede the broader health research enterprise (IOM, 2009a). In a 2007 survey, 68 percent of researchers reported that the HIPAA privacy rule had made research more difficult (Ness, 2007). The impediments arise from both actual and perceived barriers to data sharing attributed to the law and its associated regulations. In surveys, approximately half of health researchers have reported that HIPAA regulations have decreased recruitment of research participants; 80-90 percent have indicated that the regulations have increased research costs; and 50-80 percent have said they have increased the time needed to conduct research and noted that different institutional interpretations of the law and its associated regulations have impeded collaboration (Association of Academic Health Centers, 2008; Goss et al., 2009; Greene et al., 2006; IOM, 2009a; Ness, 2007). As suggested in the IOM report *Beyond the HIPAA Privacy Rule*, solving these problems will likely require a reformulation of the rule, as well as improved guidance to limit disparities in its interpretation (IOM, 2009a).

Conclusion 6-3: Regulations governing the collection and use of clinical data often create unnecessary and unintended barriers to the effectiveness and improvement of care and the derivation of research insights.

Related findings:

- *Implementation of current regulations promulgated to improve privacy offers limited protection to patients and may impede the broader health research enterprise.* In a 2007 survey, 68 percent of researchers reported that the HIPAA privacy rule had made research more difficult.
- *Current regulations have made it difficult to recruit research participants, increased the cost and time needed to conduct research, and impeded collaboration.* In surveys of researchers, approximately half have indicated that HIPAA regulations have decreased recruitment of research participants; 80-90 percent have indicated that the regulations have increased research costs; and 50-80 percent have said they have increased the time needed to conduct research.

THE LEARNING BRIDGE: FROM KNOWLEDGE TO PRACTICE

Unless the products of the nation's clinical data utility and research enterprise are disseminated and applied in practice, their results are meaningless. Current systems that generate and implement new clinical knowledge are largely disconnected and poorly coordinated. While clinical data contribute to the development of many effective, evidence-based practices, therapeutics, and interventions every year, only some of these become widely used. Many others are used only in limited ways, failing to realize their transformative potential to improve care (IOM, 2011a).

Historically, research discoveries in health care have been disseminated through the publication of study results, typically in medical journals. Clinicians are expected to set aside time to read these published results, consider how to integrate them into their practice, and change their behavior accordingly. As noted earlier in this chapter, the extraordinary number of journal articles outstrips any clinician's ability to read and process the information. Even if a clinician could read all of this information, its growth is rapidly outstripping human cognitive capacity to integrate the full body of literature when considering a specific clinical situation and a specific patient. As noted in Chapter 2, this growth in complexity can hamper a clinician's ability to make decisions. Moreover, clinicians' patterns for seeking out information have changed. Fully 86 percent of physicians now use the Internet to gather health, medical, or prescription drug information (Dolan, 2010). Of these physicians, 71 percent use a search engine to start their search for information. This change in information-seeking behavior has consequences for how medical information can be organized and publicized in a way that maximizes its chances of being implemented in clinical practice.

Unfortunately, evidence suggests that simply providing information, albeit more quickly, rarely changes clinical practice (Avorn and Fischer, 2010; Schectman et al., 2003). Multiple reasons may explain this situation. Sometimes, clinicians fail to change their behavior because they are unaware that new knowledge exists. Sometimes they may disagree that a research discovery would improve care for their patients. At other times, they do not perceive a great enough benefit to outweigh the burden of changing established practices (Cabana et al., 1999).

The challenge, therefore, is how to diffuse knowledge in ways that facilitate uptake by clinicians (McCannon and Perla, 2009). Many approaches currently are used to disseminate knowledge throughout the health care system, and these could be leveraged to increase the rate at which knowledge is disseminated. A further challenge is to disseminate knowledge that is useful for the clinical decisions faced by individual patients. To this end, traditional dissemination methods must be modified so that general research knowledge is adapted to the particular circumstances faced by each patient. While logistically demanding, this adaptation holds promise for improving the effectiveness and value of care while meeting the aim of improved patient-centeredness.

One technological tool for bringing research results into the clinical arena is clinical decision support. A clinical decision support system integrates information on a patient with a computerized database of clinical research findings and clinical guidelines. The system generates patient-specific recommendations that guide clinicians and patients in making clinical decisions (IOM, 2001a). One study, for example, found that digital decision support tools helped clinicians apply clinical guidelines, improving health outcomes for diabetics by 15 percent (Cebul et al., 2011). Tools under development may tailor the information to the individual patient, allowing the clinician to predict how an intervention would affect that patient. Further enhancing clinicians' predictive capacities are advanced informatics and simulation systems that can use data to model likely outcomes for similar patients receiving various treatments or supportive services. Clinical decision support systems also can help address cognitive errors (as discussed in Chapter 2), such as attribution, availability bias, and anchoring,[4] all of which may contribute to errors and wrong diagnoses (Blue Cross Blue Shield of Massachusetts Foundation, 2007). Greater adoption of clinical decision support could be achieved through advances in interoperability with EHR and computerized physician order entry (CPOE) systems from

---

[4]Attribution denotes a clinician's use of social stereotypes or attributes to link certain diagnoses to certain patients (Blue Cross Blue Shield of Massachusetts Foundation, 2007). Availability bias occurs when memorable cases or frequent clinical phenomena influence a clinician's diagnosis. Anchoring is a cognitive shortcut in which the first piece of clinical information heard by the clinician has an undue influence on the clinician's thought process going forward.

multiple vendors, allowing this technology to be embedded seamlessly in the standard clinical workflow (Sittig et al., 2008; Wright and Sittig, 2008).

Regardless of the channels used to distribute new clinical knowledge, the clinical research system needs to account for the many factors that promote (or inhibit) the use of this knowledge. These factors will vary in their importance according to different types of clinicians, health care organizations, geographic locations, patient populations, and other factors. In general, the dissemination of a research discovery is dependent on three broad categories of factors: attributes of the discovery, characteristics of the potentially adopting clinician or health care organization, and environmental factors. Figure 6-2 illustrates these factors and their relationships.

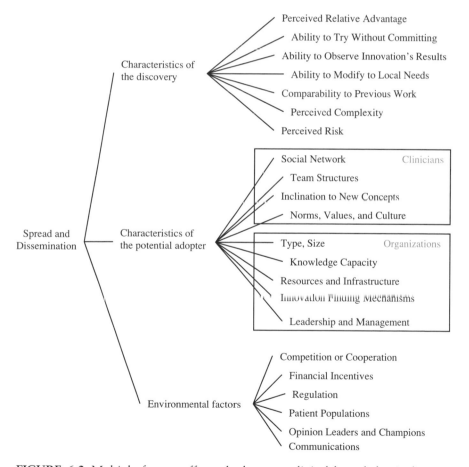

FIGURE 6-2 Multiple factors affect whether new clinical knowledge is disseminated and implemented across the health care system.

As depicted, the process of diffusion and scale-up is messy, organic, and dynamic. An individual or organization does not move linearly from research to development to implementation, but rather moves between these stages based on perceived needs and individual concerns (Greenhalgh et al., 2004).

The most obvious factor affecting the dissemination of a research discovery is its relative advantage over other competing interventions, therapeutics, or practices (Berwick, 2003; Cain and Mittman, 2002; Della Penna et al., 2009). Simply put, people are more likely to implement a new idea if they believe it can help them with a problem. In a health care context, this relative advantage could take multiple forms, from improved clinical effectiveness over existing treatments, to convenience in delivering the intervention, to reduced cost. While relative advantage is an important factor, other characteristics of a research discovery also have been found to be important, including whether the discovery's results can be observed easily and quickly, whether a potential adopter can try it without committing to it, its perceived complexity, and its ability to be modified to fit local circumstances (Rogers, 2003; Shih and Berliner, 2008; Vos et al., 2010). Many of these factors are not objective measures, but are based on the perceptions of potential adopters. This means the factors change based on the setting, the potential adopter, and time (Berwick, 2003; Greenhalgh et al., 2004).

A related cluster of factors that affect the dissemination of a research discovery encompasses the characteristics of the potentially adopting clinician. Evidence from adult learning reveals that clinicians' previous experiences and knowledge will affect their learning about new ideas and practices (Committee on Developments in the Science of Learning et al., 2000). In a related way, the dissemination of a research discovery will depend on individual clinicians' values and culture, as well as their inclination to experiment with new ideas (Bate et al., 2004; Berwick, 2003; Green and Plsek, 2002). For instance, some individuals are more willing to try new ideas, while others favor traditional methods. Dissemination will also depend on the clinician's social networks and those networks' views of the knowledge, practice, or technology (Cain and Mittman, 2002; Dopson et al., 2002; McCullough, 2008; Shih and Berliner, 2008).

This cluster of factors changes when the potential adopter is an organization instead of a clinician. For potentially adopting hospitals and health care organizations, dissemination will vary based on the type of hospital and its resources, especially whether it has resources available for implementing new ideas (McCullough, 2008). Specific capabilities that promote the adoption of new ideas are the support of the organization's leadership and management, the existence of robust channels for sharing knowledge, and the presence of structures that can discover potentially beneficial ideas from outside of the organization (Della Penna et al., 2009; Ferlie and

Shortell, 2001; Green and Plsek, 2002; Nolan et al., 2005; Norton and Mittman, 2010; Pisano et al., 2001).

Finally, environmental factors that are distinct from the previous two clusters affect the dissemination of research discoveries. Financial incentives, reimbursement, the insurance environment, and regulations all impact whether an idea is adopted (Cutler et al., 1996; Mandel, 2010; McCullough, 2008; Robinson et al., 2009; Shih and Berliner, 2008). As with the previous clusters, these factors are not absolutes, but will vary depending on the specific discovery.

The strategy used to communicate a discovery is a particularly important environmental factor. Some successful strategies have involved using in-person educational methods, providing feedback on the process, employing opinion leaders or developing champions, or outlining an overall vision (Davis and TaylorVaisey, 1997; Flodgren et al., 2011; McCannon et al., 2006; O'Connor et al., 1996; Schectman et al., 2003; Soumerai et al., 1998). Another successful communication strategy is the creation of learning or improvement networks (Podolny and Page, 1998). Such networks provide a structure for the exchange of information and include those individuals necessary for the implementation of change on a larger scale (Carnegie Foundation for the Advancement of Teaching, 2010). This type of tool may be useful for managing the high degree of variation across the health care field, because information can be shared about how to customize guidelines, practice patterns, and other knowledge to fit local conditions (McCannon and Perla, 2009). Finally, reporting of data on performance and practice variation can spur the adoption of evidence-based practices (see Chapter 8 for a discussion of the use of reporting).

The complex interplay of the above factors is illustrated by a case study on disseminating a change across a large organization. In 2005, a large, integrated health care delivery system concluded a randomized controlled trial of several palliative care models, identifying the model that improved patient satisfaction and outcomes most successfully. The next year, after the organization's national executive leadership had set the expectation that all its member hospitals would implement this care model within 1 year, the organization established a large-scale initiative to disseminate the model. Within a 2-year period, the model was in place at all 32 network hospitals, the number of palliative care consults had risen from 1,572 to 16,293, and the number of interdisciplinary palliative care teams had more than doubled. One of the more important factors responsible for this successful dissemination was the clear relative advantage of the palliative care model in terms of patient satisfaction, outcomes, and cost, as demonstrated by the randomized controlled trial. This initiative also was compatible with clinician values, which spurred an emotional pull to improve care during advanced illness. Additional reasons for the dissemination included the involvement of senior leadership and opinion leaders, existing communication channels throughout the organization, and broad social networks that shared information. While many positive factors encouraged dissemination, several impediments were faced as well, including resource constraints, the competition of preexisting palliative care models, and ambiguous accountability for implementation (Della Penna et al., 2009).

As demonstrated by this example, a considerable amount is known about the factors that contribute to successful dissemination and scale-up. For any individual case, however, it is unknown which factors will best yield widespread implementation; the success of any particular knowledge, practice, or technology is context specific and depends on local conditions and human factors (Davidoff, 2009) (see Chapter 9 for a discussion of the spread of ideas within an organization). Also unknown is how the factors that influence dissemination interact with one another to increase (or decrease) its likelihood.

A final element in understanding dissemination is customization to local conditions. As new technologies and procedures diffuse into clinical practice, health care professionals further modify and extend their application by discovering new populations, indications, and long-term effects. This observation highlights the importance of measuring the health and economic outcomes of clinical interventions in everyday practice (IOM, 2010a). The case of coronary artery bypass graft surgery offers an example of how the use of treatments changes over time: it is estimated that only 4 to 13 percent of patients who underwent this surgery a decade after its introduction would have met the eligibility criteria of the trials that determined its initial effectiveness (Hlatky et al., 1984). Similar results have been noted for other interventions; for example, slightly more than half of patients receiving the antiplatelet agent clopidogrel for vascular disease would have been eligible for the clinical trials that demonstrated its effectiveness (Choudhry et al., 2008). The ultimate use of a treatment or intervention may be very different from what its developers initially envisioned.

Conclusion 6-4: As the pace of knowledge generation accelerates, new approaches are needed to deliver the right information, in a clear and understandable format, to patients and clinicians as they partner to make clinical decisions.

Related findings:

- *The slow pace of dissemination and implementation of new knowledge in health care is harmful to patients.* For example, it took 13 years for most experts to recommend thrombolytic drugs for heart attack treatment after their first positive clinical trial (see Chapter 2).

- *Available evidence often is unused in clinical decision making.* One analysis of the use of implantable cardioverter-defibrillator (ICD) implants found that 22 percent were implanted in circumstances outside of professional society guidelines (see Chapter 3).
- *Decision support tools, which can be broadly provided in electronic health records, hold promise for improving the application of evidence.* One study found that digital decision support tools helped clinicians apply clinical guidelines, improving health outcomes for diabetics by 15 percent.

PEOPLE, PATIENTS, AND CONSUMERS AS ACTIVE STAKEHOLDERS

Given the critical role of patients and consumers in the health care system, patients need to be more fully engaged in clinical research and the data utility. The success of both enterprises depends on patient support and investment in their aims. For clinical research, this means incorporating patient perspectives and greater public participation (see also Chapter 7) to ensure that the research enterprise addresses patient needs (IOM, 2011d). For the data utility, the public has an important role in motivating its expansion to improve care and build knowledge.

Currently, public awareness of and participation in the clinical research enterprise remains limited, as exemplified by a reduced willingness to participate in clinical trials during the past decade (Woolley and Propst, 2005). In addition, national surveys from 2005 and 2010 found that approximately two-thirds of respondents had concerns about the privacy and security of their health information (Holmes and Karp, 2005; Undem, 2010). Improving this situation will require new efforts to build trust in the clinical research enterprise among patients, consumers, and the public. Building this trust will require effort on multiple fronts, including increasing trust in the results of clinical research, being open and honest about the risks and benefits of this type of research, and ensuring that appropriate privacy and security safeguards are in place for health data.

Opportunities exist for improving patient engagement in clinical research. There is some evidence that patients with complex conditions, such as cancer, may be open to sharing data for research purposes, with one study finding that 60-70 percent of cancer patients agreed their deidentified clinical data should be shared to improve clinical knowledge (Beckjord et al., 2011). Similarly, a 2004 survey found that almost 70 percent of respondents would willingly share deidentified health information to improve health care services, and a similar percentage would share their deidentified data with researchers (Research!America, 2004). A recent national survey of consumers found that almost 90 percent of respondents strongly or somewhat agreed that their health data should be used "to help improve the care of future patients who might have the same or similar condition" (Alston and Paget, 2012).

Ideally, clinical decisions should balance the health benefits of a given intervention against potential harms, taking into consideration the patient's preferences, needs, and values. Research that incorporates patient perspectives will potentially be more useful for clinicians and patients making such decisions. One means of accomplishing this is to collect information on outcomes from patients with respect to their quality of life, such as their level of function or emotional state. While important, however, it can be difficult to design instruments that can collect high-quality data reflecting a health concept of interest (Rothman et al., 2009). One promising initiative is the NIH Patient-Reported Outcomes Measurement Information System (PROMIS), which incorporates a series of items measuring different aspects of physical, mental, and social health (Cella et al., 2007, 2010). Continued improvements in the collection of this type of clinical data hold promise for improving the ability of research to help patients understand how therapies and interventions may affect their quality of life.

In addition, novel technologies allow for new means of collecting health care data directly from patients. Enabled by advances in digital technologies and informatics, patients and consumers now have the ability to be involved in collecting and sharing data on their personal condition. This vision is being actualized in biobanks operated by disease-specific organizations, in addition to social networking sites. Examples of social networking sites that aim to promote patient participation in research include PatientsLikeMe®, Love/Avon Army of Women, and Facebook health groups (see Box 6-6). While there are specific challenges for these patient-initiated approaches, due especially to bias in self-reporting, as well as issues of data quality and protection against discrimination, the prevalence of such approaches can only be expected to increase.

One major recent initiative that focuses attention on patients in clinical research is PCORI, which was established by the Patient Protection and Affordable Care Act of 2010. As noted in its mission statement, PCORI seeks to help consumers and patients make informed health care decisions by encouraging research guided by patients, caregivers, and the entire health care community (Washington and Lipstein, 2011). Because PCORI is relatively new, it is in the process of considering methods and standards for research focused on patient-centered outcomes, drafting national priorities, and developing a research agenda. This type of research holds promise for increasing the patient-centeredness of the entire clinical research enterprise.

BOX 6-6
Increased Patient Participation in Research

Patients with difficult-to-treat conditions increasingly are using websites to compare experiences and information. These patients sometimes experiment with treatments that do not yet have regulatory approval and post their data and results online. Researchers can potentially use these self-reported data to measure the effectiveness of drugs and treatments in development. While using these data has several statistical drawbacks—the selection is not blind, and self-reported data can leave room for error or fraud—a preliminary study showed the potential of this research method. Patients with amyotrophic lateral sclerosis (ALS) experimented with lithium carbonate after a small study in Italy suggested it might slow the progression of the disease, and reported their experiences on the website PatientsLikeMe. When researchers aggregated and studied these data, they determined that the lithium had no effect—the same conclusion resulting from a subsequent randomized controlled trial. This research method, even with its drawbacks, has several advantages, including speed of data collection, low cost, patient engagement, the availability of control participants, and ease of patient access (Wicks et al., 2011).

FRAMEWORK FOR ACHIEVING THE VISION[5]

Knowledge generation in the U.S. health care system presents a fundamental paradox. While the clinical research enterprise generates new insights at an ever-increasing rate, the demand for knowledge at the point of care remains unmet. The result is decisions by clinicians and patients that are inadequately informed by evidence. In addition, the data generated from every patient encounter hold tremendous promise to serve as a clinical data infrastructure that, through the use of new research techniques, can begin to meet the system's need for real-time clinical knowledge.

Given advances in computing and other technologies, the potential exists to create a clinical data utility that provides a substantial opportunity for learning (President's Information Technology Advisory Committee, 2001, 2004). The creation of this data utility will require action on the technological, clinical, research, and administrative fronts—from identifying the data that need to be captured, to encouraging broader sharing and communication of the data, to effecting the data's widespread clinical use. Recommendation 1 details the steps necessary to develop a clinical

---

[5]Note that in Chapters 6-9, the committee's recommendations are numbered according to their sequence in the taxonomy in Chapter 10.

data infrastructure that supports clinical care, improvement initiatives, and research.

Recommendation 1: The Digital Infrastructure

Improve the capacity to capture clinical, care delivery process, and financial data for better care, system improvement, and the generation of new knowledge. Data generated in the course of care delivery should be digitally collected, compiled, and protected as a reliable and accessible resource for care management, process improvement, public health, and the generation of new knowledge.

Strategies for progress toward this goal:

- *Health care delivery organizations* and *clinicians* should fully and effectively employ digital systems that capture patient care experiences reliably and consistently, and implement standards and practices that advance the interoperability of data systems.
- *The National Coordinator for Health Information Technology, digital technology developers,* and *standards organizations* should ensure that the digital infrastructure captures and delivers the core data elements and interoperability needed to support better care, system improvement, and the generation of new knowledge.
- *Payers, health care delivery organizations,* and *medical product companies* should contribute data to research and analytic consortia to support expanded use of care data to generate new insights.
- *Patients* should participate in the development of a robust data utility; use new clinical communication tools, such as personal portals, for self-management and care activities; and be involved in building new knowledge, such as through patient-reported outcomes and other knowledge processes.
- The *Secretary of Health and Human Services* should encourage the development of distributed data research networks and expand the availability of departmental health data resources for translation into accessible knowledge that can be used for improving care, lowering costs, and enhancing public health.
- *Research funding agencies and organizations,* such as the *National Institutes of Health, the Agency for Healthcare Research and Quality, the Veterans Health Administration, the Department of Defense,* and the *Patient-Centered Outcomes Research Institute,* should promote research designs and methods that draw naturally on existing care processes and that also support ongoing quality-improvement efforts.

Legal and regulatory restrictions can serve as a barrier to real-time learning and improvement. Results of previous surveys of health researchers suggest that the current formulation of the HIPAA privacy rule has increased the cost and time needed to conduct research, that different institutional interpretations of HIPAA and associated regulations have impeded collaboration, and that the rule has made it difficult to recruit subjects (Association of Academic Health Centers, 2008; Goss et al., 2009; Greene et al., 2006; IOM, 2009a; Ness, 2007). While privacy is an important societal and personal value, the current formulation of the privacy rule not only offers limited protection to patients but also may impede the broader health research enterprise (IOM, 2009a). Recommendation 2 outlines actions needed to address this challenge, drawing on the IOM report *Beyond the HIPAA Privacy Rule* (IOM, 2009a).

Recommendation 2: The Data Utility

Streamline and revise research regulations to improve care, promote the capture of clinical data, and generate knowledge. Regulatory agencies should clarify and improve regulations governing the collection and use of clinical data to ensure patient privacy but also the seamless use of clinical data for better care coordination and management, improved care, and knowledge enhancement.

Strategies for progress toward this goal:

- The *Secretary of Health and Human Services* should accelerate and expand the review of the Health Insurance Portability and Accountability Act (HIPAA) and institutional review board (IRB) policies with respect to actual or perceived regulatory impediments to the protected use of clinical data, and clarify regulations and their interpretation to support the use of clinical data as a resource for advancing science and care improvement.
- *Patient and consumer groups, clinicians, professional specialty societies, health care delivery organizations, voluntary organizations, researchers,* and *grantmakers* should develop strategies and outreach to improve understanding of the benefits and importance of accelerating the use of clinical data to improve care and health outcomes.

Further, new knowledge can be poorly integrated into regular clinical care, highlighting the need for new approaches to deliver the right information to the point of care. To ensure the availability of clinical knowledge when and where needed, Recommendation 3 outlines actions that can be taken to disseminate clinical knowledge broadly and ensure its widespread application.

Recommendation 3: Clinical Decision Support

Accelerate integration of the best clinical knowledge into care decisions. Decision support tools and knowledge management systems should be routine features of health care delivery to ensure that decisions made by clinicians and patients are informed by current best evidence.

Strategies for progress toward this goal:

- *Clinicians* and *health care organizations* should adopt tools that deliver reliable, current clinical knowledge to the point of care, and organizations should adopt incentives that encourage the use of these tools.
- *Research organizations, advocacy organizations, professional specialty societies,* and *care delivery organizations* should facilitate the development, accessibility, and use of evidence-based and harmonized clinical practice guidelines.
- *Public and private payers* should promote the adoption of decision support tools, knowledge management systems, and evidence-based clinical practice guidelines by structuring payment and contracting policies to reward effective, evidence-based care that improves patient health.
- *Health professional education programs* should teach new methods for accessing, managing, and applying evidence; engaging in lifelong learning; understanding human behavior and social science; and delivering safe care in an interdisciplinary environment.
- *Research funding agencies and organizations* should promote research into the barriers and systematic challenges to the dissemination and use of evidence at the point of care, and support research to develop strategies and methods that can improve the usefulness and accessibility of patient outcome data and scientific evidence for clinicians and patients.

Collectively, implementation of the above recommendations would increase the supply of clinical data, reduce legal and regulatory barriers to the creation of new knowledge, and improve the integration of new knowledge into regular clinical practice. Addressing the issues targeted by these recommendations can increase the knowledge available to answer relevant clinical questions while promoting the use of new clinical information in regular patient care.

REFERENCES

AHRQ (Agency for Healthcare Research and Quality). 2010. *Registries for evaluating patient outcomes: A user's guide.* 2nd ed. Rockville, MD: AHRQ.

Akhter, N., S. Milford-Beland, M. T. Roe, R. N. Piana, J. Kao, and A. Shroff. 2009. Gender differences among patients with acute coronary syndromes undergoing percutaneous coronary intervention in the American College of Cardiology-National Cardiovascular Data Registry (ACC-NCDR). *American Heart Journal* 157(1):141-148.

Alecxih, L., S. Shen, I. Chan, D. Taylor, and J. Drabek. 2010. *Individuals living in the community with chronic conditions and functional limitations: A closer look.* http://aspe.hhs.gov/daltcp/reports/2010/closerlook.pdf (accessed June 23, 2011).

Alston, C., and L. Paget. 2012. *Communicating evidence in health care: Engaging patients for improved health care decisions.* http://iom.edu/~/media/Files/Activity%20Files/Quality/VSRT/IC%20Meeting%20Docs/ECIC%2006-07-12/Lyn%20Paget%20and%20Chuck%20Alston.pdf (accessed August 31, 2012).

Association of Academic Health Centers. 2008. *HIPAA creating barriers to research and discovery: HIPAA problems widespread and unresolved since 2003.* http://www.aahcdc.org/policy/reddot/AAHC_HIPAA_Creating_Barriers.pdf (accessed June 9, 2011).

Avorn, J., and M. Fischer. 2010. "Bench to behavior": Translating comparative effectiveness research into improved clinical practice. *Health Affairs* 29(10):1891-1900.

Bastian, H., P. Glasziou, and I. Chalmers. 2010. Seventy-five trials and eleven systematic reviews a day: How will we ever keep up? *PLoS Medicine* 7(9):e1000326.

Bate, P., G. Robert, and H. Bevan. 2004. The next phase of healthcare improvement: What can we learn from social movements? *Quality & Safety in Health Care* 13(1):62-66.

Beckjord, E. B., R. Rechis, S. Nutt, L. Shulman, and B. W. Hesse. 2011. What do people affected by cancer think about electronic health information exchange? Results from the 2010 Livestrong Electronic Health Information Exchange Survey and the 2008 Health Information National Trends Survey. *Journal of Oncology Practice* 7(4):237-241.

Behrman, R. E., J. S. Benner, J. S. Brown, M. McClellan, J. Woodcock, and R. Platt. 2011. Developing the sentinel system—a national resource for evidence development. *New England Journal of Medicine* 364(6):498-499.

Berry, D. A., L. Inoue, Y. Shen, J. Venier, D. Cohen, M. Bondy, R. Theriault, and M. F. Munsell. 2006. Modeling the impact of treatment and screening on U.S. breast cancer mortality: A Bayesian approach. *Journal of the National Cancer Institute Monographs* (36):30-36.

Berwick, D. M. 2003. Disseminating innovations in health care. *Journal of the American Medical Association* 289(15):1969-1975.

Bevers, T. D., B. O. Anderson, E. Bonaccio, S. Buys, M. B. Daly, P. J. Dempsey, W. B. Farrar, I. Fleming, J. E. Garber, R. E. Harris, A. S. Heerdt, M. Helvie, J. G. Huff, N. Khakpour, S. A. Khan, H. Krontiras, G. Lyman, E. Rafferty, S. Shaw, M. L. Smith, T. N. Tsangaris, C. Williams, T. Yankeelov, T. Yaneeklov, and National Comprehensive Cancer Network. 2009. NCCN clinical practice guidelines in oncology: Breast cancer screening and diagnosis. *Journal of the National Comprehensive Cancer Network* 7(10):1060-1096.

Blue Cross Blue Shield of Massachusetts Foundation. 2007. *How doctors think—interview with Dr. Jerome Groopman.* http://bluecrossmafoundation.org/~/media/Files/Newsroom/Press%20Releases/090626PodcastPR.pdf (accessed August 31, 2012).

Blumenthal, D. 2006. Data withholding in genetics and the other life sciences: Prevalences and predictors. *Journal of Academic Medicine* 81(2):137-145.

Bocchino, C. A. 2011. Public-private partnerships: Health plans. In *Learning what works: Infrastructure required for comparative effectiveness research.* Institute of Medicine. Washington, DC: The National Academies Press. Pp. 293-300.

Boyd, C. M., J. Darer, C. Boult, L. P. Fried, L. Boult, and A. W. Wu. 2005. Clinical practice guidelines and quality of care for older patients with multiple comorbid diseases: Implications for pay for performance. *Journal of the American Medical Association* 294(6):716-724.

British Medical Journal. 2011. *Clinical evidence.* http://clinicalevidence.bmj.com/ceweb/about/knowledge.jsp (accessed October 7, 2011).

Brown, J. S., J. H. Holmes, K. Shah, K. Hall, R. Lazarus, and R. Platt. 2010. Distributed health data networks: A practical and preferred approach to multi-institutional evaluations of comparative effectiveness, safety, and quality of care. *Medical Care* 48(Suppl. 6):S45-S51.

Brownstein, J. S., S. N. Murphy, A. B. Goldfine, R. W. Grant, M. Sordo, V. Gainer, J. A. Colecchi, A. Dubey, D. M. Nathan, J. P. Glaser, and I. S. Kohane. 2010. Rapid identification of myocardial infarction risk associated with diabetes medications using electronic medical records. *Diabetes Care* 33(3):526-531.

Cabana, M. D., C. S. Rand, N. R. Powe, A. W. Wu, M. H. Wilson, P. A. Abboud, and H. R. Rubin. 1999. Why don't physicians follow clinical practice guidelines? A framework for improvement. *Journal of the American Medical Association* 282(15):1458-1465.

Cain, M., and R. Mittman. 2002. *Diffusion of innovation in health care.* Oakland: California HealthCare Foundation.

Califf, R. M. 2004. Defining the balance of risk and benefit in the era of genomics and proteomics. *Health Affairs (Millwood)* 23(1):77-87.

Campbell, M. J., A. Donner, and N. Klar. 2007. Developments in cluster randomized trials and statistics in medicine. *Statistics in Medicine* 26(1):2-19.

Carnegie Foundation for the Advancement of Teaching. 2010. *Getting ideas into action: Building networked improvement communities in education.* http://www.carnegiefoundation.org/spotlight/webinar-bryk-gomez-building-networked-improvement-communities-in-education (accessed June 17, 2011).

Cebul, R. D., T. E. Love, A. K. Jain, and C. J. Hebert. 2011. Electronic health records and quality of diabetes care. *New England Journal of Medicine* 365(9):825-833.

Cella, D., S. Yount, N. Rothrock, R. Gershon, K. Cook, B. Reeve, D. Ader, J. F. Fries, B. Bruce, M. Rose, and PROMIS Cooperative Group. 2007. The Patient-Reported Outcomes Measurement Information System (PROMIS): Progress of an NIH roadmap cooperative group during its first two years. *Medical Care* 45(5, Suppl. 1):S3-S11.

Cella, D., W. Riley, A. Stone, N. Rothrock, B. Reeve, S. Yount, D. Amtmann, R. Bode, D. Buysse, S. Choi, K. Cook, R. Devellis, D. DeWalt, J. F. Fries, R. Gershon, E. A. Hahn, J. S. Lai, P. Pilkonis, D. Revicki, M. Rose, K. Weinfurt, R. Hays, and PROMIS Cooperative Group. 2010. The Patient-Reported Outcomes Measurement Information System (PROMIS) developed and tested its first wave of adult self-reported health outcome item banks: 2005-2008. *Journal of Clinical Epidemiology* 63(11):1179-1194.

Chauhan, S. P., V. Berghella, M. Sanderson, E. F. Magann, and J. C. Morrison. 2006. American College of Obstetricians and Gynecologists practice bulletins: An overview. *American Journal of Obstetrics and Gynecology* 194(6):1564-1572.

Choudhry, N. K., R. Levin, and J. Avorn. 2008. The economic consequences of non-evidence-based clopidogrel use. *American Heart Journal* 155(5):904-909.

Chow, S. C., and M. Chang. 2008. Adaptive design methods in clinical trials—a review. *Orphanet Journal of Rare Diseases* 3:11.

Cohen, E., E. Uleryk, M. Jasuja, and P. C. Parkin. 2007. An absence of pediatric randomized controlled trials in general medical journals, 1985-2004. *Journal of Clinical Epidemiology* 60(2):118-123.

Committee on Developments in the Science of Learning, Committee on Learning Research and Educational Practice, and National Research Council. 2000. *How people learn: Brain, mind, experience, and school* (expanded edition). Washington, DC: National Academy Press.

Concato, J., N. Shah, and R. I. Horwitz. 2000. Randomized, controlled trials, observational studies, and the hierarchy of research designs. *New England Journal of Medicine* 342(25):1887-1892.

Cutler, D. M., M. B. McClellan, and National Bureau of Economic Research. 1996. The determinants of technological change in heart attack treatment. In *NBER working paper series working paper 5751.* http://www.nber.org/papers/w5751.pdf?new_window=1 (accessed August 31, 2012).

Darst, J. R., J. W. Newburger, S. Resch, R. H. Rathod, and J. E. Lock. 2010. Deciding without data. *Congenital Heart Disease* 5(4):339-342.

Davidoff, F. 2009. Heterogeneity is not always noise: Lessons from improvement. *Journal of the American Medical Association* 302(23):2580-2586.

Davis, D. A., and A. TaylorVaisey. 1997. Translating guidelines into practice—a systematic review of theoretic concepts, practical experience and research evidence in the adoption of clinical practice guidelines. *Canadian Medical Association Journal* 157(4):408-416.

Davis, R. L., D. Eastman, H. McPhillips, M. A. Raebel, S. E. Andrade, D. Smith, M. U. Yood, S. Dublin, and R. Platt. 2011. Risks of congenital malformations and perinatal events among infants exposed to calcium channel and beta-blockers during pregnancy. *Pharmacoepidemiology and Drug Safety* 20(2):138-145.

Decker, S. L., E. W. Jamoom, and J. E. Sisk. 2012. Physicians in nonprimary care and small practices and those age 55 and older lag in adopting electronic health record systems. *Health Affairs (Millwood)* 31(5):1108-1114.

Della Penna, R., H. Martel, E. B. Neuwirth, J. Rice, M. I. Filipski, J. Green, and J. Bellows. 2009. Rapid spread of complex change: A case study in inpatient palliative care. *BMC Health Services Research* 9:245.

DesRoches, C. M., C. Worzala, M. S. Joshi, P. D. Kralovec, and A. K. Jha. 2012. Small, nonteaching, and rural hospitals continue to be slow in adopting electronic health record systems. *Health Affairs (Millwood)* 31(5):1092-1099.

Detmer, D. E. 2003. Building the national health information infrastructure for personal health, health care services, public health, and research. *BMC Medical Information Decision Making* 3:1.

Dhruva, S. S., and R. F. Redberg. 2008. Variations between clinical trial participants and Medicare beneficiaries in evidence used for Medicare national coverage decisions. *Archives of Internal Medicine* 168(2):136-140.

Dolan, P. L. 2010. 86% of physicians use Internet to access health information. *American Medical News*, January 11.

Dopson, S., L. FitzGerald, E. Ferlie, J. Gabbay, and L. Locock. 2002. No magic targets! Changing clinical practice to become more evidence based. *Health Care Management Review* 27(3):35-47.

Eddy, D. M., and L. Schlessinger. 2003. Archimedes: A trial-validated model of diabetes. *Diabetes Care* 26(11):3093-3101.

Eddy, D. M., J. Adler, B. Patterson, D. Lucas, K. A. Smith, and M. Morris. 2011. Individualized guidelines: The potential for increasing quality and reducing costs. *Annals of Internal Medicine* 154(9):627-634.

Eldridge, S., D. Ashby, C. Bennett, M. Wakelin, and G. Feder. 2008. Internal and external validity of cluster randomised trials: Systematic review of recent trials. *British Medical Journal* 336(7649):876-880.

Ferlie, E. B., and S. M. Shortell. 2001. Improving the quality of health care in the United Kingdom and the United States: A framework for change. *Milbank Quarterly* 79(2):281-315.

Fiore, L. D., M. Brophy, R. E. Ferguson, L. D'Avolio, J. A. Hermos, R. A. Lew, G. Doros, C. H. Conrad, J. A. O'Neil, T. P. Sabin, J. Kaufman, S. L. Swartz, E. Lawler, M. H. Liang, J. M. Gaziano, and P. W. Lavori. 2011. A point-of-care clinical trial comparing insulin administered using a sliding scale versus a weight-based regimen. *Clinical Trials* 8(2):183-195.

Flodgren, G., E. Parmelli, G. Doumit, M. Gattellari, M. A. O'Brien, J. Grimshaw, and M. P. Eccles. 2011. Local opinion leaders: Effects on professional practice and health care outcomes. *Cochrane Database of Systematic Reviews* (8):CD000125.

Frangakis, C. 2009. The calibration of treatment effects from clinical trials to target populations. *Clinical Trials* 6(2):136-140.

Fridsma, D. 2011. Join query health in developing national standards for population queries. In *HealthITBuzz*, September 23.

Genetics and Public Policy Center. 2008. *FDA regulation of genetic tests*. http://www.dna policy.org/policy.issue.php?action=detail&issuebrief_id=11&print=1 (accessed January 4, 2010).

Gill, P., A. C. Dowell, R. D. Neal, N. Smith, P. Heywood, and A. E. Wilson. 1996. Evidence based general practice: A retrospective study of interventions in one training practice. *British Medical Journal* 312(7034):819-821.

Go, A. S., D. J. Magid, B. Wells, S. H. Sung, A. E. Cassidy-Bushrow, R. T. Greenlee, R. D. Langer, T. A. Lieu, K. L. Margolis, F. A. Masoudi, C. J. McNeal, G. H. Murata, K. M. Newton, R. Novotny, K. Reynolds, D. W. Roblin, D. H. Smith, S. Vupputuri, R. E. White, J. Olson, J. S. Rumsfeld, and J. H. Gurwitz. 2008. The Cardiovascular Research Network: A new paradigm for cardiovascular quality and outcomes research. *Circulation: Cardiovascular Quality and Outcomes* 1(2):138-147.

Goss, E., M. P. Link, S. S. Bruinooge, T. S. Lawrence, J. E. Tepper, C. D. Runowicz, and R. L. Schilsky. 2009. The impact of the privacy rule on cancer research: Variations in attitudes and application of regulatory standards. *Journal of Clinical Oncology* 27(24):4014-4020.

Grady, D., S. M. Rubin, D. B. Petitti, C. S. Fox, D. Black, B. Ettinger, V. L. Ernster, and S. R. Cummings. 1992. Hormone therapy to prevent disease and prolong life in postmenopausal women. *Annals of Internal Medicine* 117(12):1016-1037.

Green, P. L., and P. E. Plsek. 2002. Coaching and leadership for the diffusion of innovation in health care: A different type of multi-organization improvement collaborative. *Joint Commission Journal on Quality Improvement* 28(2):55-71.

Greene, S. M., A. M. Geiger, E. L. Harris, A. Altschuler, L. Nekhlyudov, M. B. Barton, S. J. Rolnick, J. G. Elmore, and S. Fletcher. 2006. Impact of IRB requirements on a multicenter survey of prophylactic mastectomy outcomes. *Annals of Epidemiology* 16(4):275-278.

Greenhalgh, T., G. Robert, F. Macfarlane, P. Bate, and O. Kyriakidou. 2004. Diffusion of innovations in service organizations: Systematic review and recommendations. *Milbank Quarterly* 82(4):581-629.

Greenhouse, J. B., E. E. Kaizar, K. Kelleher, H. Seltman, and W. Gardner. 2008. Generalizing from clinical trial data: A case study. The risk of suicidality among pediatric antidepressant users. *Statistics in Medicine* 27(11):1801-1813.

Grodstein, F., J. E. Manson, G. A. Colditz, W. C. Willett, F. E. Speizer, and M. J. Stampfer. 2000. A prospective, observational study of postmenopausal hormone therapy and primary prevention of cardiovascular disease. *Annals of Internal Medicine* 133(12):933-941.

Grodstein, F., T. B. Clarkson, and J. E. Manson. 2003. Understanding the divergent data on postmenopausal hormone therapy. *New England Journal of Medicine* 348(7):645-650.

Grodstein, F., J. E. Manson, and M. J. Stampfer. 2006. Hormone therapy and coronary heart disease: The role of time since menopause and age at hormone initiation. *Journal of Women's Health* 15(1):35-44.

Grove, A. 2011. Rethinking clinical trials. *Science* 333(6050):1679.

Grover, F. L., A. L. Shroyer, K. Hammermeister, F. H. Edwards, T. B. Ferguson, S. W. Dziuban, J. C. Cleveland, R. E. Clark, and G. McDonald. 2001. A decade's experience with quality improvement in cardiac surgery using the Veterans Affairs and Society of Thoracic Surgeons national databases. *Annals of Surgery* 234(4):464-472.

Harrison, T. R. 1962. *Principles of internal medicine.* 4th ed. New York: Blakiston Division, McGraw-Hill.

Hennekens, C. H., J. E. Buring, and S. L. Mayrent. 1987. *Epidemiology in medicine.* 1st ed. Boston, MA: Little, Brown.

Hlatky, M. A., K. L. Lee, F. E. Harrell, R. M. Califf, D. B. Pryor, D. B. Mark, and R. A. Rosati. 1984. Tying clinical research to patient-care by use of an observational database. *Statistics in Medicine* 3(4):375-384.

Holmes, B., and S. Karp. 2005. *National consumer health privacy survey 2005.* http://www.chcf.org/~/media/MEDIA%20LIBRARY%20Files/PDF/C/PDF%20ConsumersHealthInfoTechnologyNationalSurvey.pdf (accessed August 21, 2012).

Holve, E., and P. Pittman. 2009. *A first look at the volume and cost of comparative effectiveness research in the United States.* Washington, DC: AcademyHealth.

Holve, E., and P. Pittman. 2011. The cost and volume of comparative effectiveness research. In *Learning what works: Infrastructure required for comparative effectiveness research: Workshop summary.* Institute of Medicine. Washington, DC: The National Academies Press. Pp. 89-96.

Hornbrook, M. C., G. Hart, J. L. Ellis, D. J. Bachman, G. Ansell, S. M. Greene, E. H. Wagner, R. Pardee, M. M. Schmidt, A. Geiger, A. L. Butani, T. Field, H. Fouayzi, I. Miroshnik, L. Liu, R. Diseker, K. Wells, R. Krajenta, L. Lamerato, and C. N. Dudas. 2005. Building a virtual cancer research organization. *JNCI Monographs* 2005(35):12-25.

Hsiao, C.-J., E. Hing, T. C. Socey, and B. Cai. 2011. *Electronic health record systems and intent to apply for meaningful use incentives among office-based physician practices: United States, 2001-2011.* Hyattsville, MD: National Center for Health Statistics.

Ioannidis, J. P. A. 2005a. Contradicted and initially stronger effects in highly cited clinical research. *Journal of the American Medical Association* 294(2):218-228.

Ioannidis, J. P. A. 2005b. Why most published research findings are false. *PLoS Medicine* 2(8):696-701.

IOM (Institute of Medicine). 1985. *Assessing medical technologies.* Washington, DC: National Academy Press.

IOM. 2001a. *Crossing the quality chasm: A new health system for the 21st century.* Washington, DC: National Academy Press.

IOM. 2001b. *Mammography and beyond: Developing technologies for the early detection of breast cancer.* Washington, DC: National Academy Press.

IOM. 2005. *Saving women's lives: Strategies for improving breast cancer detection and diagnosis: A Breast Cancer Research Foundation and Institute of Medicine symposium.* Washington, DC: The National Academies Press.

IOM. 2008. *Knowing what works in health care: A roadmap for the nation.* Washington, DC: The National Academies Press.

IOM. 2009a. *Beyond the HIPAA privacy rule: Enhancing privacy, improving health through research.* Washington, DC: The National Academies Press.

IOM. 2009b. *Conflict of interest in medical research, education, and practice.* Washington, DC: The National Academies Press.

IOM. 2009c. *Initial national priorities for comparative effectiveness research.* Washington, DC: The National Academies Press.

IOM. 2010a. *Redesigning the clinical effectiveness research paradigm: Innovation and practice-based approaches: Workshop summary.* Washington, DC: The National Academies Press.

IOM. 2010b. *Transforming clinical research in the United States: Challenges and opportunities: Workshop summary.* Washington, DC: The National Academies Press.

IOM. 2011a. *Clinical data as the basic staple of health learning: Workshop summary.* Washington, DC: The National Academies Press.

IOM. 2011b. *Clinical practice guidelines we can trust.* Washington, DC: The National Academies Press.

IOM. 2011c. *Digital infrastructure for the learning health system: The foundation for continuous improvement in health and health care: A workshop summary.* Washington, DC: The National Academies Press.

IOM. 2011d. *Public engagement and clinical trials: New models and disruptive technologies: Workshop summary.* Washington, DC: The National Academies Press.

Kalorama Information. 2010. *Handhelds in healthcare: The world market for PDAs, tablet PCs, handheld monitors & scanners.* http://www.kaloramainformation.com/Handhelds-Healthcare-PDAs-2703662/ (accessed August 31, 2011).

Kasper, D. L., and T. R. Harrison. 2005. *Harrison's principles of internal medicine.* 16th ed., 2 vols. New York: McGraw-Hill, Medical Publications Division.

Kuperman, G. J. 2011. Health-information exchange: Why are we doing it, and what are we doing? *Journal of the American Medical Informatics Association* 18(5):678-682.

Larson, E. B. 2007. The HMO research network as a test bed. In *The learning healthcare system: Workshop summary.* Institute of Medicine. Washington, DC: The National Academies Press, Pp. 223-232.

Larsson, S., P. Lawyer, G. Garellick, B. Lindahl, and M. Lundström. 2011. Use of 13 disease registries in 5 countries demonstrates the potential to use outcome data to improve health care's value. *Health Affairs (Millwood)* 31(1):220-227.

Lauer, M. S., and S. Skarlatos. 2010. Translational research for cardiovascular diseases at the National Heart, Lung, and Blood Institute: Moving from bench to bedside and from bedside to community. *Circulation* 121(7):929-933.

Lazarus, R., K. Yih, and R. Platt. 2006. Distributed data processing for public health surveillance. *BMC Public Health* 6:235.

Lee, D. H., and O. Vielemeyer. 2011. Analysis of overall level of evidence behind Infectious Diseases Society of America practice guidelines. *Archives of Internal Medicine* 171(1):18-22.

Lee, H. Y., H. S. Ahn, J. A. Jang, Y. M. Lee, H. J. Hann, M. S. Park, and D. S. Ahn. 2005a. Comparison of evidence-based therapeutic intervention between community- and hospital-based primary care clinics. *International Journal of Clinical Practice* 59(8):975-980.

Lee, I. M., N. R. Cook, J. M. Gaziano, D. Gordon, P. M. Ridker, J. E. Manson, C. H. Hennekens, and J. E. Buring. 2005b. Vitamin E in the primary prevention of cardiovascular disease and cancer—The Women's Health Study: A randomized controlled trial. *Journal of the American Medical Association* 294(1):56-65.

Let data speak to data. 2005. *Nature* 438(7068):531.

Lohr, S. 2011. Big medical groups begin patient data-sharing project. *The New York Times,* April 6.

Luce, B. R., J. M. Kramer, S. N. Goodman, J. T. Connor, S. Tunis, D. Whicher, and J. S. Schwartz. 2009. Rethinking randomized clinical trials for comparative effectiveness research: The need for transformational change. *Annals of Internal Medicine* 151(3):206-209.

Mandel, K. E. 2010. Aligning rewards with large-scale improvement. *Journal of the American Medical Association* 303(7):663-664.

Manolio, T. A. 2010. Emerging genomic information. In *Redesigning the clinical effectiveness research paradigm: Innovation and practice-based approaches: Workshop summary.* Institute of Medicine. Washington, DC: The National Academies Press. Pp. 189-206.

Manson, J. E. 2010. Hormone replacement therapy. In *Redesigning the clinical effectiveness research paradigm: Innovation and practice-based approaches: A workshop summary.* Institute of Medicine. Washington, DC: National Academies Press. Pp. 89-104.

Manson, J. E., J. Hsia, K. C. Johnson, J. E. Rossouw, A. R. Assaf, N. L. Lasser, M. Trevisan, H. R. Black, S. R. Heckbert, R. Detrano, O. L. Strickland, N. D. Wong, J. R. Crouse, E. Stein, M. Cushman, and Women's Health Initiative Investigators. 2003. Estrogen plus progestin and the risk of coronary heart disease. *New England Journal of Medicine* 349(6):523-534.

McCannon, C. J., and R. J. Perla. 2009. Learning networks for sustainable, large-scale improvement. *Joint Commission Journal on Quality and Patient Safety* 35(5):286-291.

McCannon, C. J., M. W. Schall, D. R. Calkins, and A. G. Nazem. 2006. Saving 100,000 lives in US hospitals. *British Medical Journal* 332(7553):1328-1330.

McCullough, J. S. 2008. The adoption of hospital information systems. *Health Economics* 17(5):649-664.

Meadows, T. A., D. L. Bhatt, A. T. Hirsch, M. A. Creager, R. M. Califf, E. M. Ohman, C. P. Cannon, K. A. Eagle, M. J. Alberts, S. Goto, S. C. Smith, P. W. Wilson, K. E. Watson, P. G. Steg, and REACH Registry Investigators. 2009. Ethnic differences in the prevalence and treatment of cardiovascular risk factors in US outpatients with peripheral arterial disease: Insights from the reduction of atherothrombosis for continued health (REACH) registry. *American Heart Journal* 158(6):1038-1045.

Meier, B., and J. Roberts. 2011. Hip implant complaints suge, even as the dangers are studied. *New York Times.* http://www.nytimes.com/2011/08/23/business/complaints-soar-on-hip-implants-as-dangers-are-studied.html?pagewanted=all (accessed January 16, 2012).

Murphy, S. N., G. Weber, M. Mendis, V. Gainer, H. C. Chueh, S. Churchill, and I. Kohane. 2010. Serving the enterprise and beyond with informatics for integrating biology and the bedside (i2b2). *Journal of the American Medical Informatics Association* 17(2):124-130.

National Comprehensive Cancer Network. 2012. *NCCN clinical practice guidelines in oncology: Breast cancer.* Fort Washington, PA: National Comprehensive Cancer Network.

National Quality Forum. 2010. *Quality data model 2.1.* http://www.qualityforum.org/Projects/h/QDS_Model/Quality_Data_Model.aspx#t=2&s=&p= (accessed April 27, 2011).

Ness, R. B. 2007. Influence of the HIPAA privacy rule on health research. *Journal of the American Medical Association* 298(18):2164-2170.

Nolan, K., M. W. Schall, F. Erb, and T. Nolan. 2005. Using a framework for spread: The case of patient access in the Veterans Health Administration. *Joint Commission Journal on Quality and Patient Safety* 31(6):339-347.

Norton, W. E., and B. S. Mittman. 2010. *Scaling-up health promotion/disease prevention programs in community settings: Barriers, facilitators, and initial recommendations.* West Hartford, CT: The Patrick and Catherine Weldon Donaghue Medical Research Foundation.

O'Connor, G. T., S. K. Plume, E. M. Olmstead, J. R. Morton, C. T. Maloney, W. C. Nugent, F. Hernandez, R. Clough, B. J. Leavitt, L. H. Coffin, C. A. Marrin, D. Wennberg, J. D. Birkmeyer, D. C. Charlesworth, D. J. Malenka, H. B. Quinton, and J. F. Kasper. 1996. A regional intervention to improve the hospital mortality associated with coronary artery bypass graft surgery. The Northern New England Cardiovascular Disease Study Group. *Journal of the American Medical Association* 275(11):841-846.

Pawlson, G. 2010. Course-of-care data. In *Redesigning the clinical effectiveness research paradigm: Innovation and practice-based approaches: Workshop summary*. Institute of Medicine. Washington, DC: The National Academies Press. Pp. 325-331.

PCORI (Patient-Centered Outcomes Research Institute). 2012. *Preliminary draft methodology report: Our questions, our decisions: Standards for patient-centered outcomes research*. http://www.pcori.org/assets/PCORI-MC-Research_Methods_Framework-Review_v Finalv3.pdf (accessed July 6, 2012).

Pearson, T. A., and T. A. Manolio. 2008. How to interpret a genome-wide association study. *Journal of the American Medical Association* 299(11):1335-1344.

Physician Consortium for Performance Improvement. 2011. *Advancing health care improvement through patient registries: Moving forward*. http://www.ama-assn.org/resources/doc/cqi/registry-meeting-paper.pdf (accessed August 30, 2011).

Pisano, G. P., R. M. J. Bohmer, and A. C. Edmondson. 2001. Organizational differences in rates of learning: Evidence from the adoption of minimally invasive cardiac surgery. *Management Science* 47(6):752-768.

Piwowar, H. A., M. J. Becich, H. Bilofsky, R. S. Crowley, and on behalf of the caBIG Data Sharing and Intellectual Capital Workspace. 2008. Towards a data sharing culture: Recommendations for leadership from academic health centers. *PLoS Medicine* 5(9):1315-1319.

Platt, R. 2010. Distributed data networks. In *Redesigning the clinical effectiveness research paradigm: Innovation and practice-based approaches: Workshop summary*. Institute of Medicine. Washington, DC: The National Academies Press. Pp. 253-261.

Podolny, J., and K. Page. 1998. Network forms of organization. *Annual Review of Sociology* 24:57-76.

popHealth. 2012. *An open source quality measure reference implementation*. http://project-pophealth.org/about.html (accessed June 13, 2012).

Prasad, V., V. Gall, and A. Cifu. 2011. The frequency of medical reversal. *Archives of Internal Medicine* 171(18):1675-1676.

President's Information Technology Advisory Committee. 2001. *Transforming health care through information technology*. http://www.itrd.gov/pubs/pitac/pitac-hc-9feb01.pdf (accessed August 31, 2012).

President's Information Technology Advisory Committee. 2004. *Revolutionizing health care through information technology*. http://www.itrd.gov/pitac/meetings/2004/20040617/20040615_hit.pdf (accessed August 31, 2012).

Redberg, R. F. 2007. Evidence, appropriateness, and technology assessment in cardiology: A case study of computed tomography. *Health Affairs* 26(1):86-95.

Research!America. 2004. *Taking our pulse: The parade/research!America health poll*. http://www.researchamerica.org/uploads/poll2004parade.pdf (accessed August 21, 2012).

Robert Wood Johnson Foundation. 2010. How registries can help performance measurement improve care. In *White paper (High-Value Health Care Project)*. http://www.healthquality alliance.org/userfiles/Final%20Registries%20paper%20062110(1).pdf (accessed August 31, 2012).

Robinson, J. C., L. P. Casilino, R. R. Gillies, D. R. Rittenhouse, S. S. Shortell, and S. Fernandes-Taylor. 2009. Financial incentives, quality improvement programs, and the adoption of clinical information technology. *Medical Care* 47(4):411-417.

Rogers, E. M. 2003. *Diffusion of innovations*. 5th ed. New York: Free Press.

Rossouw, J. E., G. L. Anderson, R. L. Prentice, A. Z. LaCroix, C. Kooperberg, M. L. Stefanick, R. D. Jackson, S. A. A. Beresford, B. V. Howard, K. C. Johnson, M. Kotchen, and J. Ockene. 2002. Risks and benefits of estrogen plus progestin in healthy postmenopausal women—principal results from the Women's Health Initiative Randomized Controlled Trial. *Journal of the American Medical Association* 288(3):321-333.

Rothman, M., L. Burke, P. Erickson, N. K. Leidy, D. L. Patrick, and C. D. Petrie. 2009. Use of existing patient-reported outcome (PRO) instruments and their modification: The ISPOR good research practices for evaluating and documenting content validity for the use of existing instruments and their modification pro task force report. *Value Health* 12(8):1075-1083.

Savage, E. B., T. B. Ferguson, and V. J. DiSesa. 2003. Use of mitral valve repair: Analysis of contemporary United States experience reported to the Society of Thoracic Surgeons National Cardiac Database. *Annals Thoracic Surgery* 75(3):820-825.

Schectman, J. M., W. S. Schroth, D. Verme, and J. D. Voss. 2003. Randomized controlled trial of education and feedback for implementation of guidelines for acute low back pain. *Journal of General Internal Medicine* 18(10):773-780.

Shih, C., and E. Berliner. 2008. Diffusion of new technology and payment policies: Coronary stents. *Health Affairs* 27(6):1566-1576.

Simon, S. R., K. A. Chan, S. B. Soumerai, A. K. Wagner, S. E. Andrade, A. C. Feldstein, J. E. Lafata, R. L. Davis, and J. H. Gurwitz. 2005. Potentially inappropriate medication use by elderly persons in U.S. health maintenance organizations, 2000-2001. *Journal of the American Geriatrics Society* 53(2):227-232.

Simpson, L. A., L. Peterson, C. M. Lannon, S. B. Murphy, C. Goodman, Z. Ren, and A. Zajicek. 2010. Special challenges in comparative effectiveness research on children's and adolescents' health. *Health Affairs (Millwood)* 29(10):1849-1856.

Sittig, D. F., A. Wright, J. A. Osheroff, B. Middleton, J. M. Teich, J. S. Ash, E. Campbell, and D. W. Bates. 2008. Grand challenges in clinical decision support. *Journal of Biomedical Informatics* 41(2):387-392.

Soumerai, S. B., T. J. McLaughlin, J. H. Gurwitz, E. Guadagnoli, P. J. Hauptman, C. Borbas, N. Morris, B. McLaughlin, X. Gao, D. J. Willison, R. Asinger, and F. Gobel. 1998. Effect of local medical opinion leaders on quality of care for acute myocardial infarction: A randomized controlled trial. *Journal of the American Medical Association* 279(17):1358-1363.

Stern, M., K. Williams, D. Eddy, and R. Kahn. 2008. Validation of prediction of diabetes by the Archimedes model and comparison with other predicting models. *Diabetes Care* 31(8):1670-1671.

Stewart, W. F., N. R. Shah, M. J. Selna, R. A. Paulus, and J. M. Walker. 2007. Bridging the inferential gap: The electronic health record and clinical evidence. *Health Affairs* 26(2):w181-w191.

Tinetti, M. E., and S. A. Studenski. 2011. Comparative effectiveness research and patients with multiple chronic conditions. *New England Journal of Medicine* 364(26):2478-2481.

Tricoci, P., J. M. Allen, J. M. Kramer, R. M. Califf, and S. C. Smith. 2009. Scientific evidence underlying the ACC/AHA clinical practice guidelines. *Journal of the American Medical Association* 301(8):831-841.

Tunis, S. R., D. B. Stryer, and C. M. Clancy. 2003. Practical clinical trials: Increasing the value of clinical research for decision making in clinical and health policy. *Journal of the American Medical Association* 290(12):1624-1632.

Tunis, S. R., J. Benner, and M. McClellan. 2010. Comparative effectiveness research: Policy context, methods development and research infrastructure. *Statistics in Medicine* 29(19):1963-1976.

Undem, T. 2010. *Consumers and health information technology: A national survey.* http://www.chcf.org/~/media/MEDIA%20LIBRARY%20Files/PDF/C/PDF%20Consumers HealthInfoTechnologyNationalSurvey.pdf (accessed August 21, 2012).

Van Spall, H. G. C., A. Toren, A. Kiss, and R. A. Fowler. 2007. Eligibility criteria of randomized controlled trials published in high-impact general medical journals. *Journal of the American Medical Association* 297(11):1233-1240.

Vickers, A. J., and P. T. Scardino. 2009. The clinically-integrated randomized trial: Proposed novel method for conducting large trials at low cost. *Trials* 10:14.

Vogt, T. M., J. Elston-Lafata, D. Tolsma, and S. M. Greene. 2004. The role of research in integrated healthcare systems: The HMO research network. *American Journal of Managed Care* 10(9):643-648.

Vos, L., M. L. Dückers, C. Wagner, and G. G. van Merode. 2010. Applying the quality improvement collaborative method to process redesign: A multiple case study. *Implementation Science* 5:19.

Wagner, E. H., S. M. Greene, G. Hart, T. S. Field, S. Fletcher, A. M. Geiger, L. J. Herrinton, M. C. Hornbrook, C. C. Johnson, J. Mouchawar, S. J. Rolnick, V. J. Stevens, S. H. Taplin, D. Tolsma, and T. M. Vogt. 2005. Building a research consortium of large health systems: The Cancer Research Network. *JNCI Monographs* 2005(35):3-11.

Walach, H., T. Falkenberg, V. Fønnebø, G. Lewith, and W. B. Jonas. 2006. Circular instead of hierarchical: Methodological principles for the evaluation of complex interventions. *BMC Medical Research Methodology* 6:29.

Washington, A. E., and S. H. Lipstein. 2011. The Patient-Centered Outcomes Research Institute—promoting better information, decisions, and health. *New England Journal of Medicine* 365(15):e31.

Weber, G. M., S. N. Murphy, A. J. McMurry, D. Macfadden, D. J. Nigrin, S. Churchill, and I. S. Kohane. 2009. The Shared Health Research Information Network (SHRINE): A prototype federated query tool for clinical data repositories. *Journal of the American Medical Informatics Association* 16(5):624-630.

Wei, F., D. L. Miglioretti, M. T. Connelly, S. E. Andrade, K. M. Newton, C. L. Hartsfield, K. A. Chan, and D. S. Buist. 2005. Changes in women's use of hormones after the women's health initiative estrogen and progestin trial by race, education, and income. *Journal of the National Cancer Institute Monograph* (35):106-112.

Weisberg, H. I., V. C. Hayden, and V. P. Pontes. 2009. Selection criteria and generalizability within the counterfactual framework: Explaining the paradox of antidepressant-induced suicidality? *Clinical Trials* 6(2):109-118.

Wicks, P., T. E. Vaughan, M. P. Massagli, and J. Heywood. 2011. Accelerated clinical discovery using self-reported patient data collected online and a patient-matching algorithm. *Nature Biotechnology* 29(5):411-414.

Woolf, S. H. 2008. The meaning of translational research and why it matters. *Journal of the American Medical Association* 299(2):211-213.

Woolley, M., and S. M. Propst. 2005. Public attitudes and perceptions about health-related research. *Journal of the American Medical Association* 294(11):1380-1384.

Wright, A., and D. F. Sittig. 2008. A four-phase model of the evolution of clinical decision support architectures. *International Journal of Medical Informatics* 77(10):641-649.

Yih, W. K., B. Caldwell, R. Harmon, K. Kleinman, R. Lazarus, A. Nelson, J. Nordin, B. Rehm, B. Richter, D. Ritzwoller, E. Sherwood, and R. Platt. 2004. National bioterrorism syndromic surveillance demonstration program. *Morbidity and Mortality Weekly Report* 53(Suppl.):43-49.

Zerhouni, E. A. 2005. Translational and clinical science—time for a new vision. *New England Journal of Medicine* 353(15):1621-1623.

7

Engaging Patients, Families, and Communities

In June 2011, Alvin, a terminally ill patient with end-stage pulmonary fibrosis, was hospitalized for pneumonia. His doctor, a specialist in lung disease at a top academic medical center, gave Alvin 100 percent oxygen and powerful antibiotics and steroids, but his condition quickly deteriorated. Faced with the choice of intubation and a mechanical ventilator or palliative care, Alvin chose to forgo life support and spend his last days at home with his family. His family was given a prescription for morphine with little instruction on how to use it appropriately; when they tried to fill the prescription, several pharmacies refused. Despite the hospital's orders for oxygen to be sent home, Alvin's family found that the oxygen supplied was insufficient for his needs. The emergency medical technicians who took Alvin home offered only one solution—to bring him back to the hospital. Trying to honor his wishes, the family refused. Five hours after leaving the hospital, Alvin was in pain and struggling for breath. Since it was a Saturday evening, hospice personnel were off duty; Alvin's family had to arrange for a private-duty nurse to help them care for him in his final hours. After he passed away, a hospice nurse finally arrived, apologized, and instructed his family on how to dispose of the remaining vial of morphine correctly. Alvin's case highlights the critical importance of all members of the care team—family members, clinicians, and other health care providers—working together to overcome system complexity and poorly aligned incentives to ensure patient-centered

*care, as well as the ways in which the health care system falls short
on this critical dimension (Winakur, 2012).*

Clinicians and health care staff work tirelessly to care for their patients
in an increasingly complex, inefficient, and stressful environment. However,
the structure, incentives, and culture of the system in which they work are
often—perhaps usually—poorly aligned to support their efforts to respond
to patients' needs as their core priority. Recognizing the imperative to center
on the patient, a learning health care system is one in which patients and
their families are key drivers of the design and operation of the learning
process. When patients, their families, other caregivers, and the public are
full, active participants in care, health, the experience of care, and economic
outcomes can be substantially improved.

Crossing the Quality Chasm underscores patient-centeredness as a core
aim of the health care system, yet care often fails to meet this aim (IOM,
2001). Despite the *Quality Chasm*'s call to action more than a decade ago,
patient-centered care still is not the norm, and users continue to find the
health care system uncoordinated and stressful to navigate. As the complexity of the system continues to grow with advances in science (Chapter 2),
patient engagement takes on increased importance as a means of ensuring
that patients can find the right care for their individual characteristics,
needs, preferences, and circumstances.

In these complex situations, patients and clinicians both need to be
involved for optimal care. Clinicians supply information and advice based
on their scientific expertise in treatment and intervention options, along
with potential outcomes. Patients, their families, and other caregivers bring
personal knowledge on the suitability—or lack thereof—of different treatments for the patient's circumstances and preferences. Information from
both sources is needed to select the right care option. It is important to note
that patient-centered care does not mean simply agreeing to every patient
request. Rather, it entails meaningful engagement on the options available in order to understand the patient and establish a dialogue between
patient and clinician on the evidence and the decisions in play (Epstein et
al., 2010; Fowler et al., 2011). The provision of patient-centered care can
be complex and time-consuming, and requires broad involvement of the
patient, the family, and the care team to consider all of the issues affecting
the patient's care.

This chapter explores the ways in which a learning health care system
can fill some of the gaps in orienting and coordinating the U.S. health
care system around people's needs. First, the chapter considers what is
currently known about focusing the health care system on people's needs
and preferences, sets forth a vision for how the system could be improved

in this regard, and summarizes the benefits of moving toward that vision. The chapter then investigates how this knowledge can be applied at different levels of the health care system, from the patient care experience to the broader system. Next is a discussion of communities of care and how they can incorporate those stakeholders not normally included in the health care system. The chapter concludes with recommendations for realizing the vision of a health care system that engages patients, families, and communities. Throughout, the discussion highlights ways in which a learning health care system can better incorporate patients, families, and the public in managing health and health care.

CENTERING CARE ON PEOPLE'S NEEDS AND PREFERENCES

Informed and engaged patients, invested in their own health care as well as in the improvement of the broader health care system, are crucial to a learning system. Patients bring unique and important perspectives on their own care, on the experience in health care organizations, and on the coordination and cooperation among various elements of their care. Unfortunately, patients, their families and other caregivers, and the public all too often are not meaningfully engaged in care or as partners in its improvement. Moving to the vision of a system centered on people's needs and preferences has the potential to bring multiple benefits for patients, the health care system, and the nation.

A Focus on the Patient

As noted, more than 10 years after *Crossing the Quality Chasm* highlighted the crucial role of patient-centered care, such care still is not the norm, and patients continue to find the health care system uncoordinated and stressful to navigate. A 2011 survey of public views of the health care system found that patients have difficulty accessing care, experience poor care coordination, and want a system that is more integrated and patient-centered. Seven of 10 adults surveyed reported difficulty in making doctor's appointments when they needed them, getting advice over the phone, or receiving care after hours. Nearly half of adults reported problems with care coordination, notification of test results, and communications between primary care providers and specialists, and one-third said the health care system was poorly organized (Stremikis et al., 2011).

The lack of patient focus is particularly evident in patient communications, especially about care options. Surveys of patients who have recently made a medical decision have found that those patients often did not receive critical information about the risks and benefits of the treatment and intervention choices under consideration (Fagerlin et al., 2010; Lee et al.,

2011, 2012; Sepucha et al., 2010). These patients also reported that their clinicians stressed the benefits of interventions more than they discussed the risks, and asked patients about their preferences only half of the time (Zikmund-Fisher et al., 2010). Because modern health care often offers multiple interventions for a given condition, each with its own benefits, side effects, and costs, identifying the most valuable intervention for each patient requires both that patients be well informed about the options and that clinicians be aware of their patients' individual circumstances, preferences, and needs.

The lack of patient focus in the health care system also is evident in patient transitions between care settings. Patients often report that care transitions, such as being discharged from the hospital, are abrupt. Patients often receive little information about what the next steps are in their care, when they can resume activities, what side effects or complications they should monitor, or whom they can approach with questions about their recovery. In other cases, patients receive too much information at the time of discharge, stressing their ability to remember and apply this information over the transition period. As a result of poor transitions, almost one-fifth of hospitalized Medicare patients are rehospitalized within 30 days, often without seeing their primary care provider in the interim (Jencks et al., 2009). Communications between primary care practitioners and specialists often lack critical information, and hospitals often either do not notify primary care practitioners when their patients are discharged or relay insufficient information (Bodenheimer, 2008). Transitions may be even less effective and more complex when patients' needs extend beyond traditional health care to include a broader array of health and human services, such as long-term care; mental health and substance use care; and social, economic, and community services related to wellness and healthy lifestyles.

Foundational Elements of Patient-Centered Care

Part of the challenge is that the notion of patient-centeredness simply is not embedded in the care culture and often feels foreign, even disruptive, to clinicians unfamiliar with the concept (Berwick, 2009). Because investments in moving toward patient-centered care currently are being made on a large scale, developing a working definition of patient- or person-centered care is a matter of some urgency, especially given that patient perspectives will soon be factored into Medicare value-based payments to hospitals.[1] Absent this framework, it will be impossible to assess the progress of initiatives toward the goal of improving patient focus. The difficulty is that

---

[1] Patient Protection and Affordable Care Act, Public Law 111-148, 111th Congress (March 23, 2010).

multiple definitions of patient- or person-centered care exist, each capturing important aspects of this type of care. Moreover, the concept itself has multiple names, ranging from "patient-centered care," to "patient- and family-centered care," to "patient activation," to "patient engagement," to "public engagement."

Another challenge is determining who needs to be involved. Almost every person is a past, present, or future patient of the health care system. Moreover, each person often receives care from family caregivers, relatives, friends, and neighbors who support and assist those coping with both acute and chronic health problems, and who are vital to the patient throughout the care experience. While the term "patients" is used here for brevity, it always refers to patients, family and other caregivers, and the public. Similarly, the term "communities" includes all forms of community, such as those defined by geography, culture, disease or condition, occupation, and workplace.

Recognizing the complexity of the terms involved, several individuals and organizations have developed definitions for patient-centered care. One advocate for promoting patient-centered care defines it as "the experience (to the extent the informed, individual patient desires it) of transparency, individualization, recognition, respect, dignity, and choice in all matters, without exception, related to one's person, circumstances, and relationships in health care" (Berwick, 2009). The Institute for Patient- and Family-Centered Care outlines four concepts that underlie patient-centered care: respect and dignity, information sharing, participation, and collaboration (Institute for Patient and Family Centered Care, 2011). The National Quality Forum's National Priorities Partnership characterizes patient-centered care as health care that "honors each individual patient and family, offering voice, control, choice, skills in self-care, and total transparency, and that can and does adapt readily to individual and family circumstances, and to differing cultures, languages, and social backgrounds" (NPP, 2010).

This chapter builds on the definition of patient centered care outlined in *Crossing the Quality Chasm*: "providing care that is respectful of and responsive to individual patient preferences, needs, and values and ensuring that patient values guide all clinical decisions" (IOM, 2001, p. 40). The concept encompasses multiple dimensions, including respect for patients' values, preferences, and needs; coordination and integration of care; information, communication, and education; physical comfort; emotional support; and involvement of family and friends. *Crossing the Quality Chasm* outlines several principles to help the system provide this kind of care: care should be based on continuous healing relationships, care should be customized according to patient needs and values, the patient should be the source of control, knowledge should be shared and information should flow freely, information should be provided to patients transparently, and the patient's needs should be anticipated (IOM, 2001). In short, the patient should be considered in all aspects of care and care delivery.

Benefits of Patient-Centered Care

A growing body of evidence highlights the potential benefits of patient-centered care for clinical outcomes, health, satisfaction among health care workers, and providers' financial performance. For example, several hospitals that encourage patient-centered care by paying greater attention to patient needs and preferences, as well as care coordination, have found that adverse events decrease, employee retention increases, operating costs decrease, malpractice claims decline, lengths of stay are shorter, and the hospital's costs per case decrease (Charmel and Frampton, 2008; Epstein et al., 2010).

Patient and family involvement in decision making has been associated in primary care settings with reduced pain and discomfort, faster recovery in physical health, and improvements in emotional health (Stewart et al., 2000). Similarly, heart attack patients who did not receive patient-centered care were found to have worse long-term outcomes, such as overall health and likelihood of experiencing chest pains, than patients who received such care (Fremont et al., 2001). A study of patient-centered nursing interventions for cancer patients found that the interventions were correlated with improved patient self-representation, optimism, and sense of well-being (Radwin et al., 2009).

Patient-centered care also has been found to correlate with a patient's ability to undertake personal health maintenance and adhere to complex treatment regimens. An observational study of Commonwealth of Massachusetts employees found that physicians' knowledge of their patients and patients' trust in their physicians strongly influenced whether patients completed the recommended treatment regimen (Safran et al., 1998). Similarly, HIV patients who reported that their clinician knew them "as a person" had higher odds of receiving and completing highly active antiretroviral therapy, as well as better health outcomes, relative to other HIV patients (Beach et al., 2006). These studies underscore the potential role of patient-centered care in improving the health outcomes from a therapy or intervention that relies on patient self-management, including many therapies for chronic diseases.

In addition, patient-oriented care has been associated with decreased utilization of resources. Studies have found that patient-centered communication in primary care visits correlates with fewer diagnostic tests and referrals (Epstein et al., 2005; Stewart et al., 2000). A similar study found that patients who received less patient-centered care incurred 51 percent higher annual charges relative to patients who received more patient-centered care

(Bertakis and Azari, 2011). Further, well-informed patients often choose less aggressive and costly therapies; one study found that informed patients were up to 20 percent less likely than other patients to choose elective surgery (O'Connor et al., 2009; Stacey et al., 2011).

Yet not all care delivered in the name of patient-centeredness reduces costs or improves outcomes. For example, one study found that patient-centeredness was associated with better outcomes but also higher costs (Bechel et al., 2000). Other studies have yielded mixed results with respect to cost, quality, and value for care models that aim to implement different aspects of patient-centeredness, such as disease management and care coordination programs (Nelson, 2012; Peikes et al., 2009). This inconsistency of results stems in part from the difficulty of identifying what truly constitutes patient-centered care (Epstein and Street, 2011; Hudon et al., 2011). Confusion about the implications of patient-centered care can stymie the efforts of well-meaning individuals and organizations, producing changes that are superficial, fail to address underlying challenges, and add little value to the experience. In the name of patient-centeredness, for example, some health care organizations have adopted luxury, hotel-like amenities; added new technology; or renovated their facilities. Although some of these initiatives may enhance the patient's experience, they do not achieve the true goals of patient-centered care and may increase costs while not improving care quality or outcomes. Patient-centered care must be implemented in a way that directly addresses the patient's needs and preferences and supports those goals most important to improving quality, health, and value.

Moreover, establishing a causal link between different aspects of patient engagement and ultimate outcomes can be difficult. For example, several studies have shown a link between patient-centered care and measures of patient experience, which in turn have been linked to better health outcomes (Beach et al., 2006; Browne et al., 2010; Mead and Bower, 2002; Stewart, 1995). Yet researchers are only beginning to understand the chain of causality through which patient-centered care techniques, such as communication, contribute to better health outcomes (Epstein and Street, 2011; Street et al., 2009). Additional research is needed to understand how different patient-centered techniques produce direct and indirect outcomes—from physical and emotional health, to the ability to manage one's care, to improved decision-making ability.

Conclusion 7-1: Improved patient engagement is associated with better patient experience, health, and quality of life and better economic outcomes, yet patient and family participation in care decisions remains limited.

Related findings:

- *Patients often are insufficiently involved in care decisions.* Fewer than half of patients receive clear information on the benefits and trade-offs of the treatments for their condition, and fewer than half are satisfied with their level of control in medical decision making (see also Chapter 2).
- *Patient-centered care has been correlated with better health care outcomes and quality of life, as well as other benefits.* The use of patient-centered care in a primary care setting has been associated with reduced pain and discomfort, faster recovery in physical health, and improvements in emotional health.
- *If implemented properly, meaningful engagement of patients in their own care has the potential to reduce costs.* For example, it has been reported that informed patients are up to 20 percent less likely than other patients to choose elective surgery.

ENGAGING PATIENTS AS ACTIVE PARTICIPANTS IN THEIR CARE

Patients and the public across many diverse demographic groups have shown a desire to become more involved in their care and more informed about their health (Frosch et al., 2012; President's Commission for the Study of Ethical Problems in Medicine and Biomedical and Behavioral Research, 1982). For example, 80 percent of Internet users now seek health information online, making this the third most popular Internet activity (Fox, 2011). After a doctor's appointment, individuals seek out information on diagnoses, tests, and prescriptions to learn more (Diaz et al., 2002). While this online information is variable in quality and should be viewed with caution, this growing interest in health represents an opportunity to increase patients' involvement in their own care, in the care of their loved ones, and in the improvement of the overall system. It further highlights new roles for health professionals in partnering with patients to share reliable online sources of health information (Alston and Paget, 2012). Moreover, the development of new models of care delivery, such as patient-centered medical homes, health homes, and accountable care organizations (ACOs), offers opportunities to incorporate patient engagement. This section explores patient engagement at multiple levels—from the personal relationship of patients with their health care providers, to patients' experience while being treated in a health care organization, to the interaction of patients with the broader system, to patients' management of their own care.

Engaging Patients at the Care Delivery Level

Increased patient engagement in individual interactions with practitioners is needed. Some studies have found that patients and clinicians have differing views on the importance of different health goals and health care risks (Lee et al., 2010a,b). Other studies have found that physicians have inaccurate perceptions of their patients' health beliefs, assuming that their patients' beliefs are more aligned with their own than is actually the case. This misperception improves when patients are able to participate actively in the consultation (Johnson et al., 2010; Street and Haidet, 2011). However, studies have found that physicians tend to interrupt patients within 15 seconds of their beginning to speak at the outset of a visit, while uninterrupted patients tend to conclude their remarks in under a minute (Beckman and Frankel, 1984). These studies highlight the need to prepare health care professionals with communication skills and techniques that optimize opportunities for patient engagement.

Metrics have been developed for quantifying a patient's activation, defined as the capability to participate in the care process (Hibbard, 2004; Hibbard et al., 2004). These metrics make it possible both to assess whether interventions improve activation and to customize care based on a patient's activation level. Evidence demonstrates that increasing a patient's activation correlates with improvement in a variety of self-management behaviors (Hibbard et al., 2007; Mosen et al., 2007) and that tailoring interventions to a patient's level of activation can improve the interventions' impact (Hibbard et al., 2009). Evidence also suggests that patient activation and self-management can be enhanced through such strategies as improved communication, motivational interviewing, shared decision making, ready access to personal health information and providers, and increased focus on goals that matter to patients and their families.

Communication

Patients, their families, and other caregivers can bring useful and often critically important knowledge to bear on care if they are invited to do so. Patients often are unable to discuss all of their concerns in a single visit. Some interventions to remedy this limitation are straightforward; one study found that simply asking patients whether there was "something else" to discuss instead of "anything else" reduced the number of unmet concerns by almost 80 percent (Heritage et al., 2007). Moreover, patients bring a different perspective to the encounter than clinicians and will introduce different information. For example, patients on statin drugs were far more likely than their clinician to initiate the discussion of symptoms potentially related to the prescription (Golomb et al., 2007).

A variety of interventions are aimed at improving the state of patient-clinician communication (Maurer et al., 2012). Opportunities to improve patient-centered communication skills exist throughout all levels of health professions education, from degree to continuing education (Levinson et al., 2010). Other tools include patient coaching and question checklists, which are designed to assist patients in communicating with their clinicians. In one study, coaching and the use of checklists were shown to increase the number of questions patients asked and were associated with a modest improvement in patient health outcomes (Kinnersley et al., 2007). The implementation of these tools has yielded some success in improving clinician communication behaviors, as well as patient knowledge and satisfaction, although evidence is mixed on the ultimate impact on patient health outcomes (Coulter and Ellins, 2006).

Communication tools need to be customized to patients' circumstances, especially their health literacy. Health literacy refers to an individual's ability to obtain, understand, and apply health information to make appropriate health decisions. Given the complexity of the field, even highly educated people may have difficulty finding and understanding health information and applying it to their own care or that of their loved ones (IOM, 2004). Ensuring that patients have the tools they need to manage health information is critical, as lower levels of health literacy have been associated with increased hospitalizations, greater use of emergency rooms, lower use of preventive services, and limited ability to manage complex treatment regimens (Berkman et al., 2011). Given that effective communication requires effort from two parties, those who produce health care information for patients must consider how that information will be received and used by patients (Eckman et al., 2012). Several useful communication techniques, such as motivational interviewing, can promote certain health behaviors and adherence to treatment regimens by drawing out the patient's motivation for change (Rollnick et al., 2008). There is also a need for research on interventions that can improve a patient's ability to manage health information (Berkman et al., 2011).

Shared Decision Making

While informing patients about options is important, true patient-centered care requires a new model of decision making in which responsibility is shared between patient and clinician. Implementing this model will require a shift toward health care in which clinicians and patients work together to manage complex conditions, and make decisions on the basis of not only the best scientific evidence but also the patient's biological characteristics, preferences, values, and life circumstances. Such a decision-making model is increasingly important for the growing number of clinical situations in which there are multiple care options, each with different benefits and potential harms. In these situations, where trade-offs will have to be considered, clinicians will need to discuss the risks and benefits of competing diagnostic and treatment options with patients and their caregivers (Collins et al., 2009).

In addition to enhanced communication techniques, tools for promoting shared decision making include decision aids. Decision aids provide balanced information on diagnostic and treatment options, including risks and potential outcomes, and help patients consider what factors are most important to their decision. The goal is to help patients identify the diagnostic technology or treatment that best meets their needs, goals, and circumstances. Studies of such tools have found that they increase patients' knowledge and understanding of benefits and risks and encourage them to participate in decisions (Arterburn et al., 2011; Belkora et al., 2012; O'Connor et al., 2004, 2007a,b; Solberg et al., 2010; Stacey et al., 2011). Several organizations, including the International Patient Decision Aids Standards Collaboration, have developed standards against which to validate the quality of decision aids and ensure that they are accurate, unbiased, and understandable.

The concept of patient-centered care entails customizing care according to patient preferences along all dimensions, including the level of involvement in decision making. Some patients will be interested in playing a strong role in care decisions, while others may want to play a less active role. Evidence suggests that the system currently does not allow patients to realize their desired level of participation; in one study, fewer than half of patients reported they had achieved their preferred level of control in decision making (Degner et al., 1997). Several studies confirm that while most patients wish to be asked their opinions and be offered choices in their care, patients differ in how they would like to be involved in final care decisions (Chung et al., 2011; Deber et al., 2007; Fineberg, 2012; Levinson et al., 2005, Solberg et al., 2009). These studies illustrate the complex role of patient autonomy in the provision of patient-centered care and confirm the variability in the preferences of individual patients and patient populations in this aspect of care. They also signal that patient satisfaction requires patient-clinician communication that not only shares the appropriate clinical information for each patient, but also provides the appropriate amount of information and degree of autonomy in acting on the information. These findings suggest as well that it is important for clinicians to be working in an environment where they can function as careful listeners and coaches, as well as experts in their field.

The implementation of new communication and decision-making paradigms will need to be customized for different patient populations. For vulnerable populations, including low-income individuals, racial and ethnic minorities, and the elderly, there are multiple obstacles to achieving this type of care. For example, patients whose primary point of contact with the health care system is a hospital emergency department are unlikely to develop long-term partnerships with a clinician for making care decisions (Silow-Carroll et al., 2006). In addition, decision-making initiatives will need to be measured and rewarded routinely to ensure their regular use in clinical practice (Sepucha et al., 2004). Challenges will be faced, then, in applying shared decision-making principles to a diverse patient population. However, patient-centered care, delivered through a team approach, can be effective for patients at a range of socioeconomic levels and at a variety of health care organizations, including safety-net systems. For example, several programs have shown success in introducing patient-centered care in urban settings with populations of low socioeconomic status and in achieving long-term engagement in preventive care and improved control of chronic conditions (Jones et al., 2007; Scott et al., 2011).

Engaging Patients at the Organizational Level

Patient-centered care goes beyond direct patient-clinician interactions to the clinic, unit, and health care organization level. At this level, patient-centeredness means different things, such as creating patient and family councils, establishing portals that allow patients to access their health information, and developing policies that ensure timely access to care (Balik et al., 2011; Maurer et al., 2012). Given that patients, their families, and other caregivers are the people who actually experience care, their perspectives can contribute substantially to effective and efficient health care organizations. Leveraging their knowledge can improve the experience of care through the application of their insights to the design and delivery of care in health care organizations—from hospital design, to visiting hours, to care delivery (Bergeson and Dean, 2006; Groene, 2011; Johnson et al., 2008; Scholle et al., 2010). Thus involving patients in improvement initiatives ensures that patients' values and perspectives guide system design, in addition to keeping the teams working on these projects focused on patient priorities.

There are several successful approaches for improving the patient experience, such as those focused on reducing waiting times (Litvak and Bisognano, 2011; Litvak et al., 2005), which also can improve quality and reduce costs (see Chapter 9 for further discussion of these initiatives). To further center care on patient needs and preferences, health care organizations and systems can act on lessons learned about what patients value by engaging patients, their families, and other caregivers. For example, systems can ensure the inclusion of patient perspectives in an institution's operations by promoting patient and family participation on advisory councils, giving patients and their families direct access to the institution's decision-making structures. Case studies have shown that by working on such councils, patients may participate in institutional quality improvement projects, help redesign service delivery processes, serve on search committees for new executives, and help develop educational programs for hospital staff. They also may aid the hospital in making its procedures more efficient and patient-centered and may participate in rounds, which can lead to new suggestions for improvement (Balik et al., 2011; Conway et al., 2006; Ponte et al., 2003). Other programs have shown the potential benefits—including reduction of medical errors and increased hand hygiene—of including patients in safety initiatives, although various institutional factors may limit this potential (Davis et al., 2007; Longtin et al., 2010; Weingart et al., 2005, 2011). Using a different approach, initiatives at one health care organization, using value stream analysis and production system methods, improved care by incorporating patients in continuous improvement projects and measuring value from the patient perspective (Toussaint, 2009).

In one example, leaders at Dana-Farber Cancer Institute invited patients and family members to populate all decision-making structures and processes in the organization. Patients provided input on organizational policies, were placed on continuous improvement teams, and were invited to join search committees and develop educational programming for staff (Ponte et al., 2003). Leaders at the organizational level made the commitment to patient-centered care and communicated that vision to the organization (Shaller and The Commonwealth Fund, 2007) (see Chapter 9 for detail on the leadership and other commitments necessary to achieve a patient-centered learning health care organization). Box 7-1 presents another example of such patient and family involvement.

Another strategy for engaging patients in organizational change is routine measurement. The use of valid and reliable instruments can document the gaps between what routinely occurs and the ideal, thereby stimulating behavioral change among clinicians and patients. These tools include patient experience surveys, mechanisms for submitting complaints, and other feedback opportunities for patients. Beyond the information received, these tools convey the message that the voices of patients, families, and other caregivers are important (Shaller and The Commonwealth Fund, 2007).

Patient portals, dashboards, and other information technology-enabled devices are another avenue for bridging the gap between clinician visits and patients' ongoing information and health monitoring needs. By simplifying communication, e-mail and telephone care allow patients to reach their clinicians easily and receive information when they need it. In one organization, office visits fell by 9 percent after the implementation of electronic health records that facilitated effective patient-clinician communication via telephone (Garrido et al., 2005). Similarly, patient portals allow patients

---

BOX 7-1
Medical College of Georgia Health System

In 1993, in response to an internal assessment revealing that care focused more on the needs of clinicians than on those of patients and family members, the Medical College of Georgia (MCG) Health System in Augusta, Georgia, set out to transform its organizational culture to promote patient-centered care. To do so on both the patient and clinician sides of the care equation, MCG established a Family-Centered Care Steering Committee, which later became the Family Advisory Council—an interdisciplinary committee that provides guidance in the development of MCG programs and policies. MCG also ensured a focus on patient-centered care among its workforce by involving staff in process design, by modeling and rewarding patient-centered behaviors, and by including patient- and family-centered care attitudes and skills in position descriptions and in employee performance assessments. To monitor its efforts, MCG implemented several channels for measuring patient satisfaction, including patient and family councils, surveys, and direct feedback from patients and families to MCG leaders on their care experience. As a result of these efforts, MCG Children's Medical Center has consistently ranked in the 90th percentile in patient satisfaction among children's hospitals since opening in 1998.

SOURCES: Conway et al., 2006; Shaller and The Commonwealth Fund, 2007.

---

to communicate with their clinicians, access their health information, and monitor their own health, thereby facilitating their active participation in their care (Halamka et al., 2008; Shaller and The Commonwealth Fund, 2007). One example of the use of a patient portal in chronic care management is the Palo Alto Medical Foundation's diabetes management system, which allows patients and their clinicians to monitor key measures for the condition and highlights how the measures relate to overall health goals. Early focus group results indicate that while patients initially used the portal because they knew clinicians reviewed the results, over time they started using the system on their own to understand how different behaviors affected their health (IOM, 2011d). Likewise, Partners HealthCare's Center for Connected Health provides health information technology for patients with cardiac conditions, diabetes, and hypertension that allows them to share information with their clinicians and receive feedback. While some patients stop participating early on, 90 percent of those who remain active through the first 2 months continue to participate (IOM, 2011d). These examples demonstrate the potential of health information technologies, as well as highlight the need for these technologies to be easy for patients to use and access.

Engaging Patients at the System Level

Routine assessment of patient experience can be used to support patient-centered care across a continuum of health care settings while also providing the opportunity to promote better integration, transitions, and coordination of services. To support financial reforms and payment strategies that reward patient-centered care, it is important to develop methods for accurately measuring such care. One instrument for assessing patient experience, the Consumer Assessment of Healthcare Providers and Systems (CAHPS) suite of surveys, was developed as a nationally standardized tool for eliciting reports from patients on their experiences in interacting with the health care system (Browne et al., 2010; Charmel and Frampton, 2008). The hospital version of the survey, called Hospital CAHPS or HCAHPS, is used by hospitals to assess indicators of patient experience, including interactions with staff, information provided, overall satisfaction with the care experience, and the patient's willingness to recommend the hospital to others (Charmel and Frampton, 2008). HCAHPS results also are being used by the Centers for Medicare & Medicaid Services (CMS) to forge a link between patient experience and reimbursement. As of July 2007, hospitals had to report HCAHPS data to CMS or absorb a 2 percent reduction in reimbursement for inpatient services (Charmel and Frampton, 2008). Moreover, under recent policy initiatives, CMS will expand the use of HCAHPS when it uses the survey data as one measure in calculating value-based purchasing payments to hospitals.[2] The same focus on patient experience and patient-centered care can be applied to outpatient and non-hospital-based settings.

Despite the importance of assessing patient experience and rewarding institutions that perform well on measures of patient-centeredness, some uncertainty exists as to which aspects of the patient experience are most important to measure and best correlate with improved outcomes. Multiple terms exist for defining this aspect of the patient-centeredness of an institution, including "patient satisfaction," "patient experience," "patient perception," and "patient ratings of quality." Additionally, multiple factors affect patients' rating of their care experience, ranging from accordance with evidence-based processes, to staff care, to information availability (Gao et al., 2012; Sofaer and Firminger, 2005). Another challenge in measurement is ensuring that patient experience data are collected frequently, thereby enabling the organization to assess its improvement in patient-centeredness.

---

[2]Patient Protection and Affordable Care Act, Public Law 111-148, 111th Congress (March 23, 2010).

One study of patients' perceptions of hospital care, including inpatient care and discharge planning, suggests that higher patient satisfaction may be associated with lower 30-day readmission rates (Boulding et al., 2011). In terms of correlation with an institution's technical expertise, one study compared a hospital's overall patient satisfaction score with its clinical quality and mortality rates for heart attack patients, finding that higher satisfaction correlated with improved adherence to guidelines and lower mortality rates. Yet, high overall patient satisfaction scores showed no correlation with questions about the patient's room, meals, or wait time for tests and treatment or with the speed of the discharge process (Glickman et al., 2010). Another study of patient-centered medical homes found an association between practices rated by patients as high-quality and improved patient blood pressure control (Gray et al., 2011). Still another study found that measures of patient experience correlated with process measures of clinical quality, although they did not correlate with health outcomes (Sequist et al., 2008). Showing the relationship between patient experience and other aspects of care, another study found that patients' satisfaction with hospitals' nursing staff and with staff care influenced the patients' perceptions on overall quality of care, willingness to recommend, and willingness to return (Otani et al., 2010). On the other hand, one recent study cast doubt on the correlation between high levels of patient-centeredness and improved outcomes, finding that greater patient satisfaction was associated with higher inpatient use, higher health care costs, and increased mortality (Fenton et al., 2012). These examples highlight the range of factors that affect a patient's experience and illustrate the potential knowledge gained from these assessments, but also underscore the need for further study regarding the conclusions that can be drawn from patient satisfaction data.

Engaging Patients, Families, and Caregivers in Health Management

Refocusing the health care system on the people it serves will require renewed attention to the ways in which patients, their families, and other caregivers access health information and manage the patient's health. In some cases, patient self-management is a realistic expectation, while in other cases, family and other caregivers will be the primary managers of care. Regardless, patient engagement and support for self-management require education and interventions that enhance patients' ability to monitor and manage their own health problems (IOM, 2003). To this end, it is necessary to provide information and teach people disease-specific skills so they will understand what behavior changes they must make to improve their health prospects and will have the problem-solving skills to cope with changes in their condition. It is also necessary to recognize and assist with the reality of living with a chronic condition, provide patients with support and follow-up opportunities, and encourage patients to actively manage their disease. The horizon for these approaches is promising. Initiatives such as the Empowered Patient Coalition highlight the potential of online mechanisms to provide information and support for patients, their family and other caregivers, and their clinicians in encouraging self-management. Moreover, reviews of patient education and reminder interventions for chronic disease management have found that such interventions are associated with improved health outcomes (Deakin et al., 2005; Guevara et al., 2003; Weingarten et al., 2002). Ultimately, given the complexity of chronic disease management, engaging patients as active participants in their care is quickly becoming an imperative for the health care system.

Technology offers opportunities for clinicians to engage patients by meeting with them where they are. The use of mobile devices both to help clinicians reach out to patients and to enable people to monitor their own health holds promise for promoting patient-centered care. The advent of smartphones has led to the creation of numerous applications that enable people to become engaged more completely in their own health through greater access to health information and tracking tools such as built-in pedometers, diet management aids, and weight and blood pressure logs. A recent review of the use of mobile phones for chronic disease management found 23 articles describing interventions involving use of a mobile phone for disease prevention, diagnosis, management, and monitoring, as well as patient education. The interventions spanned a broad range of chronic illnesses, including diabetes, asthma, dementia, and hypertension. Across all interventions, high rates of user compliance and satisfaction were reported (Skinner and Finkelstein, 2008).

Early trials reveal the potential of this approach. In a trial of txt2stop, a text messaging service that sends motivational and behavioral change support messages to smokers attempting to quit, smokers who received the text messages showed significantly better cessation rates at 6 months relative to the control group (Free et al., 2011). Another study focused on IDEALL (Improving Diabetes Efforts Across Language and Literacy), an automated telephone support service for diabetics that offers targeted health education messages based on people's responses to questions about exercise, blood glucose monitoring, and other indicators. The study found that, while the service did not lead to differences in blood glucose level for participants, it did lead to increased patient participation, engagement, and self-efficacy compared with patients undergoing typical care (Schillinger et al., 2009). These trials suggest that mobile technologies represent a new avenue for engaging, educating, and activating people in their own care and that of their loved ones.

Self-care has become increasingly crucial as patients today are discharged from health care organizations more quickly and in poorer health.

As a result, postdischarge care now requires more advanced management by patients, their families, other caregivers, and the community. What used to be the purview of the health care professional now has been delegated to the patient, too often with inadequate handoff. Meeting this challenge will require new methods of education and communication; new technologies for management; and additional community supports, explored in the next section.

INTEGRATING HEALTH CARE AND THE HEALTH OF THE COMMUNITY

While patient engagement can help drive the U.S. health care system toward continuous learning and improvement, the value, quality, and care coordination challenges faced by the system cannot be met by any single platform, organization, or entity acting alone. Rather, communities and coalitions are needed to drive improvement.

Broadening the Definition of Communities

The typical definition of a community is a group located in a particular geographic area. However, communities that promote continuous learning and improvement in health care go beyond geographic boundaries to include groups linked through culture, occupation, conditions based on a common workplace, prognosis, stage in the care process, intensity of care needed, and more.

One natural community comprises people who share a particular condition or disease. The disease-specific organizations that represent these patients are a form of top-down community structure. They play a crucial role in gathering, reaching, and motivating patient constituents; funding research; advocating on behalf of patients; and conducting campaigns focused on quality improvement and patient-centered care (Conway et al., 2006). Their efforts aid patients in becoming more educated and informed consumers, and aid clinicians in staying abreast of clinical advances by disseminating clinical guidelines and decision support tools. Disease-specific affinity groups may also form organically as communities with which patients can share their experiences. Box 7-2 presents an example of how a community of patients formed around a common health care need—in this case, the need for prenatal care—can lead to improved health outcomes.

The Internet has proven key in facilitating the development and rapid growth of these communities. Examples include the New Health Partnerships, C3N, and PatientsLikeMe. Websites, blogs, and social networking platforms such as Facebook and Twitter also give patients the tools to interact with others who share their diagnosis, gain access to new expertise and

---

BOX 7-2
A Community of Patient Peers Helps Reduce Premature Births

For many patients, a community of similar patients can offer useful supports for health management. One such patient, Ruth Lopez, was referred by her physician to a CenteringPregnancy program in Washington, DC. This program provides prenatal care and education to groups of women in similar stages of pregnancy, which allows for traditional care in conjunction with peer supports. In one meeting of Ms. Lopez's program, the group worked through a focused agenda of prenatal monitoring, from reading their own urine dips to documenting their blood pressure. The group model creates opportunities for sharing advice, provides support for behavior change, and increases the time for learning at prenatal appointments. Perhaps most important, women like Ms. Lopez who receive their prenatal care through the CenteringPregnancy group health care model are 33 percent less likely to have a preterm birth, making this one of the few innovations in prenatal care shown to reduce the preterm birth rate in the United States, which now is more than 12 percent.

SOURCES: March of Dimes Perinatal Center, 2012; Norris, 2011.

---

information, query members of their network, share updates about their health status, and receive support from friends and family. For example, a group of diabetic patients at the Fargo Family Health Center decided to create a blog and listserv where they could share their diabetes treatment experiences at the center, as well as support each other in managing and living with diabetes (IOM, 2011d). In another example, a frustrated mother whose son was getting sicker and sicker despite visits to the pediatrician posted pictures of her son on Facebook, and members of her extended social network were able to relate experiences that led to a correct diagnosis of Kawasaki disease—a rare autoimmune disorder (Kogan, 2011). These examples illustrate how patients and families can utilize existing communities or create new ones to seek out information, manage their care, and gain support from others.

Another natural focal point for patient engagement is the workplace. Workplaces have several attributes that make them conducive to community-oriented health and wellness programs: they host a group of employees who share a common goal; they have social, organizational, policy, and financial supports for employee behavior change; they have open and straightforward communication channels; and they have the ability to incentivize and monitor employee participation in sponsored health programs. Over the past 40 years, increasing numbers of employers have taken advantage of these characteristics to create worksite health promotion programs designed to improve employee performance and productivity and mitigate rising health care costs associated with preventable, lifestyle, and behavior-based chronic diseases. According to some studies, well-designed workplace health programs have the potential to produce strong returns on investment, although there are outstanding questions on the returns generated and the generalizability of the results (Chapman, 2005; Goetzel et al., 1999; IOM, 2010). According to a 2008 study, however, only 6.9 percent of health promotion programs offered by employers are evidence-based and include five essential elements: health education, employee screenings, supportive physical and social environments, integration of health promotion into the organizational culture, and links to employee services (Linnan et al., 2008). Recent policy support for evidence-based workplace health programs includes technical assistance and assessment, federal grants to small businesses, and policy changes that allow employers to offer financial incentives to encourage employee participation in wellness programs (Kaiser Family Foundation, 2011).

Such workplace communities do face challenges. One of these challenges lies in the tension between the goals of employers and employees, some of which will differ. Another is the need to build trust, as well as to operate transparently (Berry et al., 2010; Goetzel et al., 2007).

Recognition of the potential of communities to achieve better outcomes at lower cost has led to a number of initiatives aimed at bringing coalitions together to improve health care. One example is the Aligning Forces for Quality project, which has brought together coalitions of clinicians, patients, employers, insurers, and others in 16 communities to focus on improving health care quality, reducing disparities, and developing new models with the potential to be diffused nationally (Aligning Forces for Quality, 2012; Hurley et al., 2009).

Coordinating Patient Care Throughout the Health Care System and Community

Opportunities exist for bridging the gaps between patients, their care, and the broader community. One example is care transitions—changes in the set of clinicians delivering care or in the setting of care that patients must navigate. In the current health care system, both the incentives that encourage health care spending and the increasing specialization of clinicians have led to a situation in which a growing number of patients are seeing an array of clinicians in a variety of care settings. This increase in the number of clinicians and settings involved in a patient's care has led to a corresponding increase in hospitalizations, adverse events, errors, and breakdowns in communication across the care team, and has left patients in the precarious position of coordinating their own care without the knowledge or resources to do so. Further, the rising prevalence of chronic conditions in the United States, with 27 percent of Americans having multiple such conditions, necessitates coordinated care interventions, because chronically ill people experience frequent changes in their health status that require transitions between multiple care providers. Such transitions require successful interactions among the multiple clinicians, organizations, and community-based resources involved in the patient's care and support (HHS, 2010; Naylor et al., 2011).

New innovations in care delivery, such as the patient-centered medical home, are aimed at coordinating a patient's care across specialists, hospitals, home health agencies, nursing homes, the patient's family and other caregivers, and community-based services (AAFP et al., 2007; Fields et al., 2010). Multiple initiatives have been developed to increase opportunities to engage patients and their families in care processes, practice improvement, and the design of medical homes (Scholle et al., 2010). Another example is the Patient Protection and Affordable Care Act's creation of ACOs—collaboratives of health care professionals and institutions that provide coordinated health care services to a defined panel of Medicare patients in exchange for a share of the resultant cost savings (Merlis, 2010). Because they will share primary care, hospital, and other organizational resources, ACOs have the potential to develop into integrated, de facto communities of clinicians and patients. Although it remains to be seen whether ACOs will deliver on their promise of better-coordinated care at lower cost, their formation represents a key opportunity for community engagement. Involving patients in the design, formation, and evaluation of ACOs would help ensure that these organizations will adhere to the principles of patient-centered care (Springgate and Brook, 2011).

Achieving the elements of effective care transitions represents a crucial challenge—and opportunity—that can be met only in an environment of collaborative patient-centeredness where patients, families, clinicians, and health and social institutions work together to accomplish quality care transitions. Still, successful models demonstrate that effective care transitions are indeed possible. For example, the Care Transitions Model has been shown to reduce hospital admissions by 17 percent and costs by 50 percent (Naylor et al., 1999). A review of 21 randomized controlled trials focused on improving care transitions for chronically ill adults found that, despite substantial heterogeneity among the populations and care transition interventions studied, all but one of the trials yielded positive findings with respect to health outcomes, quality of life, patient satisfaction, resource use, and costs. Nine of the trials showed reductions in readmissions, and eight of those showed reductions in all-cause readmissions in the 30 days after discharge (Naylor et al., 2011). These findings suggest that effective care transition models hold great potential for bridging gaps between care settings and community-based organizations.

Several more recent initiatives have been undertaken to improve care coordination and transitions. One is the Department of Health and Human Services' strategic framework for multiple chronic conditions, initiated in 2010, which is designed to facilitate home- and community-based services (HHS, 2010). Similarly, Massachusetts has established a strategic plan for improving care transitions in the state. In developing this plan, it was found that seven principles of effective care transitions were necessary: transfer of clinical information, a communication infrastructure that supports care transitions, patient and family engagement, clinical responsibility for the patient and accountability on the part of clinicians with no lapses in care, clinician and practice engagement, assessment of transitions using standardized process and outcome measures, and payment incentives that promote effective transitions and minimize adverse events (Bonner et al., 2010). Many other initiatives are under way nationally to improve the coordination of patients' care. Although initiatives on care coordination are important for improving patient health, however, achieving cost savings from these programs can be difficult in many cases (Nelson, 2012; Peikes et al., 2009).

Leveraging Resources Beyond the Traditional Health Care Enterprise

Although historical commonalities exist between the health care system and public health, the two have evolved into distinct sectors, with the health care system focusing on care of individual patients and the public health sector concentrating on populations, prevention, and social determinants of health. Both perspectives are needed to improve the health of Americans and to confront the problems of increased prevalence of chronic diseases, which is often due to biological and social factors, and rising health care costs (IOM, 2011b,c, 2012a). Moreover, synergies can be realized in improving the quality and value of care by applying a population perspective to traditional medical practice, using clinical practice to identify and address community health problems, strengthening health promotion and health protection by mobilizing community campaigns, and improving health care by coordinating services for individuals (Lasker and Committee on Medicine and Public Health, 1997). Indeed, these sectors have important potential overlap in health surveillance, health promotion, and prevention (Rowan et al., 2007).

Several initiatives have been aimed at increasing coordination on this front in the United States and in an international context. Most reported outcomes from these initiatives have been positive, including improved population health, health care delivery processes, and partnership and team functioning. However, evidence on how best to accomplish this integration, as well as how to sustain such initiatives, is limited (Martin-Misener et al., 2009). An Institute of Medicine (IOM) committee recently explored in depth the opportunities for integrating the primary care and public health sectors (IOM, 2012b).

Important examples exist of leveraging resources beyond the traditional health care system to promote the provision of services to people whose health and social needs are intertwined (Craig et al., 2011). New initiatives have linked community health centers and community development financial institutions to support community improvements, such as addressing food deserts,[3] reducing childhood exposure to allergens and irritants, and increasing the supply of affordable housing and community supports to allow older adults to age in the community (Braunstein and Lavizzo-Mourey, 2011; Erickson and Andrews, 2011; Kotelchuck et al., 2011). These initiatives reflect a recognition of the many determinants of health that can be harnessed to promote patients' health and well-being (IOM, 1997, 2011a; Madden et al., 2007; McGinnis and Foege, 1993; McGinnis et al., 2002). Most determinants of the health status of individuals and populations lie not in health care—medical care accounts for only 10 to 20 percent of overall health prospects—but in such factors as behavior, social circumstances, and environment. Thus, protecting and improving health requires close clinical-community coordination (McGinnis et al., 2002). Such initiatives also reflect a recognition that health is not merely a biological descriptor; rather, it represents patients' and populations' ability to detect and respond to their illnesses; improve their current and future functional capacity; and achieve physical, emotional, and social well-being (IOM, 1997). Further, these initiatives address the increasing burden of chronic disease on the health care and public health systems, on health care expenditures, and on the U.S. population as a whole (Lasker and Committee on Medicine and Public Health, 1997).

Other new initiatives encourage coordination among health care services and community resources. Successful care coordination initiatives identify community needs and assets and system-level stakeholders and institutions that define parameters for community action (Craig et al., 2011; McKnight, 1978). They utilize patient stratification techniques to target patients whose needs are not being met by the primary care system—patients who visit emergency rooms more frequently than others, whose illnesses require inpatient care, and whose health care costs are among the highest in the community. Using these criteria, such initiatives develop panels of patients for whom they assume responsibility and harness resources—family members, religious groups, and others—as partners in those patients' care. These

---

[3]The term *food desert* refers to neighborhoods and communities where access to affordable and nutritious foods is limited (IOM, 2009).

initiatives also have skilled leaders who can coordinate the interests of stake-holders, including hospital administrators and state and local health, housing, and mental health departments, at the system level (Craig et al., 2011). Box 7-3 describes an example of a community initiative aimed at improving care delivery and health outcomes through better care coordination.

BOX 7-3
Vermont Blueprint for Health

Communities of integrated health services, spanning organizations and clinicians, are an example of the evolving definition of communities—in this case focused on care coordination. Community-based teams support patient-centered services, helping to better coordinate and more seamlessly transition care across a spectrum of services in a community. One example is the Vermont Blueprint for Health, a statewide public-private initiative that seeks to transform care delivery; improve health outcomes; and expand access to seamless, well-coordinated care. As a key component of Vermont's Multi-Player Advanced Primary Care Practice Demonstration, a pilot program sponsored by the Centers for Medicare & Medicaid Services, the Vermont Blueprint for Health operates through a network of integrated medical homes, each supported by an integrated information technology infrastructure and community health teams. These teams are typically composed of nurse coordinators, social workers, and behavioral health counselors working to improve health outcomes while containing costs through the provision of coordinated care.

By extending health care delivery to services not typically provided in the primary care setting, these community health teams are able to provide individual care coordination, health and wellness coaching, and behavioral health counseling as an integrated and coordinated set of services. Nurse coordinators primarily track patient activities within physician practices by following up on overdue appointments or tests, ensuring proper refilling of and adherence to prescriptions, working with patients to achieve their personal health management goals, and overseeing short-term care for high-need patients. Behavioral health coordinators also work within physician practices, monitoring patients for any untreated mental health conditions and ensuring speedy follow-up for those who require it. Outside of the primary care practices, community health workers assist patients in applying for insurance, adhering to treatment plans, managing stress, and progressing toward their personal wellness goals. Public health specialists facilitate closer coordination between the community health team and public health initiatives, while dietitians provide nutrition education and work with diabetic patients to manage their conditions. This team approach to better self-management has yielded many successes for the Blueprint initiative, including a 31 percent decrease in emergency department use and a 36 percent decrease in associated costs per person per month.

SOURCE: Bielaszka-DuVernay, 2011.

Successful care coordination models also utilize care coordinators to work with identified patients in formulating care plans that advance the patients' life and health goals and to coordinate services, including social services and health provider services, to meet those goals. Care coordinators may be nurses, social workers, other health workers, or lay people as long as they have the skills to communicate with and motivate their patients, coordinate a broad range of services, and do all that is necessary to prevent negative outcomes (Bradway et al., 2011). New types of health care professionals also have been introduced to coordinate care in many health care settings; an example is the increasing use of hospitalists to coordinate care in inpatient visits (Meltzer and Chung, 2010; Meltzer et al., 2002).

Conclusion 7-2: Coordination and integration of patient services currently are poor. Improvement in this area will require strong and sustained avenues of communication and cooperation between and among clinical and community stewards of services.

Related findings:

- *Care often is poorly coordinated across different settings and providers.* In one survey, roughly 25 percent of patients noted that a test had to be repeated because the results from another provider had not been shared (see also Chapter 3).
- *Inadequate, sometimes absent, continuity of care endangers patients.* Almost one-fifth of hospitalized Medicare patients are rehospitalized within 30 days, often without seeing their primary care provider in the interim (see also Chapter 3).
- *Although results for care coordination programs are mixed, there are effective interventions for improving care transitions.* For example, the Care Transitions Model has been shown to reduce readmissions by 17 percent and costs by 50 percent.
- *Comprehensive health care requires accounting for factors typically outside of the traditional health care system.* Most determinants of health lie outside of health care, with health care accounting for only 10 to 20 percent of health prospects. Thus there is a clear need for close clinical-community coordination.

FRAMEWORK FOR ACHIEVING THE VISION[4]

As discussed in this chapter, neither patients nor clinicians can perform their tasks alone. While clinicians supply their scientific expertise on the benefits and risks of different options, patients contribute their knowledge about the suitability of different options for their needs, goals, and circumstances. Both are necessary to providing the right care. Given that patient-centered care is not simply agreeing to every patient request, many tools are needed to communicate information, create partnerships, and improve decision-making models (Maurer et al., 2012). Further, involving patients meaningfully at the organizational and system levels requires changes in organizational structures and measurement tools and an expanded focus on the patient in all aspects of care. Recommendation 4 highlights the broad aims that different stakeholder groups need to pursue if health care's focus on patients is to increase.

Recommendation 4: Patient-Centered Care

Involve patients and families in decisions regarding health and health care, tailored to fit their preferences. Patients and families should be given the opportunity to be fully engaged participants at all levels, including individual care decisions, health system learning and improvement activities, and community-based interventions to promote health.

Strategies for progress toward this goal:

- *Patients and families* should expect to be offered full participation in their own care and health and encouraged to partner, according to their preference, with clinicians in fulfilling those expectations.
- *Clinicians* should employ high-quality, reliable tools and skills for informed shared decision making with patients and families, tailored to clinical needs, patient goals, social circumstances, and the degree of control patients prefer.
- *Health care delivery organizations,* including programs operated by the *Department of Defense, the Veterans Health Administration,* and *Health Resources and Services Administration,* should monitor and assess patient perspectives and use the insights thus gained to improve care processes; establish patient portals to facilitate data sharing and communication among clinicians, patients, and

---

[4]Note that in Chapters 6-9, the committee's recommendations are numbered according to their sequence in the taxonomy in Chapter 10.

families; and make high-quality, reliable tools available for shared decision making with patients at different levels of health literacy.

- The *Agency for Healthcare Research and Quality,* partnering with the *Centers for Medicare & Medicaid Services, other payers,* and *stakeholder organizations,* should support the development and testing of an accurate and reliable core set of measures of patient-centeredness for consistent use across the health care system.
- The *Centers for Medicare & Medicaid Services* and *other public and private payers* should promote and measure patient-centered care through payment models, contracting policies, and public reporting programs.
- *Digital technology developers* and *health product innovators* should develop tools to assist individuals in managing their health and health care, in addition to providing patient supports in new forms of communities.

Beyond patient-centered care, this chapter has described how integrating services among and across health care organizations and community-based organizations can improve health and address complex care needs. Further, partnerships between health care organizations and public health systems can advance community health goals. Recommendation 5 describes the broad actions that different stakeholders need to take to improve co-ordination and partnerships between and among the health care system, community resources, and public health bodies. Further, the recommendation introduces two specific actions that can be taken to produce change immediately by rewarding care that improves population health and by increasing the accuracy of metrics that measure population health.

Recommendation 5: Community Links

Promote community-clinical partnerships and services aimed at man aging and improving health at the community level. Care delivery and community-based organizations and agencies should partner with each other to develop cooperative strategies for the design, implementation, and accountability of services aimed at improving individual and population health.

Strategies for progress toward this goal:

- *Health care delivery organizations* and *clinicians* should partner with *community-based organizations* and *public health agencies* to leverage and coordinate prevention, health promotion, and community-based interventions to improve health outcomes, including strategies related to the assessment and use of web-based tools.

- *Public and private payers* should incorporate population health improvement into their health care payment and contracting policies and accountability measures.
- *Health economists, health service researchers, professional specialty societies,* and *measure development organizations* should continue to improve measures that can readily be applied to assess performance on both individual and population health.

For many patients, care can be fragmented and uncoordinated, whether they are transitioning from the hospital to a community setting or between two different clinicians. As patient needs have grown more complex, focusing on coordination and communication across all of a patient's health care providers has become increasingly crucial. These coordination and communication needs may be more acute when patients require services beyond the traditional health care system, such as social and community services, for managing their condition. Recommendation 6 outlines actions that need to be taken to improve care transitions and coordination to provide seamless care for patients.

Recommendation 6: Care Continuity

Improve coordination and communication within and across organizations. Payers should structure payment and contracting to reward effective communication and coordination between and among members of a patient's care team.

Strategies for progress toward this goal:

- *Health care delivery organizations* and *clinicians,* partnering with *patients, families,* and *community organizations,* should develop coordination and transition processes, data sharing capabilities, and communication tools to ensure safe, seamless patient care.
- *Health economists, health service researchers, professional specialty societies,* and *measure development organizations* should develop and test metrics with which to monitor and evaluate the effectiveness of care transitions in improving patient health outcomes.
- *Public and private payers* should promote effective care transitions that improve patient health through their payment and contracting policies.

Given the advantages that accrue from involving patients and communities in health care, their inclusion is a goal for a learning health care system. Challenges are entailed in promoting this involvement, from changing the existing culture of medicine to creating metrics that accurately measure involvement. As noted in this chapter, there are differences between patient involvement in care and measures such as patient satisfaction. However, these challenges do not prevent a focus on patients in care, and each can be overcome to allow for a health care system that continually improves patient care.

REFERENCES

AAFP (American Academy of Family Physicians, AAP (American Academy of Pediatrics), ACP (American College of Physicians), and (AOA) American Osteopathic Association. 2007. *Joint principles of the patient-centered medical home.* http://www.pcpcc.net/content/joint-principles-patient-centered-medical-home (accessed August 31, 2012).

Aligning Forces for Quality. 2012. *AF4Q alliance overview.* http://forces4quality.org/af4q-alliances-overview (accessed May 15, 2012).

Alston, C., and L. Paget. 2012. *Communicating evidence in health care: Engaging patients for improved health care decisions.* http://iom.edu/~/media/Files/Activity%20Files/Quality/VSRT/IC%20Meeting%20Docs/ECIC%2006-07-12/Lyn%20Paget%20and%20Chuck%20Alston.pdf (accessed August 31, 2012).

Arterburn, D. E., E. O. Westbrook, T. A. Bogart, K. R. Sepucha, S. N. Bock, and W. G. Weppner. 2011. Randomized trial of a video-based patient decision aid for bariatric surgery. *Obesity (Silver Spring)* 19(8):1669-1675.

Balik, B., J. Conway, L. Zipperer, and J. Watson. 2011. *Achieving an exceptional patient and family experience of inpatient hospital care.* Cambridge, MA: Institute for Healthcare Improvement.

Beach, M. C., J. Keruly, and R. D. Moore. 2006. Is the quality of the patient provider relationship associated with better adherence and health outcomes for patients with HIV? *Journal of General Internal Medicine* 21(6):661-665.

Bechel, D. L., W. A. Myers, and D. G. Smith. 2000. Does patient-centered care pay off? *Joint Commission Journal on Quality Improvement* 26(7):400-409.

Beckman, H. B., and R. M. Frankel. 1984. The effect of physician behavior on the collection of data. *Annals of Internal Medicine* 101(5):692-696.

Belkora, J. K., S. Volz, A. E. Teng, D. H. Moore, M. K. Loth, and K. R. Sepucha. 2012. Impact of decision aids in a sustained implementation at a breast care center. *Patient Education and Counseling* 86(2):195-204.

Bergeson, S. C., and J. D. Dean. 2006. A systems approach to patient-centered care. *Journal of the American Medical Association* 296(23):2848-2851.

Berkman, N. D., S. L. Sheridan, K. E. Donahue, D. J. Halpern, A. Viera, K. Crotty, A. Holland, M. Brasure, K. N. Lohr, E. Harden, E. Tant, I. Wallace, and M. Viswanathan. 2011. *Health literacy interventions and outcomes: An updated systematic review.* Rockville, MD: RTI International/University of North Carolina Evidence-based Practice Center.

Berry, L. L., A. M. Mirabito, and W. B. Baun. 2010. What's the hard return on employee wellness programs? *Harvard Business Review* 88(12):104-112, 142.

Bertakis, K. D., and R. Azari. 2011. Patient-centered care is associated with decreased health care utilization. *Journal of the American Board of Family Medicine* 24(3):229-239.

Berwick, D. M. 2009. What "patient-centered" should mean: Confessions of an extremist. *Health Affairs (Millwood)* 28(4):w555-w565.

Bielaszka-DuVernay, C. 2011. Vermont's blueprint for medical homes, community health teams, and better health at lower cost. *Health Affairs (Millwood)* 30(3):383-386.

Bodenheimer, T. 2008. Coordinating care—a perilous journey through the health care system. *New England Journal of Medicine* 358(10):1064-1071.

Bonner, A., C. Schneider, and J. S. Weissman. 2010. *Massachusetts strategic plan for care transitions.* Boston, MA: Massachusetts State Quality Improvement Institute.

Boulding, W., S. W. Glickman, M. P. Manary, K. A. Schulman, and R. Staelin. 2011. Relationship between patient satisfaction with inpatient care and hospital readmission within 30 days. *The American Journal of Managed Care* 17(1):41-48.

Bradway, C., R. Trotta, M. B. Bixby, E. McPartland, M. C. Wollman, H. Kapustka, K. McCauley, and M. D. Naylor. 2011. A qualitative analysis of an advanced practice nurse-directed transitional care model intervention. *Gerontologist* 52(3):394-407.

Braunstein, S., and R. Lavizzo-Mourey. 2011. How the health and community development sectors are combining forces to improve health and well-being. *Health Affairs (Millwood)* 30(11):2042-2051.

Browne, K., D. Roseman, D. Shaller, and S. Edgman-Levitan. 2010. Analysis & commentary. Measuring patient experience as a strategy for improving primary care. *Health Affairs (Project Hope)* 29(5):921-925.

Chapman, L. S. 2005. *Meta-evaluation of worksite health promotion economic return studies: 2005 update.* http://www.inspirationaljourneys.org/wp-content/uploads/2010/04/Meta-evaluation-of-worksite-health-promotion-economic-return-studies-2005-update.pdf (accessed August 31, 2012).

Charmel, P. A., and S. B. Frampton. 2008. Building the business case for patient-centered care. *Healthcare Financial Management* 62(3):80-85.

Chung, G. S., R. E. Lawrence, F. A. Curlin, V. Arora, and D. O. Meltzer. 2011. Predictors of hospitalised patients' preferences for physician-directed medical decision-making. *Journal of Medical Ethics* 38(2):77-82.

Collins, E. D., C. P. Moore, K. F. Clay, S. A. Kearing, A. M. O'Connor, H. A. Llewellyn-Thomas, R. J. Barth, Jr., and K. R. Sepucha. 2009. Can women with early-stage breast cancer make an informed decision for mastectomy? *Journal of Clinical Oncology* 27(4):519-525.

Conway, J., B. Johnson, S. Edgman-Levitan, J. Schlucter, D. Ford, P. Sodomka, and L. Simmons. 2006. *Partnering with patients and families to design a patient- and family-centered health care system.* Bethesda, MD: Institute for Family-Centered Care with Institute for Healthcare Improvement.

Coulter, A., and J. Ellins. 2006. *Patient-focused interventions: A review of the evidence.* http://www.health.org.uk/publications/research_reports/patientfocused.html (accessed June 11, 2010).

Craig, C., D. Eby, and J. Whittington. 2011. *Care coordination model: Better care at lower cost for people with multiple health and social needs.* Cambridge, MA: Institute for Healthcare Improvement.

Davis, R. E., R. Jacklin, N. Sevdalis, and C. A. Vincent. 2007. Patient involvement in patient safety: What factors influence patient participation and engagement? *Health Expectations* 10(3):259-267.

Deakin, T., C. McShane, J. Cade, and R. Williams. 2005. Group based training for self-management strategies in people with type 2 diabetes mellitus. *Cochrane Database of Systematic Reviews* 2:CD003417.

Deber, R. B., N. Kraetschmer, S. Urowitz, and N. Sharpe. 2007. Do people want to be autonomous patients? Preferred roles in treatment decision-making in several patient populations. *Health Expectations* 10(3):248-258.

Degner, L. F., L. J. Kristjanson, D. Bowman, J. A. Sloan, K. C. Carriere, J. O'Neil, B. Bilodeau, P. Watson, and B. Mueller. 1997. Information needs and decisional preferences in women with breast cancer. *Journal of the American Medical Association* 277(18):1485-1492.

Diaz, J. A., R. A. Griffith, J. J. Ng, S. E. Reinert, P. D. Friedmann, and A. W. Moulton. 2002. Patients' use of the Internet for medical information. *Journal of General Internal Medicine* 17(3):180-185.

Eckman, M. H., R. Wise, A. C. Leonard, E. Dixon, C. Burrows, F. Khan, and E. Warm. 2012. Impact of health literacy on outcomes and effectiveness of an educational intervention in patients with chronic diseases. *Patient Education and Counseling* 87(2):143-151.

Epstein, R. M., and R. L. Street, Jr. 2011. The values and value of patient-centered care. *Annals of Family Medicine* 9(2):100-103.

Epstein, R. M., P. Franks, C. G. Shields, S. C. Meldrum, K. N. Miller, T. L. Campbell, and K. Fiscella. 2005. Patient-centered communication and diagnostic testing. *Annals of Family Medicine* 3(5):415-421.

Epstein, R. M., K. Fiscella, C. S. Lesser, and K. C. Stange. 2010. Why the nation needs a policy push on patient-centered health care. *Health Affairs (Millwood)* 29(8):1489-1495.

Erickson, D., and N. Andrews. 2011. Partnerships among community development, public health, and health care could improve the well-being of low-income people. *Health Affairs (Millwood)* 30(11):2056-2063.

Fagerlin, A., K. R. Sepucha, M. P. Couper, C. A. Levin, E. Singer, and B. J. Zikmund-Fisher. 2010. Patients' knowledge about 9 common health conditions: The decisions survey. *Medical Decision Making* 30(Suppl. 5):S35-S52.

Fenton, J. J., A. F. Jerant, K. D. Bertakis, and P. Franks. 2012. The cost of satisfaction: A national study of patient satisfaction, health care utilization, expenditures, and mortality. *Archives of Internal Medicine* 172(5):405-411.

Fields, D., E. Leshen, and K. Patel. 2010. Analysis & commentary. Driving quality gains and cost savings through adoption of medical homes. *Health Affairs (Millwood)* 29(5):819-826.

Fineberg, H. 2012. From shared decision making to patient-centered decision making. *Israel Journal of Health Policy Research* 1(1):6.

Fowler, F. J., Jr., C. A. Levin, and K. R. Sepucha. 2011. Informing and involving patients to improve the quality of medical decisions. *Health Affairs (Millwood)* 30(4):699-706.

Fox, S. 2011. *Health topics: 80% of Internet users look for health information online*. Washington, DC: Pew Research Center.

Free, C., R. Knight, S. Robertson, R. Whittaker, P. Edwards, W. Zhou, A. Rodgers, J. Cairns, M. G. Kenward, and I. Roberts. 2011. Smoking cessation support delivered via mobile phone text messaging (txt2stop): A single-blind, randomised trial. *Lancet* 378(9785):49-55.

Fremont, A. M., P. D. Cleary, J. Lee Hargraves, R. M. Rowe, N. B. Jacobson, and J. Z. Ayanian. 2001. Patient centered processes of care and long term outcomes of myocardial infarction. *Journal of General Internal Medicine* 16(12):800-808.

Frosch, D. L., S. G. May, K. A. Rendle, C. Tietbohl, and G. Elwyn. 2012. Authoritarian physicians and patients' fear of being labeled 'difficult' among key obstacles to shared decision making. *Health Affairs (Millwood)* 31(5):1030-1038.

Gao, G. G., J. S. McCullough, R. Agarwal, and A. K. Jha. 2012. A changing landscape of physician quality reporting: Analysis of patients' online ratings of their physicians over a 5-year period. *Journal of Medical Internet Research* 14(1):e38.

Garrido, T., L. Jamieson, Y. Zhou, A. Wiesenthal, and L. Liang. 2005. Effect of electronic health records in ambulatory care: Retrospective, serial, cross sectional study. *British Medical Journal* 330(7491):581.

Glickman, S. W., W. Boulding, M. Manary, R. Staelin, M. T. Roe, R. J. Wolosin, E. M. Ohman, E. D. Peterson, and K. A. Schulman. 2010. Patient satisfaction and its relationship with clinical quality and inpatient mortality in acute myocardial infarction. *Circulation: Cardiovascular Quality and Outcomes* 3(2):188-195.

Goetzel, R. Z., T. R. Juday, and R. J. Ozminkowski. 1999. What's the ROI? A systematic review of return on investment (ROI) studies of corporate health and productivity management initiatives. *AWHP's Worksite Health* 6(3):12-21.

Goetzel, R. Z., D. Shechter, R. J. Ozminkowski, P. F. Marmet, M. J. Tabrizi, and E. C. Roemer. 2007. Promising practices in employer health and productivity management efforts: Findings from a benchmarking study. *Journal of Occupational and Environmental Medicine* 49(2):111-130.

Golomb, B. A., J. J. McGraw, M. A. Evans, and J. E. Dimsdale. 2007. Physician response to patient reports of adverse drug effects: Implications for patient-targeted adverse effect surveillance. *Drug Safety* 30(8):669-675.

Gray, B. M., W. Weng, and E. S. Holmboe. 2011. An assessment of patient-based and practice infrastructure-based measures of the patient-centered medical home: Do we need to ask the patient? *Health Services Research* 47(1, Pt. 1):4-21.

Groene, O. 2011. Patient centeredness and quality improvement efforts in hospitals: Rationale, measurement, implementation. *International Journal for Quality in Health Care* 23(5):531-537.

Guevara, J. P., F. M. Wolf, C. M. Grum, and N. M. Clark. 2003. Effects of educational interventions for self management of asthma in children and adolescents: Systematic review and meta-analysis. *British Medical Journal* 326(7402):1308.

Halamka, J. D., K. D. Mandl, and P. C. Tang. 2008. Early experiences with personal health records. *Journal of the American Medical Informatics Association* 15(1):1-7.

Heritage, J., J. D. Robinson, M. N. Elliott, M. Beckett, and M. Wilkes. 2007. Reducing patients' unmet concerns in primary care: The difference one word can make. *Journal of General Internal Medicine* 22(10):1429-1433.

HHS (U.S. Department of Health and Human Services). 2010. *Multiple chronic conditions—a strategic framework: Optimum health and quality of life for individuals with multiple chronic conditions*. Washington, DC: HHS.

Hibbard, J. H. 2004. Moving toward a more patient-centered health care delivery system. *Health Affairs (Millwood)* (Suppl. Variation):VAR133-135.

Hibbard, J. H., J. Stockard, E. R. Mahoney, and M. Tusler. 2004. Development of the Patient Activation Measure (PAM): Conceptualizing and measuring activation in patients and consumers. *Health Services Research* 39(4, Pt. 1):1005-1026.

Hibbard, J. H., E. R. Mahoney, R. Stock, and M. Tusler. 2007. Do increases in patient activation result in improved self-management behaviors? *Health Services Research* 42(4):1443-1463.

Hibbard, J. H., J. Greene, and M. Tusler. 2009. Improving the outcomes of disease management by tailoring care to the patient's level of activation. *American Journal of Managed Care* 15(6):353-360.

Hudon, C., M. Fortin, J. L. Haggerty, M. Lambert, and M. E. Poitras. 2011. Measuring patients' perceptions of patient-centered care: A systematic review of tools for family medicine. *Annals of Family Medicine* 9(2):155-164.

Hurley, R. E., P. S. Keenan, G. R. Martsolf, D. D. Maeng, and D. P. Scanlon. 2009. Early experiences with consumer engagement initiatives to improve chronic care. *Health Affairs (Millwood)* 28(1):277-283.

Institute for Patient- and Family-Centered Care. 2011. *Frequently asked questions.* http://www.ipfcc.org/faq.html (accessed November 11, 2011).

IOM (Institute of Medicine). 1997. *Improving health in the community: A role for performance monitoring.* Washington, DC: National Academy Press.

IOM. 2001. *Crossing the quality chasm: A new health system for the 21st century.* Washington, DC: National Academy Press.

IOM. 2003. *Priority areas for national action: Transforming health care quality.* Washington, DC: The National Academies Press.

IOM. 2004. *Health literacy: A prescription to end confusion.* Washington, DC: The National Academies Press.

IOM. 2009. *The public health effects of food deserts: Workshop summary.* Washington, DC: The National Academies Press.

IOM. 2010. *Value in health care: Accounting for cost, quality, safety, outcomes, and innovation: Workshop summary.* Washington, DC: The National Academies Press.

IOM. 2011a. *Clinical data as the basic staple of health learning: Workshop summary.* Washington, DC: The National Academies Press.

IOM. 2011b. *For the public's health: The role of measurement in action and accountability.* Washington, DC: The National Academies Press.

IOM. 2011c. *For the public's health: Revitalizing law and policy to meet new challenges.* Washington, DC: The National Academies Press.

IOM. 2011d. *Patients charting the course: Citizen engagement in the learning health system: Workshop summary.* Washington, DC: The National Academies Press.

IOM. 2012a. *For the public's health: Investing in a healthier future.* Washington, DC: The National Academies Press.

IOM. 2012b. *Primary care and public health: Exploring integration to improve population health.* Washington, DC: The National Academies Press.

Jencks, S. F., M. V. Williams, and F. A. Coleman. 2009. Rehospitalizations among patients in the Medicare fee-for-service program. *New England Journal of Medicine* 360(14):1418-1428.

Johnson, B., M. Abraham, J. Conway, L. Simmons, S. Edgman-Levitan, P. Sodomka, J. Schlucter, and D. Ford. 2008. *Partnering with patients and families to design a patient- and family-centered health care system: Recommendations and promising practices.* Bethesda, MD: Institute for Family-Centered Care and Institute for Healthcare Improvement.

Johnson, F. R., B. Hauber, S. Ozdemir, C. A. Siegel, S. Hass, and B. E. Sands. 2010. Are gastroenterologists less tolerant of treatment risks than patients? Benefit-risk preferences in Crohn's disease management. *Journal of Managed Care Pharmacy* 16(8):616-628.

Jones, C. A., L. T. Clement, T. Morphew, K. Y. Kwong, J. Hanley-Lopez, F. Lifson, L. Opas, and J. J. Guterman. 2007. Achieving and maintaining asthma control in an urban pediatric disease management program: The breathmobile program. *Journal of Allergy and Clinical Immunology* 119(6):1445-1453.

Kaiser Family Foundation. 2011. *Summary of new health reform law.* 2011. Menlo Park, CA: Kaiser Family Foundation.

Kinnersley, P., A. Edwards, K. Hood, N. Cadbury, R. Ryan, H. Prout, D. Owen, F. MacBeth, P. Butow, and C. Butler. 2007. Interventions before consultations for helping patients address their information needs. *Cochrane Database Systematic Reviews* 3(3).

Kogan, D. C. 2011. How Facebook saved my son's life. *Slate.* http://www.slate.com/articles/double_x/doublex/2011/07/how_facebook_saved_my_sons_life.html (accessed May 15, 2012).

Kotelchuck, R., D. Lowenstein, and J. N. Tobin. 2011. Community health centers and community development financial institutions: Joining forces to address determinants of health. *Health Affairs (Millwood)* 30(11):2090-2097.

Lasker, R. D., and Committee on Medicine and Public Health. 1997. *Medicine & public health: The power of collaboration.* New York: The New York Academy of Medicine.

Lee, C. N., R. Dominik, C. A. Levin, M. J. Barry, C. Cosenza, A. M. O'Connor, A. G. Mulley, Jr., and K. R. Sepucha. 2010a. Development of instruments to measure the quality of breast cancer treatment decisions. *Health Expectations* 13(3):258-272.

Lee, C. N., C. S. Hultman, and K. Sepucha. 2010b. Do patients and providers agree about the most important facts and goals for breast reconstruction decisions? *Annals of Plastic Surgery* 64(5):563-566.

Lee, C. N., J. Belkora, Y. Chang, B. Moy, A. Partridge, and K. Sepucha. 2011. Are patients making high-quality decisions about breast reconstruction after mastectomy? *Plastic and Reconstructive Surgery* 127(1):18-26.

Lee, C. N., Y. Chang, N. Adimorah, J. K. Belkora, B. Moy, A. H. Partridge, D. W. Ollila, and K. R. Sepucha. 2012. Decision making about surgery for early-stage breast cancer. *Journal of the American College of Surgeons* 214(1):1-10.

Levinson, W., A. Kao, A. Kuby, and R. A. Thisted. 2005. Not all patients want to participate in decision making. A national study of public preferences. *Journal of General Internal Medicine* 20(6):531-535.

Levinson, W., C. S. Lesser, and R. M. Epstein. 2010. Developing physician communication skills for patient-centered care. *Health Affairs (Millwood)* 29(7):1310-1318.

Linnan, L., M. Bowling, J. Childress, G. Lindsay, C. Blakey, S. Pronk, S. Wieker, and P. Royall. 2008. Results of the 2004 National Worksite Health Promotion Survey. *American Journal of Public Health* 98(8):1503-1509.

Litvak, E., and M. Bisognano. 2011. More patients, less payment: Increasing hospital efficiency in the aftermath of health reform. *Health Affairs (Millwood)* 30(1):76-80.

Litvak, E., P. I. Buerhaus, F. Davidoff, M. C. Long, M. L. McManus, and D. M. Berwick. 2005. Managing unnecessary variability in patient demand to reduce nursing stress and improve patient safety. *Joint Commission Journal on Quality and Patient Safety* 31(6):330-338.

Longtin, Y., H. Sax, L. L. Leape, S. E. Sheridan, L. Donaldson, and D. Pittet. 2010. Patient participation: Current knowledge and applicability to patient safety. *Mayo Clinic Proceedings* 85(1):53-62.

Madden, R., C. Sykes, and T. B. Ustun. 2007. *World Health Organization family of international classifications: Definition, scope and purpose.* Geneva, Switzerland: World Health Organization.

March of Dimes Perinatal Center. 2012. *Peristats.* http://www.marchofdimes.com/peristats/default.aspx (accessed May 15, 2012).

Martin-Misener, R., R. Valaitis, and Strengthening Primary Health Care through Primary Care and Public Health Collaboration Research Team. 2009. *A scoping literature review of collaboration between primary care and public health.* Hamilton, ON: McMaster University.

Maurer, M., P. Dardess, K. L. Carman, K. Frazier, and L. Smeeding. 2012. *Guide to patient and family engagement: Environmental scan report.* Rockville, MD: Agency for Healthcare Research and Quality.

McGinnis, J. M., and W. H. Foege. 1993. Actual causes of death in the United States. *Journal of the American Medical Association* 270(18):2207-2212.

McGinnis, J. M., P. Williams-Russo, and J. R. Knickman. 2002. The case for more active policy attention to health promotion. *Health Affairs (Millwood)* 21(2):78-93.

McKnight, J. L. 1978. Politicizing health care. *Social Policy* 9(3):36-39.

Mead, N., and P. Bower. 2002. Patient-centered consultations and outcomes in primary care: A review of the literature. *Patient Education and Counseling* 48(1):51-61.

Meltzer, D. O., and J. W. Chung. 2010. U.S. trends in hospitalization and generalist physician workforce and the emergence of hospitalists. *Journal of General Internal Medicine* 25(5):453-459.

Meltzer, D., W. G. Manning, J. Morrison, M. N. Shah, L. Jin, T. Guth, and W. Levinson. 2002. Effects of physician experience on costs and outcomes on an academic general medicine service: Results of a trial of hospitalists. *Annals of Internal Medicine* 137(11):866-874.

Merlis, M. 2010. *Accountable care organizations.* http://healthaffairs.org/healthpolicybriefs/brief_pdfs/healthpolicybrief_23.pdf (accessed August 31, 2012).

Mosen, D. M., J. Schmittdiel, J. Hibbard, D. Sobel, C. Remmers, and J. Bellows. 2007. Is patient activation associated with outcomes of care for adults with chronic conditions? *Journal of Ambulatory Care Management* 30(1):21-29.

Naylor, M. D., D. Brooten, R. Campbell, B. S. Jacobsen, M. D. Mezey, M. V. Pauly, and J. S. Schwartz. 1999. Comprehensive discharge planning and home follow-up of hospitalized elders: A randomized clinical trial. *Journal of the American Medical Association* 281(7):613-620.

Naylor, M. D., L. H. Aiken, E. T. Kurtzman, D. M. Olds, and K. B. Hirschman. 2011. The care span: The importance of transitional care in achieving health reform. *Health Affairs (Project Hope)* 30(4):746-754.

Nelson, L. 2012. *Lessons from Medicare's demonstration projects on disease management and care coordination.* Washington, DC: Congressional Budget Office.

Norris, M. 2011. Group prenatal care: Finding strength in numbers. *National Public Radio,* July 13.

NPP (National Priorities Partnership). 2010. *Patient and family engagement.* http://www.nationalprioritiespartnership.org/PriorityDetails.aspx?id=596 (accessed February 18, 2011).

O'Connor, A. M., H. A. Llewellyn-Thomas, and A. B. Flood. 2004. Modifying unwarranted variations in health care: Shared decision making using patient decision aids. *Health Affairs (Millwood)* (Suppl. Variation):VAR63-72.

O'Connor, A. M., D. Stacey, M. J. Barry, N. F. Col, K. B. Eden, V. Entwistle, V. Fiset, M. Holmes-Rovner, S. Khangura, H. Llewellyn-Thomas, and D. R. Rovner. 2007a. Do patient decision aids meet effectiveness criteria of the international patient decision aid standards collaboration? A systematic review and meta-analysis. *Medical Decision Making* 27(5):554-574.

O'Connor, A. M., J. E. Wennberg, F. Legare, H. A. Llewellyn-Thomas, B. W. Moulton, K. R. Sepucha, A. G. Sodano, and J. S. King. 2007b. Toward the "tipping point": Decision aids and informed patient choice. *Health Affairs* 26(3):716-725.

O'Connor, A. M., C. L. Bennett, D. Stacey, M. Barry, N. F. Col, K. B. Eden, V. A. Entwistle, V. Fiset, M. Holmes-Rovner, S. Khangura, H. Llewellyn-Thomas, and D. Rovner. 2009. Decision aids for people facing health treatment or screening decisions. *Cochrane Database of Systematic Reviews* (3):CD001431.

Otani, K., B. Waterman, K. M. Faulkner, S. Boslaugh, and W. C. Dunagan. 2010. How patient reactions to hospital care attributes affect the evaluation of overall quality of care, willingness to recommend, and willingness to return. *Journal of Healthcare Management American College of Healthcare Executives* 55(1):25-37; discussion 38.

Peikes, D., A. Chen, J. Schore, and R. Brown. 2009. Effects of care coordination on hospitalization, quality of care, and health care expenditures among Medicare beneficiaries: 15 randomized trials. *Journal of the American Medical Association* 301(6):603-618.

Ponte, P. R., G. Conlin, J. B. Conway, S. Grant, C. Medeiros, J. Nies, L. Shulman, P. Branowicki, and K. Conley. 2003. Making patient-centered care come alive: Achieving full integration of the patient's perspective. *Journal of Nursing Administration* 33(2):82-90.

President's Commission for the Study of Ethical Problems in Medicine and Biomedical and Behavioral Research. 1982. *Making healthcare decisions*. 6 vols. Vol. 1. Buffalo, NY: W.S. Hein.

Radwin, L. E., H. J. Cabral, and G. Wilkes. 2009. Relationships between patient-centered cancer nursing interventions and desired health outcomes in the context of the health care system. *Research in Nursing & Health* 32(1):4-17.

Rollnick, S., W. R. Miller, and C. Butler. 2008. *Motivational interviewing in health care: Helping patients change behavior (applications of motivational interviewing)*. New York: Guilford Press.

Rowan, M. S., W. Hogg, and P. Huston. 2007. Integrating public health and primary care. *Healthcare Policy* 3(1):e160.

Safran, D. G., D. A. Taira, W. H. Rogers, M. Kosinski, J. E. Ware, Jr., and A. R. Tarlov. 1998. Linking primary care performance to outcomes of care. *Journal of Family Practice* 47(3):213-220.

Schillinger, D., M. Handley, F. Wang, and H. Hammer. 2009. Effects of self-management support on structure, process, and outcomes among vulnerable patients with diabetes. *Diabetes Care* 32(4):559.

Scholle, S. H., P. Torda, D. Peikes, E. Han, and J. Genevro. 2010. *Engaging patients and families in the medical home* (prepared by Mathematica Policy Research under contract no. HHSA290200900019i to2). Rockville, MD: Agency for Healthcare Research and Quality.

Scott, L., T. Morphew, M. E. Bollinger, S. Samuelson, S. Galant, L. Clement, K. O'Cull, F. Jones, and C. A. Jones. 2011. Achieving and maintaining asthma control in inner-city children. *Journal of Allergy and Clinical Immunology* 128(1):56-63.

Sepucha, K. R., F. J. Fowler, and A. G. Mulley. 2004. Policy support for patient-centered care: The need for measurable improvements in decision quality. *Health Affairs (Millwood)* (Suppl. Variation):VAR54-62.

Sepucha, K. R., A. Fagerlin, M. P. Couper, C. A. Levin, E. Singer, and B. J. Zikmund-Fisher. 2010. How does feeling informed relate to being informed? The decisions survey. *Medical Decision Making* 30(Suppl. 5):S77-S84.

Sequist, T. D., E. C. Schneider, M. Anastario, E. G. Odigie, R. Marshall, W. H. Rogers, and D. G. Safran. 2008. Quality monitoring of physicians: Linking patients' experiences of care to clinical quality and outcomes. *Journal of General Internal Medicine* 23(11):1784-1790.

Shaller, D., and The Commonwealth Fund. 2007. *Patient-centered care What does it take?* New York: The Commonwealth Fund.

Silow-Carroll, S., T. Alteras, and L. Stepnick. 2006. *Patient-centered care for underserved populations: Definition and best practices*. Washington, DC: Economic and Social Research Institute.

Skinner, C., and J. Finkelstein. 2008. *Review of mobile phone use in preventive medicine and disease management*. Anaheim, CA: ACTA Press.

Sofaer, S., and K. Firminger. 2005. Patient perceptions of the quality of health services. *Annual Review of Public Health* 26:513-559.

Solberg, L. I., S. E. Asche, L. H. Anderson, K. Sepucha, N. M. Thygeson, J. E. Madden, L. Morrissey, and K. K. Kraemer. 2009. Evaluating preference-sensitive care for uterine fibroids: It's not so simple. *Journal of Women's Health* 18(7):1071-1079.

Solberg, L. I., S. E. Asche, K. Sepucha, N. M. Thygeson, J. E. Madden, L. Morrissey, K. K. Kraemer, and L. H. Anderson. 2010. Informed choice assistance for women making uterine fibroid treatment decisions: A practical clinical trial. *Medical Decision Making* 30(4):444-452.

Springgate, B. F., and R. H. Brook. 2011. Accountable care organizations and community empowerment. *Journal of the American Medical Association* 305(17):1800-1801.

Stacey, D., C. L. Bennett, M. J. Barry, N. F. Col, K. B. Eden, M. Holmes-Rovner, H. Llewellyn-Thomas, A. Lyddiatt, F. Legare, and R. Thomson. 2011. Decision aids for people facing health treatment or screening decisions. *Cochrane Database of Systematic Reviews* (10):CD001431.

Stewart, M. A. 1995. Effective physician-patient communication and health outcomes: A review. *Canadian Medical Association Journal* 152(9):1423.

Stewart, M., J. B. Brown, A. Donner, I. R. McWhinney, J. Oates, W. W. Weston, and J. Jordan. 2000. The impact of patient-centered care on outcomes. *Journal of Family Practice* 49(9):796-804.

Street, R. L., Jr., and P. Haidet. 2011. How well do doctors know their patients? Factors affecting physician understanding of patients' health beliefs. *Journal of General Internal Medicine* 26(1):21-27.

Street, R. L., Jr., G. Makoul, N. K. Arora, and R. M. Epstein. 2009. How does communication heal? Pathways linking clinician-patient communication to health outcomes. *Patient Education and Counseling* 74(3):295-301.

Stremikis, K., C. Schoen, and A.-K. Fryer. 2011. *A call for change: The 2011 Commonwealth Fund survey of public views of the U.S. healthcare system.* Washington, DC: The Commonwealth Fund.

Toussaint, J. 2009. Writing the new playbook for U.S. health care: Lessons from Wisconsin. *Health Affairs (Millwood)* 28(5):1343-1350.

Weingart, S. N., O. Pagovich, D. Z. Sands, J. M. Li, M. D. Aronson, R. B. Davis, D. W. Bates, and R. S. Phillips. 2005. What can hospitalized patients tell us about adverse events? Learning from patient-reported incidents. *Journal of General Internal Medicine* 20(9):830-836.

Weingart, S. N., J. Zhu, L. Chiappetta, S. O. Stuver, E. C. Schneider, A. M. Epstein, J. A. David-Kasdan, C. L. Annas, F. J. Fowler, Jr., and J. S. Weissman. 2011. Hospitalized patients' participation and its impact on quality of care and patient safety. *International Journal for Quality in Health Care* 23(3):269-277.

Weingarten, S. R., J. M. Henning, E. Badamgarav, K. Knight, and V. Hasselblad. 2002. Interventions used in disease management programmes for patients with chronic illness which ones work? Meta-analysis of published reports. *British Medical Journal* 325(7370):925.

Winakur, J. 2012. The transition abyss. *Health Affairs Blog*, June 18. http://healthaffairs.org/blog/2012/01/18/the-transition-abyss/ (accessed August 31, 2012).

Zikmund-Fisher, B. J., M. P. Couper, E. Singer, P. A. Ubel, S. Ziniel, F. J. Fowler, Jr., C. A. Levin, and A. Fagerlin. 2010. Deficits and variations in patients' experience with making 9 common medical decisions: The decisions survey. *Medical Decision Making* 30(Suppl. 5):S85-S95.

8

Achieving and Rewarding
High-Value Care

After starting to feel chest pains, a 52-year-old female nurse went to her primary care physician to be evaluated. Even though her initial physical exam and diagnostic tests indicated there was little probability she had a serious cardiac disease, she received a cardiac computed tomography (CT) scan and coronary angiography for reassurance. During the cardiac catheterization for angiography, her left main coronary artery was torn after the second contrast injection, which required immediate coronary bypass surgery. Following a long hospital stay, the patient's heart was not pumping normally, and she was discharged home to undergo intensive cardiac rehabilitation. After a difficult clinical experience over 6 months, her condition deteriorated, and she underwent coronary angioplasty and therapies to prevent blood clots. Eight weeks later, she was having severe heart problems related to her previous surgeries and required an emergency heart transplant. This case highlights the fact that all tests and interventions have the potential to lead to harm, and illustrates the need for measurement, transparency, and alignment of incentives focused on value (Becker et al., 2011; Redberg, 2011).

Health care payment policies strongly influence how care is delivered, whether new scientific insights and knowledge about best care are diffused broadly, and whether improvement initiatives succeed. As with most aspects of the health care enterprise, a variety of financial incentives and payment models currently are in use. However, most of these models tend to pay clinicians and health care organizations without a specific focus on patient health and value, which has contributed to waste and inefficiency.

Opportunities exist to eliminate wasteful spending while maintaining or enhancing health care quality and improving overall health outcomes. Several health care organizations and health insurers have been leveraging these opportunities to test new models of paying for care and organizing care delivery. Many individual initiatives have demonstrated success, but systematic reviews and studies continue to find conflicting evidence as to which payment models might work best and under what circumstances. While there will likely continue to be a diversity of payment systems, then, the opportunity exists for additional learning on the relative effectiveness of different payment systems with respect to learning. It is clear, however, that high-value care—the best care for the patient, with the optimal result for the circumstances, delivered at the right price—requires that incentives be structured to reward the best outcomes for the patient.

This chapter begins by describing the obstacles that constrain the delivery of high-value care. Next it addresses in turn the measurement of results and value and strategies for achieving transparency. Methods for transitioning to a system that rewards continuous improvement are then discussed. The final section presents recommendations for realizing the vision of a health care system that achieves and rewards high-value care.

OBSTACLES TO HIGH-VALUE CARE

Expenditures on health care are imposing an increasing burden on the budgets of the federal government, state governments, and families without producing commensurate improvements in health or the quality of care. Rather, much of the money spent on health care is wasted, in some cases causing harm. As detailed in Chapter 3, the total amount of waste falls into six broad categories, illustrated in Figure 8-1. Many factors are responsible for this lack of value, from misaligned incentives to a lack of transparency on cost and quality. Overcoming these obstacles will require a determined effort to understand the results achieved from health care; improvements in the structure of and incentives for care; engagement strategies, such as shared decision making, that focus care on patient needs and goals (see Chapter 7); and changes in health care culture needed to support these initiatives (the subject of Chapter 9).

Financial incentives play an important role in the way the health care system learns (see Chapter 6 for a discussion of the factors affecting the spread of knowledge in health care). They create the economic reality for providers and strongly influence how care is delivered (Flodgren et al., 2011; Halvorson, 2009; Hillman, 1991; IOM, 2001). For example,

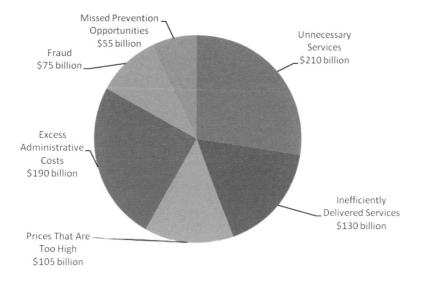

FIGURE 8-1 Sources of waste and excess costs in health care.
SOURCE: Data derived from IOM, 2010b.

clinicians who are paid for each service tend to recommend more visits and services than clinicians who are paid under other methods (Gosden et al., 2000; Helmchen and Lo Sasso, 2010; Hickson et al., 1987). In one study, when primary care physicians began to be paid for each procedure and encounter, the number of procedures increased, and the number of encounters increased from 11 to 61 percent depending on the specialty (Helmchen and Lo Sasso, 2010).

As with many other aspects of the health care enterprise, a variety of financial incentives and payment models are currently in use. Some are modeled on a fee-for-service structure and some on a capitated or global payment system; other models exist as well. The most common models for both public and private plans tend to pay clinicians based on the volume of individual procedures and tests. Higher-quality care rarely is rewarded by payment and contracting policies, so there is little relationship between the cost or price of care and the quality and outcomes of the care provided (Fisher et al., 2003; Office of Attorney General of Massachusetts, 2011; Yasaitis et al., 2009). One study found, on average, only a 4.3 percent correlation (as measured by a coefficient of determination) between the quality of care delivered and the price of the medical service; indeed, higher prices often were associated with lower quality (Office of Attorney General of Massachusetts, 2011).

Several common payment systems can promote greater use of care. When each service generates additional revenue, there is a strong economic incentive for clinicians and health care organizations to provide more interventions and diagnostic procedures, treat with greater intensity, and care for more patients. At the same time, focusing payment on services discourages providers from undertaking other important activities that could improve a patient's health, such as spending more time talking with the patient, counseling about prevention, communicating by e-mail or telephone, coordinating care across providers, and spending time with family members.

Financial incentives can either aid or inhibit the success of organizational initiatives to improve quality and value (Mandel, 2010; Robinson et al., 2009). Many current payment models can serve as a disincentive for provider organizations seeking to implement high-quality care protocols, given that they may see lower revenues as a result of performing fewer services. This trade-off is exemplified by the experience of one nonprofit health care organization that implemented a program to improve care for back pain. Under its improvement program, the organization changed the care it delivered at its spine clinic to begin with physical therapy, reserving magnetic resonance imaging (MRI) and intensive evaluation for patients with complex cases. The protocol accorded with several evidence-based guidelines; imaging for lower back pain often is overused as an early diagnostic tool when it is unlikely to improve outcomes (Good Stewardship Working Group, 2011). After implementing the protocol, the organization found that patient waiting times were reduced, outcomes improved, and overall costs were low. Under the current payment system, however, the institution was paid for high-cost imaging studies, which it was conducting less frequently, but it was not paid for inexpensive follow-up care such as telephone consultations, which it was conducting more often. As a result, the organization began to lose money. To sustain the improvement initiative, it had to negotiate with local insurers and employers to establish a new payment system for back pain (Blackmore et al., 2011; Fuhrmans, 2007). Box 8-1 provides another example of the disjunction between evidence-based practice and current payment models.

Finally, most current incentive structures fail to distinguish among those treatments that are highly effective for patients with a particular condition, such as aspirin for heart attack patients or antibiotics for treating bacterial infections; those that are effective for some patients but are administered to patients for whom they are ineffective; and those of questionable effectiveness for most patients. Whereas treatments that are generally effective and applied appropriately account for a small fraction of the health care system's total cost growth, the latter two categories of treatments incur substantial costs (Baicker and Chandra, 2011; Chandra and Skinner, 2011).

BOX 8-1
Waste in Health Care:
The Underuse and Overuse of Screening Colonoscopy

The case of colonoscopy screening illustrates the disjunction between evidence and current payment models. Summarizing the current evidence on colorectal cancer screening, the U.S. Preventive Services Task Force (USPSTF) recommends regular screening for colorectal cancer for adults aged 50 to 75, using a fecal occult blood test (FOBT), sigmoidoscopy, or colonoscopy. The USPSTF notes that routine colonoscopies should be repeated only every 10 years, advises against routine screening of adults aged 76 to 85, and discourages any screening for patients older than 85 (USPSTF, 2008). These recommendations reflect the balance between clinical benefits of screening and the potential for the procedure to result in serious harm, such as colon perforation and adverse cardiovascular events, especially among older patients (Warren et al., 2009).

However, current use of colonoscopy frequently strays from these evidence-based recommendations. Only 65 percent of adults aged 50 to 75 receive the recommended colorectal cancer screenings (CDC, 2011). Yet, overuse occurs as well. Among Medicare patients, almost one-quarter repeat the test within 7 years instead of the recommended 10, with no demonstrated clinical rationale for doing so. The portion of patients repeating the test early remains high for those older than 75, 17 percent of whom repeat the test within 7 years without a clinical indication. These trends occur despite the USPSTF recommendations, as well as Medicare regulations that limit payment for screening colonoscopy to once every 10 years (Goodwin et al., 2011).

Conclusion 8-1: The prevailing approach to paying for health care, based predominantly on individual services and products, encourages wasteful and ineffective care.

Related findings.

- *Clinicians who are paid for each service tend to recommend more visits and services than those who are paid under other payment methods.* In one study, the initiation of encounter- and procedure-based payment for primary care led to an increased number of encounters and procedures, with visits increasing from 11 to 61 percent depending on the specialty.
- *The current payment model does not reward quality.* One study found, on average, only a 4.3 percent correlation between the quality of care delivered and the price of the medical service; indeed, higher prices often were associated with lower quality.

MEASUREMENT OF RESULTS AND VALUE

One important tool for improving the value of health care is having a reliable method for defining the value of different interventions, innovations, and care practices. In simple terms, value is the level of benefit achieved for a given cost. However, this concept is complicated by the fact that the perceived benefits of a particular intervention, diagnostic technology, or process will vary for each stakeholder in the health care system (Hussey et al., 2009; IOM, 2010b). Given the system's clear imperative to focus on the patient (see Chapter 7), value measurement for a particular intervention needs to consider improvements in patient health (length of life, health status), patient quality of life, the patient's sense of well-being, quality of care (technical and with respect to compassion), and population health (overall and among different groups). In considering the cost component, a comprehensive measure of value would include all financial resources devoted to the particular treatment for the patient's medical condition, as well as potential adverse outcomes. The definition of cost is further complicated by the fact that different stakeholders have different perspectives on costs—patients may consider out-of-pocket costs, hospitals may look at production costs, and payers may review the medical loss ratio—and each perspective raises additional methodological issues (Fishman and Hornbrook, 2009; Hussey et al., 2009; IOM, 2010b).

One major difficulty in measuring value is finding metrics that can accurately quantify performance with available data. These performance measurement challenges range from providing adequate statistical accuracy to adjusting the measures to account for differences in patient populations (see Table 8-1). Another issue is ensuring the availability of adequate high-quality data with which to calculate the performance metric. Current measures often rely on administrative and claims data; unfortunately, administrative data sources frequently lack information identifying the patient's underlying clinical condition and indicating whether patient care was delivered according to best practices (Devoe et al., 2011; Tang et al., 2007). The increasing use of interoperable electronic health records, which contain detailed information on care processes, may address these shortcomings and yield further improvements in clinical performance measurement.

Another challenge to performance measurement is the fact that individual clinicians often see few patients for any given performance measure, which can cause two similar clinicians to have very different performance scores. The statistical accuracy of these measurements can be further reduced if they are calculated from claims data, because each health plan collects and maintains its claims data separately (Landon and Normand, 2008; Landon et al., 2003; Scholle et al., 2008, 2009). One strategy for improving the reliability of performance metrics is to combine data from multiple

TABLE 8-1 Challenges Faced in Developing Metrics for Assessing Value

Measurement Challenge	Questions to Consider
Attribution	How can patient health outcomes be attributed to a specific provider or health care organization, especially for chronic care management?
Data sources	Can this metric be calculated from existing electronic health records or related clinical data sources?
Statistical accuracy	For the average provider or health care organization, will there be a sufficient number of patients with which to estimate this performance metric with adequate confidence for use in a payment mechanism?
Tailoring of care	Does the metric exclude patients who, based on clinical practice guidelines, should not receive the care?
Risk adjustment	Can the performance metrics be properly adjusted for different patient populations with different risk factors, demographics, and health conditions?
Setting benchmarks	Do sufficient data exist with which to establish a performance benchmark for this metric?

SOURCE: Adapted with permission from Schneider et al., 2011.

health plans, which has shown success in pilot experiments conducted in Colorado, Florida, and Wisconsin (Higgins et al., 2011b; Toussaint et al., 2011). Further efforts to ensure accuracy are necessary to build buy-in from providers and organizations for the goals of these measures.

Another outstanding issue is the need to ensure that performance metrics are linked to patient health outcomes. In some cases, process measures have been found to correlate poorly with clinical outcomes, such as in the case of heart failure (Fonarow et al., 2007). Moreover, there is concern that if performance metrics were applied, providers would focus on the specific processes that were defined as high-quality to the exclusion of other important, but difficult to measure, aspects of care (IOM, 2007; Werner and Asch, 2007). Effective metrics that drive improvement are defined by four characteristics: solid evidence that the measured process leads to improved health outcomes, certainty that the metric records whether the desired care has been delivered, close linkage between the process and the desired health outcome, and limited adverse consequences (Chassin et al., 2010). Metrics also must be updated frequently to accord with changes in knowledge over time; the goal is to ensure that metrics reward clinical care that agrees with the currently available evidence. Standards-setting organizations, such as the National Quality Forum (NQF), and measurement organizations, such as the National Committee for Quality Assurance (NCQA), are currently working to improve the accuracy, utility, and application of performance metrics.

Instead of focusing on processes, some metrics are drawn directly from patient health outcomes. A motivation for this strategy is the fact that what matters to patients is the outcome of their care—the effect of their care on the length of their life, their quality of life, and their overall functioning and well-being. One of the difficulties of this model is accurately measuring outcomes that are relevant for patients rather than limiting assessments to what can be easily measured and ensuring that care decisions flow from patient needs, goals, and circumstances (see Chapter 7 for a discussion of patients' perceptions and needs in maintaining their health and shared decision-making frameworks). For instance, while mortality can be quantified simply, it provides only a limited picture of the total value a patient receives from a given intervention.

After identifying the metrics that best quantify health outcomes, the next challenge is attributing the effect of a given treatment or the actions of a given provider to these metrics. Some treatments, such as surgical procedures, often allow for closer linkages between a procedure and its outcomes, while others, notably chronic care management, have longer time lags between the provision of care and its ultimate outcomes. For chronic care, the patient's health depends on years, or even decades, of medical treatments, with many providers being involved in the care process. In addition, worse health outcomes often are associated with factors outside the traditional health care system, such as diet and smoking (McGinnis and Foege, 1993). Assessing the value of care based on outcomes for patients with chronic conditions will therefore require a hybrid strategy that involves evaluating both care processes and health outcomes so value metrics can accurately assess the care provided.

STRATEGIES FOR ACHIEVING TRANSPARENCY

Measurement itself is only part of the improvement process. Transparency on results supplies data that clinicians can use for improvement initiatives, provides information that patients and consumers can use to select care and providers, and draws attention to high-value health care providers and organizations (IOM, 2006, 2010a). Some of the earliest such efforts include New York State's initiative to report the mortality and complications associated with coronary artery bypass graft surgery and the Health Care Financing Administration's (HCFA's) reporting of hospital mortality (Berwick and Wald, 1990; Hannan et al., 1994). Since these initial efforts, multiple reporting systems have been introduced, from the Healthcare

Effectiveness Data and Information Set (HEDIS) for health plans to the Centers for Medicare & Medicaid Services' (CMS') initiatives on comparing the quality of hospitals and health care providers (Friedberg and Damberg, 2012; NCQA, 2011; O'Neil et al., 2010).

Public reporting has been correlated with improved performance on those measures reported and has encouraged organizations to undertake improvement activities (Hafner et al., 2011; Hibbard et al., 2003, 2005a). For instance, the Joint Commission found that compliance with best practices, such as the administration and discontinuation of prophylactic antibiotics for selected surgical patients, increased dramatically after the metric was publicly reported (Chassin et al., 2010); the rates of compliance with the Joint Commission's pneumonia care composite metric rose from 72 percent to 95 percent in 8 years (Joint Commission, 2011). Similarly, after CMS released measurements of the quality of heart attack care, improvements such as lower mortality, reduced lengths of stay, and reduced readmissions soon followed (Werner and Bradlow, 2006, 2010). Based on these and related successes, many health care opinion leaders believe increased transparency is an important factor in improving the overall performance of the health care system (Stremikis et al., 2010).

One channel through which transparency can improve health care quality and value is by affecting the selection of providers and health care organizations. In every community, hospitals and physician practices are delivering both high- and low-value care. Patients, however, are not equipped with the tools needed to identify organizations that provide high-quality, high-value care. The public often has more information when making decisions about purchasing consumer goods, such as refrigerators or televisions, than when making decisions about health care.

An aim of public reporting and improved transparency is to remedy this lack of information. By drawing attention to high-value providers and organizations, public reporting can affect the number of patients who choose to visit a given clinician or health care organization, thereby providing a business case for improving value (IOM, 2006, 2010a; Werner et al., 2010). One tool for drawing additional attention to high-value providers and organizations is the use of tiered benefit plans, which have lower patient cost sharing for those providers deemed to be of higher quality (an example is described in Box 8-2). By coupling reporting with financial incentives, these types of plans may drive greater patient volume to providers and organizations that offer higher-value care. Such benefit structures highlight the need for accurate measurement of care value.

Today, however, few consumers use publicly reported information to make decisions about clinicians or health care organizations; a 2008 survey found that only 14 percent of respondents had seen and used comparative quality information about health plans, clinicians, or health care

---

BOX 8-2
Making Information on Quality Accessible to Consumers

Although accessible information exists to support consumer purchasing for most goods and services, few comprehensive resources are available for comparing the quality of health care providers and hospitals. One effort aimed at expanding the amount of such information is the getbettermaine.org initiative, sponsored by the Maine Health Management Coalition in partnership with the Maine Quality Forum, Maine Quality Counts, the Maine Health Access Foundation, and the Robert Wood Johnson Foundation. The goal of this initiative is to provide patients and consumers with easily accessible information on care quality for various providers and hospitals in the state. Provider and hospital participation, which is voluntary, has been high, with all Maine hospitals and about 70 percent of the state's physicians participating. This information is being leveraged in the design of health insurance benefits through value-based insurance design. Insurance benefits for state employees provide lower deductibles and copays for the use of providers and care settings deemed of high quality by the initiative, which can encourage providers and hospitals to consider their care quality measures (Richardson, 2011).

---

organizations in the past year (Kaiser Family Foundation, 2008). Many Americans choose health care providers based on the advice of friends, relatives, and coworkers or on recommendations from a current provider or their health plan (Blendon et al., 2011; Kaiser Family Foundation, 2011; Tu and Lauer, 2008). One reason for the low usage of publicly reported information is that many consumers believe care quality does not vary significantly among different health care organizations and different clinicians, which limits their motivation to make use of independent quality assessments. Moreover, many current reporting efforts use language and presentation formats that impede consumers' ability to use them for making decisions (Hibbard and Peters, 2003; Hibbard and Sofaer, 2010; Hibbard et al., 2002; Vaiana and McGlynn, 2002). Finally, consumers are heterogeneous in their use of publicly reported information, with usage varying based on demographic and socioeconomic factors. Thus the presentation and content of public reports need to be tailored to individual characteristics (Kolstad and Chernew, 2009).

Reporting also offers opportunities for clinicians to improve the quality of the care they provide by giving them more information on their current performance (Berwick et al., 2003). This type of information fills a critical need, because most physicians lack data on the care provided in their own practice, from their own rates of hospital readmissions to when their patients return to work. Without a baseline, clinicians cannot know whether their practices are improving. Reporting this type of information focuses attention on a specific quality issue and may support physicians and organizations in efforts to improve their practices (Porter, 2010). Other efforts, using voluntary reporting initiatives, sponsored by medical specialty societies or an integrated delivery system, have shown promise in providing information that clinicians can use for quality improvement activities (Ferguson et al., 2003; Grover et al., 2001).

A final means by which transparency may lead to improvement is by impacting a provider's or health care organization's reputation (Hibbard et al., 2005b). In a hospital reporting initiative in Wisconsin, hospitals indicated their belief that the report would affect their public reputation, although not patient volume (Hibbard et al., 2003). This concern appeared to motivate hospitals to undertake quality improvement initiatives.

Although reporting and transparency have had demonstrated impacts on clinical behavior, limited evidence exists about their overall impact on value. Studies and systematic reviews of the public reporting literature suggest that reporting of performance data stimulates quality improvement activities, especially at hospitals, but the impact on effectiveness, safety, and patient-centeredness remains unknown (Fung et al., 2008; Smith et al., 2012). Moreover, recent studies have shown limited effects of public reporting on the quality of care processes or health outcomes, such as mortality, suggesting that there are opportunities for improvement in designing and implementing transparency initiatives to produce optimal results (Ryan et al., 2012; Tu et al., 2009).

Improving transparency initiatives will require action on multiple fronts. First, there is a need to increase alignment among different transparency initiatives. Many reporting efforts are currently under way, each measuring different aspects of care delivery; this multiplicity can confuse consumers and limit impact (Rothberg et al., 2008). Second, there is concern that transparency initiatives may exacerbate health care disparities, as organizations and providers in geographic areas with limited resources may have less ability to undertake improvement efforts (Casalino et al., 2007). Finally, reporting requires that health care practices incur costs for establishing metrics in their data systems, for maintaining the data, and for entering data during each patient visit (Halladay et al., 2009). Although further work is needed to improve the practical implementation of transparency and minimize negative consequences, greater transparency is necessary to provide the information needed to promote continuous learning and improvement.

There also are specific issues to consider when transparency initiatives focus on cost, seeking to increase public knowledge and allow consumers to engage in cost-conscious shopping and thereby stimulate competition on cost and quality (Sinaiko and Rosenthal, 2011). The health care market is unusual in that the prices for services are largely confidential. Several aspects of the health care market make cost information difficult to obtain. These include health care factors such as the fragmented billing of different providers for an episode of care, the difficulty of predicting the services that will be provided during an episode of care, and varying insurance benefit structures, as well as legal factors such as antitrust law, contractual obligations between insurers and providers, and hesitancy to disclose negotiated rates (Government Accountability Office, 2011a).

Additional challenges facing this type of reporting include the common perception that higher-cost care is higher-quality, limited provider competition in some geographic areas, and differences between prices for procedures and overall health care costs (Ginsburg, 2007; Hibbard et al., 2012; Tu and Lauer, 2009). While there is significant interest in overcoming these barriers to improve the transparency of cost information, such transparency initiatives have been implemented in few places, and their effectiveness remains unclear (Government Accountability Office, 2011a). Nonetheless, evidence demonstrates that transparency can focus employer and policy attention on price differences (Tu and Lauer, 2009). Increased penetration of high-deductible health plans also may encourage greater use of reported information, although this will require that the information be available in an understandable format and customizable for a particular patient's situation.

Conclusion 8-2: Transparency of process, outcome, price, and cost information, both within health care and with patients and the public, has untapped potential to support continuous learning and improvement in patient experience, outcomes, and cost and the delivery of high-value care.

Related findings:

- *Reporting and transparency improve performance in certain circumstances.* Following public reporting of pneumonia care measures, for example, rates of compliance rose from 72 percent to 95 percent in 8 years.
- *Reporting and transparency provide clinicians with information they want and need.* Results of one initiative indicated that coupling financial incentives with assistance to clinicians in monitoring their practice patterns against those of others decreased spending growth by 2 percent per quarter while improving overall care quality.

THE PATH TO A SYSTEM THAT PAYS FOR
CONTINUOUS IMPROVEMENT

To address the current flawed payment system, it is necessary to ensure that financial incentives promote quality care and patient health. Health care organizations and private health plans have been testing new models of care delivery; many of these innovations have shown initial success in improving quality and value (Higgins et al., 2011a; Milstein and Gilbertson, 2009; Song et al., 2011). Similarly, the Patient Protection and Affordable Care Act of 2010 has created opportunities to explore pilot delivery models, such as through the Center for Medicare & Medicaid Innovation, and established several new models for Medicare and Medicaid payment, such as the formation of accountable care organizations (Thorpe and Ogden, 2010). Both private and public innovations in health care payment offer opportunities to transition the health care system toward one characterized by continuous improvement. One example is described in Box 8-3.

There are multiple methods for transitioning health care incentives from the current system toward one that rewards value (Table 8-2). These methods may build on existing models, such as by adding incentives for care coordination or shared decision making to procedure-based payment. Another approach entails policies on coverage with evidence development, which are focused on incorporating new treatments and technologies into payment policies while building an evidence base on their effectiveness. More fundamental shifts include global payment systems that provide clinicians with a single payment for all the care needed by a given patient (with some versions adjusting for patient health status and other factors, as well as including incentives for improved patient outcomes). These incentive models also differ in whether they target changing provider or consumer behavior. Table 8-2 does not include all strategies for improving value; for instance, conditions of participation in an insurance plan could be a strong motivation for changing provider behavior. However, the table does highlight the breadth of payment and delivery system organization models currently under consideration.

Properly designed financial incentives can improve the quality of care and its outcomes (Conrad and Perry, 2009). As noted in the Institute of Medicine (IOM) report *Rewarding Provider Performance: Aligning Incentives in Medicare,* however, an evidence base does not yet exist for determining which type of payment strategy would best improve care quality (IOM, 2007). Since the publication of that report, systematic reviews and studies have continued to find conflicting evidence on which payment models best improve the quality and value of care delivered by individual clinicians and through health care organizations (Government Accountability Office, 2011b; Petersen et al., 2006; Rosenthal, 2008; Scott et al., 2011;

BOX 8-3
Innovations in Health Care Payment:
The Alternative Quality Contract

Blue Cross Blue Shield of Massachusetts established the Alternative Quality Contract (AQC) in January 2009, combining two forms of payment to providers. The program provides a global payment to cover all care services for a given patient—primary care, specialty care, hospital care, prescription drugs, and other services. The global payment, adjusted for age, sex, and health status, is negotiated in a 5-year contract. This time frame, which is longer than that of most payment contracts, allows providers to make investments that permit them to change their care practices over time. Additionally, the program includes payment incentives of up to 10 percent of the global budget tied to performance measures.

The provider groups in the program receive technical support, such as reports on spending, utilization, and quality. As noted earlier in this chapter, providers often lack such information about their panel of patients, which hinders many improvement efforts and limits the ability to manage a patient's care. The program also shares data on variations in practice patterns for many common conditions, such as back pain and gastroesophageal reflux disease, and use of procedures, such as advanced imaging, allowing individual providers to learn how other clinicians are treating similar conditions.

Currently, the AQC includes only patients in health maintenance organization (HMO) or point of service (POS) plans. Initial results suggest that the program was associated with modest reductions in the growth of medical costs (2 percent per quarter) and improved quality in its first year. Further, all of the groups participating in the AQC earned quality bonuses in the first year. In interviews, the participating medical groups said they have focused on building their infrastructure for primary care providers, managing referrals, and improving their data management capabilities. While initial results are promising, further research will be needed to understand whether this type of plan can reduce long-term growth in health spending while improving overall care quality.

SOURCES: Chernew et al., 2011; Mechanic et al., 2011; Song et al., 2011.

Werner et al., 2011). Because the ideal payment model is unknown, there is an opportunity for additional learning and for building an evidence base on what works best.

As part of the learning process for discovering the ideal payment model, it is important to consider the differing impacts of a particular value initiative on different organizations and clinicians. Because organizations vary, a given intervention will work better in some environments than in others (Government Accountability Office, 2011b). For instance, some providers can bear greater levels of financial risk than others, which impacts their ability to accept payment methods such as bundled and global payments

TABLE 8-2 Selected List of Payment Policies and Delivery System Reforms That Change the Method for Recognizing High-Value Care

Payment Strategy	Program	Summary
Incentives for Process	Payment for shared decision making	Incentive payments are provided for clinicians that use validated patient decision aids and other shared decision-making tools, with the aim of encouraging the consideration of patient needs, values, goals, and preferences in clinical decisions.
	Incentives for disease management/ incentives for coordination	A payer makes additional payments to a provider for care coordination activities.
Penalties for Unwanted Outcomes	Penalties for health care–acquired conditions	A payer applies financial disincentives to clinicians or hospitals for conditions that are acquired in the course of care, such as infections or "never" events (e.g., preventable falls, medical errors).
	Penalties for potential preventable hospital readmissions	A payer financially penalizes a hospital for potentially avoidable readmissions within a set time frame (such as 30 days).
Payment Methods That Share Accountability	Value-based purchasing/pay for performance	Providers or hospitals are rewarded based on performance, which can be defined in multiple ways, including adhering to a specified process, avoiding overuse, or improving a given health outcome.
	Gain sharing/ performance-based risk sharing	Savings (and potentially excess costs) are shared between stakeholder groups, such as hospitals and physicians, hospitals and payers, physicians and payers, or other combinations.
	Bundled payment	For a given condition or clinical episode, the payment is bundled into a single, comprehensive payment that covers all services involved in the patient's care.
	Global payment	A single payment covers all services provided to a patient population during a defined time period. This model shares features of capitation, although it often includes adjustments for performance and patient risk.

continued

TABLE 8-2 Continued

Payment Strategy	Program	Summary
	Accountable care organizations	Groups of providers voluntarily assume responsibility for the care of a population of patients and share savings if they meet specified quality and cost performance benchmarks.
	Medical homes	A medical home provides comprehensive primary care services to a population of patients, with responsibilities to coordinate care, provide whole-person care, and ensure timely access to care.
Consumer-Directed Payment Methods	Value-based insurance design	The premise of this type of insurance design is to align benefits (coverage levels, co-payments, deductibles) with the demonstrated value of treatments and diagnostics. Most current plans of this type have been limited to prescription drugs.
	Tiered networks	A variant of value-based insurance design, a tiered network plan varies the cost sharing for providers and hospitals based on their tier. Tiers are determined according to providers' quality or value as measured or determined by the health plan.
	Consumer-directed health plans	Consumer-directed plans generally couple high deductibles with a health savings account, with the goal of increasing consumer price sensitivity.

(Office of Attorney General of Massachusetts, 2011). Similarly, it is important to understand potential adverse effects of a given incentive structure on clinicians (Kurtzman et al., 2011).

A second challenge is the need to understand how different incentive structures affect patients. Many payers have developed financial incentives specifically focused on patients and consumers, including consumer-directed health plans, employer wellness programs, and value-based insurance design. As an example, value-based insurance design models configure benefit design (such as co-payments, clinician networks, and deductibles) to encourage patient and consumer use of high-value services. Such models have shown potential in several cases, although obstacles still exist to their widespread adoption (Chernew et al., 2010; Fendrick et al., 2009, 2010). For these types of models to be successful, it is necessary to understand how patients actually respond to financial incentives. Current evidence shows that increasing overall cost sharing for patients often lowers the consumption of both effective and ineffective care (Baicker and Goldman, 2011; Beeuwkes Buntin et al., 2011; Chandra et al., 2010; Chernew et al., 2008; Choudhry et al., 2010b; Hsu et al., 2006; Manning et al., 1987).

One field of study that has substantial relevance to understanding the effect of different incentive structures is behavioral economics (Volpp et al., 2008a). This field has shown that people's responses to different incentive structures may depart, sometimes dramatically so, from the predictions of traditional economics and its conception of the ideal decision maker (Loewenstein et al., 2012). While people respond differently from traditional theories, however, they do react according to several common pathways, including loss aversion, optimism bias, and a bias toward the present (Volpp et al., 2009b). To translate the impact of one of these factors, the fact that most people focus on the present means that incentives with the same frequency as the desired actions are more likely to be effective; a monthly or yearly incentive, for example, will not effectively motivate daily action (Volpp et al., 2008b, 2011). In applying these principles to practice, special consideration should be given to customizing incentives to different populations to ensure their effectiveness (Choudhry et al., 2010a, 2011; Volpp et al., 2009a).

Another challenge faced in developing patient incentives is ensuring that patients have the tools necessary to take advantage of the incentives. Many consumer-focused payment models require that consumers estimate their out-of-pocket costs for their specific situation and under different benefit plans. New tools, such as calculators supplied by large employers and health plans, have been developed to make this task easier. Ensuring that information on health care costs is understandable to a broad audience is key to several new initiatives, such as the proposed standardized summary of insurance benefits (Quincy, 2011).

Payment policies and incentives may need to take into account the heterogeneity of patient health care usage. In 2008, the half of the population with the lowest expenditures accounted for 3.1 percent of total health care costs, while (as noted in Chapter 2) the 5 percent of patients with the highest expenditures accounted for 50 percent of the total (Cohen and Yu, 2011). This concentration of care among a small number of patients has encouraged new initiatives designed to focus efforts on patients with the greatest health care needs, given the potential to improve outcomes and value for that population. Box 8-4 highlights one example. Other initiatives likewise have shown statistically significant cost reductions, with one site realizing a 12 to 16 percent reduction in monthly expenditure growth by focusing on its medically complex patients (McCall et al., 2010).

BOX 8-4
Tailoring Care for Medically Complex Patients:
The AtlantiCare Special Care Center

Tailoring of care for medically complex patients can lead to improved care quality and patient health. One clinic using this model is the AtlantiCare Special Care Center—a clinic established to serve the small percentage of patients with multiple chronic diseases that accounted for the majority of the health care spending of the Local 54 Health and Welfare Fund, a union providing benefits to Atlantic City hospitality industry workers. The benefits of focusing on patients with multiple conditions can be seen in the case of Vibha Gandhi. Vibha, struggling with diabetes, obesity, and heart disease, was confined to her wheelchair and had just suffered her third heart attack. Her physicians had described her advanced coronary artery disease as inoperable just before she visited the Special Care Center for the first time.

Upon checking in, Vibha met with a health coach, Jayshree, who provided support and could connect with Gujarati-speaking patients like Vibhali while care was specially coordinated among the clinic's doctors, nurses, other clinicians, and health coaches. With Jayshree's encouragement, Vibha's health began to improve. She changed her dietary habits, committed to exercise, closely monitored her diabetes, and even took up yoga every Tuesday. Now capable of walking for a quarter mile without losing her breath, Vibha is able to live a sustainable life as a result of intensive monitoring, coaching, and personalized care.

In addition to cases of patients like Vibha, the broad results of the Special Care Center approach have been encouraging. Fully 93 percent of patients offered positive remarks on care coordination, compared with 51 percent under the previous care model. Moreover, 93 percent of patients reported that their clinic doctor seemed to know all the important information about their medical history, compared with 56 percent previously. At the same time, the clinic has increased its patients' rate of prescription drug compliance, lowered patients' smoking rates below the national average through its smoking cessation program, and helped patients lower their LDL (low-density lipoprotein) cholesterol levels by 10 percentage points in just 1 year.

SOURCES: Blash et al., 2010; Gawande, 2011.

For all payment models, it is necessary to ensure that they support patient-centered care. One concern is ensuring that incentive structures do not penalize clinicians who customize their care to patient needs, goals, and circumstances even when that care departs from guidelines (Keirns and Goold, 2009). Furthermore, some types of payment models can exacerbate disparities in health care (Blustein et al., 2011). These considerations are important to minimizing unintended consequences.

Another challenge in implementing new models is aligning incentives in the current multipayer environment. Different payers, including private health insurance plans, Medicaid, and Medicare, often use different measures to assess and reward provider performance (Lee et al., 2010). As a result, practices and hospitals must have multiple incentive models for their patients. Yet most clinicians tend to provide similar care for all of their patients, regardless of the type of insurance they hold (Baker, 1999; Glied and Zivin, 2002). The lack of alignment limits opportunities for learning by reducing the potential for a given incentive model to change medical practice in a fundamental way.

Finally, it is important to note that financial incentives do not operate in a vacuum. They are one factor, although an important one, in moving the system toward high-value care. In addition to financial incentives, other factors, such as the use of electronic health records and the organizational structure of health care (Chapter 9), play significant and important roles (Conrad and Perry, 2009; IOM, 2007). Nonetheless, payment is a crucial element for accomplishing widespread change.

FRAMEWORK FOR ACHIEVING THE VISION[1]

Rising health care costs in the United States are straining the budgets of federal and state payers, employers, and patients. Yet many of these expenditures are wasted and do not improve patient health. Continuously improving the value achieved by health care, thereby continually reducing waste, requires greater availability of information on health care performance in terms of patient experience, outcomes, and cost.

Health care payment practices also play an important role in determining the value achieved by the health care system. While current payment practices often reward service volume over value, a continuously learning health care system aligns its incentives to reward evidence-based, high-quality care. Recommendation 8 describes actions necessary to encourage incentives for continuous learning and improvement, as well as to develop the metrics needed to measure value.

Recommendation 8: Financial Incentives

Structure payment to reward continuous learning and improvement in the provision of best care at lower cost. Payers should structure payment models, contracting policies, and benefit designs to reward care that is effective and efficient and continuously learns and improves.

---

[1]Note that in Chapters 6-9, the committee's recommendations are numbered according to their sequence in the taxonomy in Chapter 10.

Strategies for progress toward this goal:

- *Public and private payers* should reward continuous learning and improvement through outcome- and value-oriented payment models, contracting policies, and benefit designs. Payment models should adequately incentivize and support high-quality team-based care focused on the needs and goals of patients and families.
- *Health care delivery organizations* should reward continuous learning and improvement through the use of internal practice incentives.
- *Health economists, health service researchers, professional specialty societies,* and *measure development organizations* should partner with *public and private payers* to develop and evaluate metrics, payment models, contracting policies, and benefit designs that reward high-value care that improves health outcomes.

Also necessary for continuous learning and improvement is transparency. Recommendation 9 outlines broad measures needed to increase the transparency of information in health care along multiple dimensions of performance. Further, the recommendation encompasses actions by public and private payers to supply such data and an increase in these transparency initiatives.

Recommendation 9: Performance Transparency

Increase transparency on health care system performance. Health care delivery organizations, clinicians, and payers should increase the availability of information on the quality, prices and cost, and outcomes of care to help inform care decisions and guide improvement efforts.

Strategies for progress toward this goal:

- *Health care delivery organizations* should collect and expand the availability of information on the safety, quality, prices and cost, and health outcomes of care.
- *Professional specialty societies* should encourage transparency on the quality, value, and outcomes of the care provided by their members.
- *Public and private payers* should promote transparency in quality, value, and outcomes to aid plan members in their care decision making.

- *Consumer and patient organizations* should disseminate this information to facilitate discussion, informed decision making, and care improvement.

Recommendations 8 and 9 are intended to promote continuous learning with respect to the value achieved by the health care system. They build on the successes realized by health care organizations and insurers in developing new models of paying for care and organizing care delivery. While a diversity of payment systems is likely to persist, these successes highlight the opportunity for incentives designed to encourage learning and improvement. By aligning incentives to focus on the patient, new payment and incentive methods can promote high-value care that reduces waste and fosters a sustainable health care system for the future.

REFERENCES

Baicker, K., and A. Chandra. 2011, August 8. *Aspirin, angioplasty, and proton beam therapy: The economics of smarter health care spending.* Paper presented at Jackson Hole Economic Policy Symposium, Jackson Hole, Wyoming.

Baicker, K., and D. Goldman. 2011. Patient cost-sharing and healthcare spending growth. *Journal of Economic Perspectives* 25(2):47-68.

Baker, L. C. 1999. Association of managed care market share and health expenditures for fee-for-service Medicare patients. *Journal of the American Medical Association* 281(5):432-437.

Becker, M. C., J. M. Galla, and S. E. Nissen. 2011. Left main trunk coronary artery dissection as a consequence of inaccurate coronary computed tomographic angiography. *Archives of Internal Medicine* 171(7):698-701.

Beeuwkes Buntin, M., A. M. Haviland, R. McDevitt, and N. Sood. 2011. Healthcare spending and preventive care in high-deductible and consumer-directed health plans. *American Journal of Managed Care* 17(3):222-230.

Berwick, D. M., and D. L. Wald. 1990. Hospital leaders' opinions of the HCFA mortality data. *Journal of the American Medical Association* 263(2):247-249.

Berwick, D. M., B. James, and M. J. Coye. 2003. Connections between quality measurement and improvement. *Medical Care* 41(Suppl. 1):I30-I38.

Blackmore, C. C., R. S. Mecklenburg, and G. S. Kaplan. 2011. At Virginia Mason, collaboration among providers, employers, and health plans to transform care cut costs and improved quality. *Health Affairs* 30(9):1680-1687.

Blash, L., S. Chapman, and C. Dower. 2010. *The special care center: A joint venture to address chronic disease.* San Francisco, CA: Center for the Health Professions.

Blendon, R. J., J. M. Benson, G. K. SteelFisher, and K. J. Weldon. 2011. *Report on Americans' views on the quality of health care.* Cambridge, MA: Robert Wood Johnson Foundation and the Harvard School of Public Health.

Blustein, J., J. S. Weissman, A. M. Ryan, T. Doran, and R. Hasnain-Wynia. 2011. Analysis raises questions on whether pay-for-performance in Medicaid can efficiently reduce racial and ethnic disparities. *Health Affairs (Millwood)* 30(6):1165-1175.

Casalino, L. P., A. Elster, A. Eisenberg, E. Lewis, J. Montgomery, and D. Ramos. 2007. Will pay-for-performance and quality reporting affect health care disparities? *Health Affairs (Millwood)* 26(3):w405-w414.

CDC (Centers for Disease Control and Prevention). 2011. Vital signs: Colorectal cancer screening, incidence, and mortality—United States, 2002-2010. *Morbidity and Mortality Weekly Report* 60(26):884-889.

Chandra, A., and J. S. Skinner. 2011. *Technology growth and expenditure growth in health care.* Cambridge, MA: National Bureau of Economic Research.

Chandra, A., J. Gruber, and R. McKnight. 2010. Patient cost-sharing and hospitalization offsets in the elderly. *American Economic Review* 100(1):193-213.

Chassin, M. R., J. M. Loeb, S. P. Schmaltz, and R. M. Wachter. 2010. Accountability measures—using measurement to promote quality improvement. *New England Journal of Medicine* 363(7):683-688.

Chernew, M. E., M. R. Shah, A. Wegh, S. N. Rosenberg, I. A. Juster, A. B. Rosen, M. C. Sokol, K. Yu-Isenberg, and A. M. Fendrick. 2008. Impact of decreasing copayments on medication adherence within a disease management environment. *Health Affairs (Millwood)* 27(1):103-112.

Chernew, M. E., I. A. Juster, M. Shah, A. Wegh, S. Rosenberg, A. B. Rosen, M. C. Sokol, K. Yu-Isenberg, and A. M. Fendrick. 2010. Evidence that value-based insurance can be effective. *Health Affairs (Millwood)* 29(3):530-536.

Chernew, M. E., R. E. Mechanic, B. E. Landon, and D. G. Safran. 2011. Private-payer innovation in Massachusetts: The "alternative quality contract." *Health Affairs (Millwood)* 30(1):51-61.

Choudhry, N. K., M. A. Fischer, J. Avorn, S. Schneeweiss, D. H. Solomon, C. Berman, S. Jan, J. Liu, J. Lii, M. A. Brookhart, J. J. Mahoney, and W. H. Shrank. 2010a. At Pitney Bowes, value-based insurance design cut copayments and increased drug adherence. *Health Affairs (Millwood)* 29(11):1995-2001.

Choudhry, N. K., M. B. Rosenthal, and A. Milstein. 2010b. Assessing the evidence for value-based insurance design. *Health Affairs (Millwood)* 29(11):1988-1994.

Choudhry, N. K., J. Avorn, R. J. Glynn, E. M. Antman, S. Schneeweiss, M. Toscano, L. Reisman, J. Fernandes, C. Spettell, J. L. Lee, R. Levin, T. Brennan, and W. H. Shrank. 2011. Full coverage for preventive medications after myocardial infarction. *New England Journal of Medicine* 365(22):2088-2097.

Cohen, S. B., and W. Yu. 2011. *The concentration and persistence in the level of health expenditures over time: Estimates for the U.S. population, 2008-2009.* Rockville, MD: Agency for Healthcare Research and Quality.

Conrad, D. A., and L. Perry. 2009. Quality-based financial incentives in health care: Can we improve quality by paying for it? *Annual Review of Public Health* 30:357-371.

Devoe, J. E., R. Gold, P. McIntire, J. Puro, S. Chauvie, and C. A. Gallia. 2011. Electronic health records vs. Medicaid claims: Completeness of diabetes preventive care data in community health centers. *Annals of Family Medicine* 9(4):351-358.

Fendrick, A. M., M. E. Chernew, and G. W. Levi. 2009. Value-based insurance design: Embracing value over cost alone. *American Journal of Managed Care* 15(Suppl. 10):S277-S283.

Fendrick, A. M., D. G. Smith, and M. E. Chernew. 2010. Applying value-based insurance design to low-value health services. *Health Affairs (Millwood)* 29(11):2017-2021.

Ferguson, T. B., E. D. Peterson, L. P. Coombs, M. C. Eiken, M. L. Carey, F. L. Grover, E. R. DeLong, and Society of Thoracic Surgeons and the National Cardiac Database. 2003. Use of continuous quality improvement to increase use of process measures in patients undergoing coronary artery bypass graft surgery: A randomized controlled trial. *Journal of the American Medical Association* 290(1):49-56.

Fisher, E. S., D. E. Wennberg, T. A. Stukel, D. J. Gottlieb, F. L. Lucas, and E. L. Pinder. 2003. The implications of regional variations in Medicare spending. Part 1: The content, quality, and accessibility of care. *Annals of Internal Medicine* 138(4):273-287.

Fishman, P. A., and M. C. Hornbrook. 2009. Assigning resources to health care use for health services research: Options and consequences. *Medical Care* 47(7 Suppl. 1):S70-S75.

Flodgren, G., M. P. Eccles, S. Shepperd, A. Scott, E. Parmelli, and F. R. Beyer. 2011. An overview of reviews evaluating the effectiveness of financial incentives in changing healthcare professional behaviours and patient outcomes. *Cochrane Database of Systematic Reviews* (7):CD009255.

Fonarow, G. C., W. T. Abraham, N. M. Albert, W. G. Stough, M. Gheorghiade, B. H. Greenberg, C. M. O'Connor, K. Pieper, J. L. Sun, C. Yancy, J. B. Young, and OPTIMIZE-HF Investigators and Hospitals. 2007. Association between performance measures and clinical outcomes for patients hospitalized with heart failure. *Journal of the American Medical Association* 297(1):61-70.

Friedberg, M. W., and C. L. Damberg. 2012. A five-point checklist to help performance reports incentivize improvement and effectively guide patients. *Health Affairs* 31(3):612-618.

Fuhrmans, V. 2007. A novel plan helps hospital wean itself off pricey tests. *Wall Street Journal*, January 12.

Fung, C. H., Y. W. Lim, S. Mattke, C. Damberg, and P. G. Shekelle. 2008. Systematic review: The evidence that publishing patient care performance data improves quality of care. *Annals of Internal Medicine* 148(2):111-123.

Gawande, A. 2011. The hot spotters: Can we lower medical costs by giving the neediest patients better care. *New Yorker* 40-51.

Ginsburg, P. B. 2007. Shopping for price in medical care. *Health Affairs (Millwood)* 26(2):w208-w216.

Glied, S., and J. G. Zivin. 2002. How do doctors behave when some (but not all) of their patients are in managed care? *Journal of Health Economics* 21(2):337-353.

Good Stewardship Working Group. 2011. The "top 5" lists in primary care: Meeting the responsibility of professionalism. *Archives of Internal Medicine* 171(15):1385-1390.

Goodwin, J. S., A. Singh, N. Reddy, T. S. Riall, and Y. F. Kuo. 2011. Overuse of screening colonoscopy in the Medicare population. *Archives of Internal Medicine* 171(15):1335-1343.

Gosden, T., F. Forland, I. S. Kristiansen, M. Sutton, B. Leese, A. Giuffrida, M. Sergison, and L. Pedersen. 2000. Capitation, salary, fee-for-service and mixed systems of payment: Effects on the behaviour of primary care physicians. *Cochrane Database of Systematic Reviews* (3):CD002215.

Government Accountability Office. 2011a. *Health care price transparency: Meaningful price information is difficult for consumers to obtain prior to receiving care.* Washington, DC: Government Accountability Office.

Government Accountability Office. 2011b. *Value in health care: Key information for policymakers to assess efforts to improve quality while reducing costs.* Washington, DC: Government Accountability Office.

Grover, F. L., A. L. Shroyer, K. Hammermeister, F. H. Edwards, T. B. Ferguson, S. W. Dziuban, J. C. Cleveland, R. E. Clark, and G. McDonald. 2001. A decade's experience with quality improvement in cardiac surgery using the Veterans Affairs and Society of Thoracic Surgeons national databases. *Annals of Surgery* 234(4):464-472.

Hafner, J. M., S. C. Williams, R. G. Koss, B. A. Tschurtz, S. P. Schmaltz, and J. M. Loeb. 2011. The perceived impact of public reporting hospital performance data: Interviews with hospital staff. *International Journal for Quality in Health Care* 23(6):697-704.

Halladay, J. R., S. C. Stearns, T. Wroth, L. Spragens, S. Hofstetter, S. Zimmerman, and P. D. Sloane. 2009. Cost to primary care practices of responding to payer requests for quality and performance data. *Annals of Family Medicine* 7(6):495-503.

Halvorson, G. C. 2009. *Health care will not reform itself: A user's guide to refocusing and reforming American health care.* New York: CRC Press.

Hannan, E. L., H. Kilburn, M. Racz, E. Shields, and M. R. Chassin. 1994. Improving the outcomes of coronary artery bypass surgery in New York state. *Journal of the American Medical Association* 271(10):761-766.

Helmchen, L. A., and A. T. Lo Sasso. 2010. How sensitive is physician performance to alternative compensation schedules? Evidence from a large network of primary care clinics. *Health Economics* 19(11):1300-1317.

Hibbard, J. H., and E. Peters. 2003. Supporting informed consumer health care decisions: Data presentation approaches that facilitate the use of information in choice. *Annual Review of Public Health* 24:413-433.

Hibbard, J. H., and S. Sofaer. 2010. *Best practices in public reporting no. 1: How to effectively present health care performance data to consumers.* Rockville, MD: Agency for Healthcare Research and Quality.

Hibbard, J. H., P. Slovic, E. Peters, and M. L. Finucane. 2002. Strategies for reporting health plan performance information to consumers: Evidence from controlled studies. *Health Services Research* 37(2):291-313.

Hibbard, J. H., J. Stockard, and M. Tusler. 2003. Does publicizing hospital performance stimulate quality improvement efforts? *Health Affairs (Millwood)* 22(2):84-94.

Hibbard, J. H., J. Stockard, and M. Tusler. 2005a. Hospital performance reports: Impact on quality, market share, and reputation. *Health Affairs (Millwood)* 24(4):1150-1160.

Hibbard, J. H., J. Stockard, and M. Tusler. 2005b. It isn't just about choice: The potential of a public performance report to affect the public image of hospitals. *Medical Care Research and Review* 62(3):358-371.

Hibbard, J. H., J. Greene, S. Sofaer, K. Firminger, and J. Hirsh. 2012. An experiment shows that a well-designed report on costs and quality can help consumers choose high-value health care. *Health Affairs (Millwood)* 31(3):560-568.

Hickson, G. B., W. A. Altemeier, and J. M. Perrin. 1987. Physician reimbursement by salary or fee-for-service: Effect on physician practice behavior in a randomized prospective study. *Pediatrics* 80(3):344-350.

Higgins, A., K. Stewart, K. Dawson, and C. Bocchino. 2011a. Early lessons from accountable care models in the private sector: Partnerships between health plans and providers. *Health Affairs (Millwood)* 30(9):1718-1727.

Higgins, A., T. Zeddies, and S. D. Pearson. 2011b. Measuring the performance of individual physicians by collecting data from multiple health plans: The results of a two-state test. *Health Affairs (Millwood)* 30(4):673-681.

Hillman, A. L. 1991. Managing the physician: Rules versus incentives. *Health Affairs* 10(4):138-146.

Hsu, J., M. Price, J. Huang, R. Brand, V. Fung, R. Hui, B. Fireman, J. P. Newhouse, and J. V. Selby. 2006. Unintended consequences of caps on Medicare drug benefits. *New England Journal of Medicine* 354(22):2349-2359.

Hussey, P. S., H. de Vries, J. Romley, M. C. Wang, S. S. Chen, P. G. Shekelle, and E. A. McGlynn. 2009. A systematic review of health care efficiency measures. *Health Services Research* 44(3):784-805.

IOM (Institute of Medicine). 2001. *Crossing the quality chasm: A new health system for the 21st century.* Washington, DC: National Academy Press.

IOM. 2006. *Performance measurement: Accelerating improvement.* Washington, DC: The National Academies Press.

IOM. 2007. *Rewarding provider performance: Aligning incentives in Medicare.* Washington, DC: The National Academies Press.

IOM. 2010a. *The healthcare imperative: Lowering costs and improving outcomes: Workshop series summary.* Washington, DC: The National Academies Press.

IOM. 2010b. *Value in health care: Accounting for cost, quality, safety, outcomes, and innovation: Workshop summary.* Washington, DC: The National Academies Press.

Joint Commission. 2011. *Improving America's hospitals: The Joint Commission's annual report on quality and safety.* http://www.jointcommission.org/assets/1/6/TJC_Annual_Report_2011_9_13_11_.pdf (accessed September 25, 2011).

Kaiser Family Foundation. 2008. *2008 update on consumers' views of patient safety and quality information.* Menlo Park, CA: Kaiser Family Fundation.

Kaiser Family Foundation. 2011. *Trends in the use of hospital and provider quality ratings.* Menlo Park, CA: Kaiser Family Foundation.

Keirns, C. C., and S. D. Goold. 2009. Patient-centered care and preference-sensitive decision making. *Journal of the American Medical Association* 302(16):1805-1806.

Kolstad, J. T., and M. E. Chernew. 2009. Quality and consumer decision making in the market for health insurance and health care services. *Medical Care Research and Review* 66(Suppl. 1):S28-S52.

Kurtzman, E. T., D. O'Leary, B. H. Sheingold, K. J. Devers, E. M. Dawson, and J. E. Johnson. 2011. Performance-based payment incentives increase burden and blame for hospital nurses. *Health Affairs* 30(2):211-218.

Landon, B. E., and S. L. Normand. 2008. Performance measurement in the small office practice: Challenges and potential solutions. *Annals of Internal Medicine* 148(5):353-357.

Landon, B. E., S. L. Normand, D. Blumenthal, and J. Daley. 2003. Physician clinical performance assessment: Prospects and barriers. *Journal of the American Medical Association* 290(9):1183-1189.

Lee, P. V., R. A. Berenson, and J. Tooker. 2010. Payment reform—the need to harmonize approaches in Medicare and the private sector. *New England Journal of Medicine* 362(1):3-5.

Loewenstein, G., K. G. Volpp, and D. A. Asch. 2012. Incentives in health: Different prescriptions for physicians and patients. *Journal of the American Medical Association* 307(13):1375-1376.

Mandel, K. E. 2010. Aligning rewards with large-scale improvement. *Journal of the American Medical Association* 303(7):663-664.

Manning, W. G., J. P. Newhouse, N. Duan, E. B. Keeler, A. Leibowitz, and M. S. Marquis. 1987. Health insurance and the demand for medical care: Evidence from a randomized experiment. *American Economic Review* 77(3):251-277.

McCall, N., J. Cromwell, and C. Urato. 2010. *Evaluation of Medicare Care Management for High Cost Beneficiaries (CMHCB) demonstration: Massachusetts General Hospital and Massachusetts General Physicians Organization (MGH).* Research Triangle Park, NC: RTI International.

McGinnis, J. M., and W. H. Foege. 1993. Actual causes of death in the United States. *Journal of the American Medical Association* 270(18):2207-2212.

Mechanic, R. E., P. Santos, B. E. Landon, and M. E. Chernew. 2011. Medical group responses to global payment: Early lessons from the "alternative quality contract" in Massachusetts. *Health Affairs (Millwood)* 30(9):1734-1742.

Milstein, A., and E. Gilbertson. 2009. American medical home runs. *Health Affairs (Millwood)* 28(5):1317-1326.

NCQA (National Committee for Quality Assurance). 2011. *HEDIS & quality measurement.* http://www.ncqa.org/tabid/59/Default.aspx (accessed September 24, 2011).

Office of Attorney General of Massachusetts. 2011. *Examination of health care cost trends and cost drivers.* Boston, MA: Massachusetts Attorney General.

O'Neil, S., J. Schurrer, and S. Simon. 2010. *Environmental scan of public reporting programs and analysis.* Cambridge, MA: Mathematica Policy Research.

Petersen, L. A., L. D. Woodard, T. Urech, C. Daw, and S. Sookanan. 2006. Does pay-for-performance improve the quality of health care? *Annals of Internal Medicine* 145(4): 265-272.

Porter, M. E. 2010. What is value in health care? *New England Journal of Medicine* 363(26):2477-2481.

Quincy, L. 2011. *Making health insurance cost-sharing clear to consumers: Challenges in implementing health reform's insurance disclosure requirements.* New York: The Commonwealth Fund.

Redberg, R. F. 2011. PCI for late reperfusion after myocardial infarction continues despite negative OAT trial: Less is more. *Archives of Internal Medicine* 171(18):1645.

Richardson, J. 2011. New website helps patients find quality care. *Morning Centinal*, August 27.

Robinson, J. C., L. P. Casilino, R. R. Gillies, D. R. Rittenhouse, S. S. Shortell, and S. Fernandes-Taylor. 2009. Financial incentives, quality improvement programs, and the adoption of clinical information technology. *Medical Care* 47(4):411-417.

Rosenthal, M. B. 2008. Beyond pay for performance—emerging models of provider-payment reform. *New England Journal of Medicine* 359(12):1197-1200.

Rothberg, M. B., E. Morsi, E. M. Benjamin, P. S. Pekow, and P. K. Lindenauer. 2008. Choosing the best hospital: The limitations of public quality reporting. *Health Affairs (Millwood)* 27(6):1680-1687.

Ryan, A. M., B. K. Nallamothu, and J. B. Dimick. 2012. Medicare's public reporting initiative on hospital quality had modest or no impact on mortality from three key conditions. *Health Affairs (Millwood)* 31(3):585-592.

Schneider, E. C., P. S. Hussey, and C. Schnyer. 2011. *Payment reform: Analysis of models and performance measurement implications.* Santa Monica, CA: RAND Corporation.

Scholle, S. H., J. Roski, J. L. Adams, D. L. Dunn, E. A. Kerr, D. P. Dugan, and R. E. Jensen. 2008. Benchmarking physician performance: Reliability of individual and composite measures. *American Journal of Managed Care* 14(12):833-838.

Scholle, S. H., J. Roski, D. L. Dunn, J. L. Adams, D. P. Dugan, L. G. Pawlson, and E. A. Kerr. 2009. Availability of data for measuring physician quality performance. *American Journal of Managed Care* 15(1):67-72.

Scott, A., P. Sivey, D. Ait Ouakrim, L. Willenberg, L. Naccarella, J. Furler, and D. Young. 2011. The effect of financial incentives on the quality of health care provided by primary care physicians. *Cochrane Database of Systematic Reviews* 9:CD008451.

Sinaiko, A. D., and M. B. Rosenthal. 2011. Increased price transparency in health care—challenges and potential effects. *New England Journal of Medicine* 364(10):891-894.

Smith, M. A., A. Wright, C. Queram, and G. C. Lamb. 2012. Public reporting helped drive quality improvement in outpatient diabetes care among Wisconsin physician groups. *Health Affairs (Millwood)* 31(3):570-577.

Song, Z., D. G. Safran, B. E. Landon, Y. He, R. P. Ellis, R. E. Mechanic, M. P. Day, and M. E. Chernew. 2011. Health care spending and quality in year 1 of the alternative quality contract. *New England Journal of Medicine* 365(10):909-918.

Stremikis, K., K. Davis, and S. Guterman. 2010. *Health care opinion leaders' views on transparency and pricing.* New York: The Commonwealth Fund.

Tang, P. C., M. Ralston, M. F. Arrigotti, L. Qureshi, and J. Graham. 2007. Comparison of methodologies for calculating quality measures based on administrative data versus clinical data from an electronic health record system: Implications for performance measures. *Journal of the American Medical Informatics Association* 14(1):10-15.

Thorpe, K. E., and L. L. Ogden. 2010. Analysis & commentary. The foundation that health reform lays for improved payment, care coordination, and prevention. *Health Affairs (Millwood)* 29(6):1183-1187.

Toussaint, J. S., C. Queram, and J. W. Musser. 2011. Connecting statewide health information technology strategy to payment reform. *American Journal of Managed Care* 17(3):e80-88.

Tu, H. T., and J. Lauer. 2008. *Word of mouth and physician referrals still drive health care provider choice.* Washington, DC: Center for Studying Health System Change.

Tu, H. T., and J. Lauer. 2009. *Impact of health care price transparency on price variation: The New Hampshire experience.* Washington, DC: Center for Studying Health System Change.

Tu, J. V., L. R. Donovan, D. S. Lee, J. T. Wang, P. C. Austin, D. A. Alter, and D. T. Ko. 2009. Effectiveness of public report cards for improving the quality of cardiac care: The effect study: A randomized trial. *Journal of the American Medical Association* 302(21):2330-2337.

USPSTF (U.S. Preventive Services Task Force). 2008. Screening for colorectal cancer: U.S. Preventive Services Task Force recommendation statement. *Annals of Internal Medicine* 149(9):627-637.

Vaiana, M. E., and E. A. McGlynn. 2002. What cognitive science tells us about the design of reports for consumers. *Medical Care Research and Review* 59(1):3-35.

Volpp, K. G., L. K. John, A. B. Troxel, L. Norton, J. Fassbender, and G. Loewenstein. 2008a. Financial incentive-based approaches for weight loss: A randomized trial. *Journal of the American Medical Association* 300(22):2631-2637.

Volpp, K. G., G. Loewenstein, A. B. Troxel, J. Doshi, M. Price, M. Laskin, and S. E. Kimmel. 2008b. A test of financial incentives to improve warfarin adherence. *BMC Health Services Research* 8:272.

Volpp, K., A. Troxel, J. Long, D. Frosch, S. Kumanyika, R. Townsend, A. Reed, J. Smith, M. Helweg-Larsen, K. Enge, and S. Kimmel. 2009a. *Impact of financial incentives on blood pressure: Results from the collaboration to reduce disparities in hypertension study.* Paper presented at Society of General Internal Medicine Annual Meeting, Miami Beach, FL.

Volpp, K. G., M. V. Pauly, G. Loewenstein, and D. Bangsberg. 2009b. P4P4P: An agenda for research on pay-for-performance for patients. *Health Affairs (Millwood)* 28(1):206-214.

Volpp, K. G., D. A. Asch, R. Galvin, and G. Loewenstein. 2011. Redesigning employee health incentives—lessons from behavioral economics. *New England Journal of Medicine* 365(5):388-390.

Warren, J. L., C. N. Klabunde, A. B. Mariotto, A. Meekins, M. Topor, M. L. Brown, and D. F. Ransohoff. 2009. Adverse events after outpatient colonoscopy in the Medicare population. *Annals of Internal Medicine* 150(12):849-857, w152.

Werner, R. M., and D. A. Asch. 2007. Clinical concerns about clinical performance measurement. *Annals of Family Medicine* 5(2):159-163.

Werner, R. M., and E. T. Bradlow. 2006. Relationship between Medicare's hospital compare performance measures and mortality rates. *Journal of the American Medical Association* 296(22):2694-2702.

Werner, R. M., and E. T. Bradlow. 2010. Public reporting on hospital process improvements is linked to better patient outcomes. *Health Affairs (Millwood)* 29(7):1319-1324.

Werner, R., E. Stuart, and D. Polsky. 2010. Public reporting drove quality gains at nursing homes. *Health Affairs (Millwood)* 29(9):1706-1713.

Werner, R. M., J. T. Kolstad, E. A. Stuart, and D. Polsky. 2011. The effect of pay-for-performance in hospitals: Lessons for quality improvement. *Health Affairs (Millwood)* 30(4):690-698.

Yasaitis, L., E. S. Fisher, J. S. Skinner, and A. Chandra. 2009. Hospital quality and intensity of spending: Is there an association? *Health Affairs (Millwood)* 28(4):w566-w572.

9

Creating a New Culture of Care

In July 2000, Mr. Q., a 50-year-old man, was admitted to a local hospital for surgery on his right ankle to correct hemophilia-related arthritis. Arriving at the surgical check-in center at 6:00 AM, Mr. and Mrs. Q. found the waiting room filled with more than 100 other patients and family members, all attempting to reach the one staff member handling the check-in process. After checking in, they found that the hematology nurse had not arrived; instead, Mr. and Mrs. Q. were responsible for ensuring that Mr. Q. received the requisite blood clotting factor before undergoing anesthesia. At 7:20 AM, Mr. Q. was wheeled to his operating room, while Mrs. Q. proceeded to the waiting room. Mr. Q's surgery was finished at 9:30 AM, but it took until 3:30 PM for him to be assigned a room in the hospital. Because of unanticipated bed demands, he was not assigned to the orthopedics ward, but to another ward that had space. Yet, when Mrs. Q. proceeded to the designated room, she found it empty and had to search the ward to find her husband's room. Mr. Q. required regular medication to control his pain, and although he requested additional medication to control his pain on his first night, he was forced to wait until the next morning for a resident to fill his request. When Mr. Q. was ready to be discharged, Mrs. Q had to take the initiative to ensure that her husband had the right prescriptions and could retain a wheelchair. While Mr. and Mrs. Q. both felt the doctors who provided Mr. Q.'s care were excellent, they agreed that the only efficiency

they experienced throughout this ordeal was receipt of Mr. Q.'s
bill (Cleary, 2003).

As with many other aspects of the health care enterprise, there is great diversity in the organizations that deliver care, from small group practices, to independent practice associations, to individual hospitals, to large integrated delivery systems. Each brings different strengths and weaknesses, and each plays a significant and important role in delivering high-quality, high-value care. Because of their size and care capacities, however, health care organizations can set an example for improvement in the health care system by using new practice methods, setting standards, and sharing resources and information with smaller practices.

The role of health care organizations is especially important in a learning health care system, because organizational factors have been shown to have an impact on care quality and patient outcomes. One study found that high-performing organizations in heart attack care, as measured by improved mortality rates, generally had features such as good communication and coordination, shared values and culture, and experience with problem solving and learning (Curry et al., 2011). Similarly, another study found that staff engagement and hospital leadership influenced the success of a program designed to prevent hospital-acquired infections (Sinkowitz-Cochran et al., 2011). And numerous studies have shown that engagement of hospital boards and other leaders in quality improvement has a significant effect on quality and outcomes (IHI, 2007; Jiang et al., 2008, 2009; Vaughn et al., 2006).

Given the importance of health care organizations to the broader learning enterprise and the impact of organizational factors on care, it is critical that health care organizations increase their learning capacity. A learning health care organization harnesses its internal wisdom—staff expertise, patient feedback, financial data, and other knowledge—to improve its operations. It engages in a continuous feedback loop of monitoring internal practices, assessing what can be improved, testing and adjusting in response to data, and implementing its findings both locally and across the organization. Although the particular policy elements that will encourage well-led, continuously learning organizations while discouraging those that are poorly run are unknown, it is evident that organizations engaged in continuous improvement efforts are more nimble and better suited to weathering changes in the market and in the practice of medicine.

Simply put, an organization that promotes continuous learning and improvement is one that "make[s] the right thing easy to do" (Halvorson, 2009). Its environment reduces stress on front-line staff, improves job satisfaction, and prevents staff burnout (Boan and Funderburk, 2003). Its environment simplifies procedures and workflows so that providers can operate at peak performance to care for patients, and embraces cognitive supports such as checklists and reminders that make providers' jobs easier. In this environment, internal processes and procedures align with the organization's aim or mission and with leaders' vision and actions.

Many institutions still struggle to implement sustainable, transformational system changes (Leape and Berwick, 2005; Lukas et al., 2007; Wachter, 2010). They face both external obstacles, such as financial incentives that emphasize quantity of services over quality, and internal challenges to achieving improvement. To overcome these obstacles and challenges and become entities that continuously learn and improve, health care organizations must adopt systematic problem-solving techniques, build operational models that encourage and reward sustained quality, become transparent on cost and outcomes, and foster leadership and a culture that support improvement efforts. Finally, the lessons learned by pioneer organizations must be diffused more broadly so the whole system can benefit. This chapter examines the common elements necessary to build organizations that continuously learn and improve, including organizational leadership for care transformation; teaming, partnership, and continuity; consistency, reliability, and transparency of results; and alignment of incentives within and across organizations. The chapter ends with recommendations for achieving the vision of a new culture of care.

ORGANIZATIONAL LEADERSHIP FOR CARE TRANSFORMATION

An organization's leadership sets the tone for the entire system. Leaders' visibility makes them uniquely positioned to define the organization's quality goals, communicate these goals and gain acceptance from staff, make learning a priority, and marshal the resources necessary for the vision to become reality. Furthermore, leadership has the ability to align activities to ensure that individuals have the necessary resources, time, and energy to accomplish the organization's goals. By defining and visibly emphasizing a vision that encourages and rewards learning and improvement, leadership at all levels of the organization prompt its disparate elements to work together toward a common end.

Leadership at All Levels

If the aim is to build an organization that maximizes effectiveness and efficiency through continuous learning, an effective leader is one that defines continuous learning and improvement as central to the organization's overall mission (Boan and Funderburk, 2003; Denison and Mishrah, 1995; Fisher and Alford, 2000; Garvin et al., 2008). Leaders at all levels of the organization, from the chief executive officer (CEO) and the board to middle managers and front-line staff, have a role to play in translating the organization's learning aim to practice. Beyond orienting the organization's staff toward a common goal, a leader's definition and communication of this mission can have a positive impact on the quality of care delivered (IOM, 2001; Weiner et al., 1996, 1997). A survey of hospital leaders found that those hospitals whose leader was heavily engaged in quality improvement efforts tended to provide higher-quality care (Vaughn et al., 2006). Another study showed that hospitals with better outcomes from their heart attack care tended to have senior management involvement (Curry et al., 2011).

At the helm of the organization, effective CEOs disseminate their vision so that all employees can see their role in the overall mission (Ford and Angermeier, 2008; IOM, 2001). Executive leadership can align internal policies with this mission and marshal the resources necessary to drive continuous improvement efforts. Other strategies employed by successful CEOs include establishing compacts that outline what clinicians and the organization can expect of one another, embodying a sense of realistic optimism that encourages the organization to pursue its aim at the highest level while acknowledging the likely challenges, harnessing "creative tension" to highlight the difference between their vision and the current state of the organization, directing the organization away from the status quo, and directing the organization toward learning by making the benefits of a learning system attractive (IHI, 2006; Menkes, 2011; Senge, 1990; Silversin and Kornacki, 2000).

As highly visible members of the organization's leadership team, CEOs and other executives are uniquely positioned to serve as role models who embody the organization's aim. Executives' high visibility has even led to the development of formal methods of "rounding to influence," where leaders are seen engaging with staff and asking specific questions to monitor and evaluate the implementation of specific patient safety initiatives (Reinertsen and Johnson, 2010). Executives also can mentor internal networks of the front-line leaders who are the key changemakers in the organization and provide the resources, support, and incentives these leaders need to drive change. In this way, senior leaders can acknowledge that their role is to set the stage for continuous learning and step back while other organizational leaders—clinical leaders and other front-line providers—work in teams to accomplish the organization's goals (Carroll and Edmondson, 2002; Government Accountability Office, 2011).

Thus while senior leadership is responsible for setting and advancing the aim of the organization, a continuously learning organization also requires leadership on the part of the managers and front-line workers who translate that aim into practice. Middle managers play a crucial role in on-the-ground, day-to-day management of a hospital's departments and services—the units that, collectively, make up the organization. These managers form the critical bridge between senior leaders and front-line staff and bear primary responsibility for translating executives' vision into action by aligning department goals with the strategic goals of the organization (Federico and Bonacum, 2010). Unit leaders therefore must challenge the prevailing mental models—deep-seated assumptions and ways of thinking about problems—and refocus attention on the barriers to learning and improvement (Senge, 1990). To this end, middle managers must be able to set priorities for improvement efforts, establish and implement continuous learning cycles, and generate enthusiasm for continuous learning among staff by fostering a culture of respect that empowers staff to undertake improvements.

Accomplishing these goals often requires understanding continuous improvement methods, the design of learning cycles, and improvement metrics and measurement. Leaders at all levels need to practice evidence-based management, which calls for demanding data from continuous learning cycles, logically interpreting these data to effect changes, and encouraging experimentation (Pfeffer and Sutton, 2006). Finally, leaders must be adept at coaching and empowering staff to take on continuous improvement projects successfully (Federico and Bonacum, 2010; Pfeffer and Sutton, 2006). Furthermore, these changes require both technical and adaptive leadership styles to manage the different types of challenges facing health care organizations (Heifetz and Laurie, 2001). To ensure that clinical leaders have the tools needed to support large-scale improvement, additional opportunities are needed to educate health care workers about organizational management, systematic problem-solving techniques, and process improvement. Initiatives such as the Institute for Healthcare Improvement (IHI) Open School have been developed to address these needs, and the Accreditation Council for Graduate Medical Education (ACGME) recently announced a shift to an outcomes-based accreditation system encompassing core competencies that include practice-based learning and improvement and systems-based practice (Nasca et al., 2012). However, additional efforts are needed to cultivate the leadership, process improvement, and problem-solving skills necessary for the transition to a continuously learning health care system. Box 9-1 presents an example of leadership commitment to creating a learning organization.

Governance

Like CEOs and other executives, hospital boards play an important role in guiding the organization toward continuous learning and improvement. Under federal regulations and accreditation standards, hospital boards are

---

BOX 9-1
An Example of Leadership Commitment to
Creating a Learning Organization

In 2004, ThedaCare, a community health system in Wisconsin, first began the process of incorporating lean engineering principles for continuous improvement across its entire system to increase productivity and improve outcomes. As a first step, a project team representing a range of ThedaCare operations managers was assembled to identify the core components and goals of an ideal management system. Most of the managers highlighted the need for a structured management reporting system and clear performance expectations if improvements were to be realized. The organization's leadership thus became aware that the lack of a distinct management system was the direct cause of the hospital's inability to sustain process improvements and productivity gains. Simultaneously, leaders realized that they could not simply transplant a predefined system into their operations, and the focus thus shifted to developing standard strategies for identifying and solving problems, including such tasks as preparing daily stat sheets to keep track of ongoing safety and quality defects, managing daily huddles, teaching, coaching and mentoring, and collecting data for monthly performance review meetings.

Two pilot sites—Appleton Medical Center and Theda Clark Medical Center—applied these lessons to their operations. By doing so, the Appleton Medical Center's medical/surgical unit was able to increase its productivity by 11 percent between 2008 and 2009, and the radiation oncology unit achieved a productivity increase of 5 percent. In addition to productivity, patient safety improved—the Appleton inpatient oncology unit and the Theda Clark neuro/surgical unit were able to reduce falls by 70 percent and 35 percent, respectively. Similar successes were seen with other follow-up programs, which has encouraged further work to eliminate wasteful processes and process variations (Barnas, 2011).

---

accountable for the quality of care provided by their organization (Belmont et al., 2011). They also are responsible not only for ensuring the organization's financial health and reputation, but also for overseeing its executives and shaping the organization's mission (Conway, 2008).

Studies have demonstrated that greater board involvement in the organization's activities is associated with improved quality of care and patient health outcomes. For instance, when boards spend time examining health care quality issues, set a quality agenda, formally monitor quality performance metrics, and reward executive leadership on the basis of measured progress toward quality and safety goals, better outcomes tend to result (IHI, 2007; Jiang et al., 2009; Vaughn et al., 2006). One survey found that hospitals governed by boards with a committee dedicated to quality were associated with more than 25 percent lower risk-adjusted mortality rates for three common medical conditions (Jiang et al., 2008).

Interventions that boards can undertake to improve quality and safety include setting goals for improving performance, gathering qualitative and quantitative data to shed light on current practices, establishing and monitoring system measures, focusing on the hospital's culture, learning from other high-performing boards, and establishing accountability measures for the board and hospital executives (Conway, 2008; Conway et al., 2011). If implemented, these system-based practices can provide boards with the capability not only to meet regulatory standards in terms of care quality and public reporting, but also to accomplish the broader aim of steering their organization toward continuous learning and improvement.

TEAMING, PARTNERSHIP, AND CONTINUITY

If leadership provides the top-down mission of an organization, the organization's culture represents the social scaffolding that empowers system transformation. Simply defined, organizational culture is the pattern of prevailing attitudes, beliefs, and assumptions among leaders and staff (Parmelli et al., 2011; Schein, 2004). Organizational culture can foster strong communication and coordination among providers, provide the kind of psychological safety that encourages the reporting of errors, and support innovation and creativity. An organization's underlying culture therefore is fundamental to the implementation and sustainability of its learning and improvement initiatives (Garvin et al., 2008; Klein and Sorra, 1996).

Several examples demonstrate the way in which an organization's culture affects care quality and patient outcomes. A study of hospitals ranked in the top 5 percent for heart attack outcomes found that those hospitals had cultures that shared a commitment to organizational learning, innovation, creativity, and trial and error and had nonpunitive approaches to problem solving (see Box 9-2) (Curry et al., 2011). Other studies have found that cultural factors, such as empowering all members of the team to speak up when they see problems and placing priority on patient safety, are critical to reducing catheter-related blood stream infections in intensive care units (Pronovost et al., 2006a,b; Vigorito et al., 2011). Still other studies have linked an organization's patient safety culture with lower rates of in-hospital complications and adverse events (Mardon et al., 2010).

A first step toward improving an organization's culture is to measure it. A variety of instruments exist with which to measure different aspects of culture, including the Veterans Health Administration Patient Safety Culture Questionnaire and the Agency for Healthcare Research and Quality's (AHRQ's) surveys on patient safety. The appropriate instrument for a given set of circumstances depends on the goals of the organization and the

---

BOX 9-2
Nonpunitive Reporting as a Tool for Culture Change

In 1995, two incidences of chemotherapy overdose occurred at Dana-Farber Cancer Institute, spurring a period of self-assessment characterized by a culture of blame. The errors led to low morale among the staff, a loss of trust among patients and their families, the loss of deemed status from Medicare, and the designation of conditional accreditation by the Joint Commission.

After these incidents, Dana-Farber endeavored to investigate how the errors occurred. Leaders engaged the staff to gain an understanding of the organization's approach to reporting and responding to errors, finding that the Institute had a culture in which the response to errors was disciplining staff. At the same time, system analyses were not conducted to investigate the root cause of those errors. As a result of these findings, leaders gathered to develop a set of principles that would define a fair and just culture. The principles centered on the belief that staff should feel safe in talking about mistakes and noted the core values of respect, impact, excellence, and discovery. They also acknowledged the difference between individual accountability and system failures and highlighted Dana-Farber's responsibility to ensure the competency of its staff. As a result of these efforts, managers now use a systems approach to investigate errors before disciplining staff, and staff surveys indicate improved perceptions of respect among clinical and nonclinical staff members.

SOURCE: Connor et al., 2007.

---

elements of culture it wishes to modify (AHRQ, 2010; Colla et al., 2005; Scott et al., 2003). Following measurement, a variety of interventions—many of which were developed outside of the health care enterprise—can be undertaken to change the organization's culture to support high performance, although questions remain about which intervention is most effective for a given health care organization (Parmelli et al., 2011).

A culture of teamwork is fundamental to building a learning organization and ensuring the continuity of care that yields better outcomes for patients. Initiatives that promote teamwork have been found to correlate positively with quality of care. In a large, multifacility integrated health care system, an intervention that focused on teamwork training, coaching, and communication skills saw an 18 percent reduction in annual mortality among participating facilities, with adverse events continuing to decrease, versus only a 7 percent reduction among nonparticipating facilities (Neily et al., 2010, 2011). In another initiative, implementing collaborative care protocols with a care team resulted in a 34 percent increase in patient satisfaction, 32 percent lower average costs per case compared with units not participating in the collaborative care process, and a 30 percentage point improvement in adherence to guidelines on door-to-balloon times (Toussaint, 2009). Alternatively, failure to provide this type of team environment can have real negative consequences for patients, because adverse events often occur when health care professionals are afraid to speak up. In one study, 58 percent of nurses surveyed said a safety tool warned them of a problem, but they felt unsafe in speaking up or were unable to get the attention of their clinical colleagues (Maxfield et al., 2005).

One challenge to promoting partnership across disciplines is that it requires providers to shed elements of their traditional roles in favor of new roles as members of a care team. Unfortunately, the increased specialization of health care professionals has led to a situation in which practitioners receive little training in coordinating across specialties to manage care delivery (IOM, 2001). Clear lines of communication may help break down barriers between units, as well as between front-line staff and managers. One tool for building improved communication is promoting a common language and terminology within the organization. Other important factors for successful teams include an environment of psychological safety that allows all team members to speak up and participate, effective conflict management processes, and leadership that effectively frames the quality challenges the team will address (Edmondson et al., 2001; IOM, 2001).

CONSISTENCY, RELIABILITY, AND TRANSPARENCY OF RESULTS

Although supportive leadership and culture are necessary elements for an organization to undertake continuous learning, these elements alone are not sufficient to create sustainable, transformational change. Continuous learning cannot proceed without concrete learning processes—that is, mechanisms that help the organization continuously capture knowledge and implement improvements (Pisano et al., 2001). These mechanisms can take many forms and may even be borrowed from leaders in other industries, but they share some essential elements: conducting systematic problem solving and experimentation, transferring knowledge throughout the organization, learning from past experience and from others, and using internal transparency as a tool to motivate further improvements (Garvin, 1993; Garvin et al., 2008; Young et al., 2004).

Engineering of Reliable Performance

As noted above, to learn and improve continuously, organizations must undertake problem solving in a systematic way. Too often, ambiguity exists with respect to who has responsibility for certain tasks or how work should be done, leading to errors, inefficiencies, and wide variations in how tasks are carried out. These ambiguities are compounded by the natural tendency to work around problems rather than engage in problem solving to address the underlying causes (Senge, 1990; Spear and Schmidhofer, 2005). Systematic problem solving, grounded in the scientific method, requires that staff work in teams to identify a problem, discover the underlying factors behind the problem, create a plan to address those factors, implement the solution thus generated, and measure whether the solution is achieving the desired results (Furman and Caplan, 2007; Spear, 2005; Young et al., 2004). Sometimes a team's first approximation of a solution to an identified problem will fail, but this, too, presents a learning opportunity. Through multiple iterations, these closed-loop learning cycles have the potential to yield answers as to how the unit, the department, and ultimately the whole institution can standardize complex processes for optimal effectiveness and efficiency and the highest quality of care (Garvin, 1993; Lukas et al., 2007; Spear, 2006; Toussaint, 2009). They represent a tool organizations can use to learn from errors and inefficiencies to drive improvement. The benefits can be substantial. For example, Denver Health introduced Lean process improvement across the organization in 2006 and by 2012 had realized $151 million in financial benefits, as well as the lowest observed-to-expected hospital mortality rate in the University Healthsystem Consortium, a consortium of academic medical centers and affiliated hospitals (Cosgrove et al., 2012).

This sort of systems-based problem solving requires that employees be willing to experiment, seek out new knowledge, and anticipate problems instead of addressing only problems immediately at hand. It requires an organizational culture that incentivizes experimentation among staff—one that recognizes failure as key to the learning process and does not penalize employees if their experiments are unsuccessful. Further, because these projects are undertaken by employees, they require that employees possess skills that include experiment design, workflow analysis, storyboarding, and statistical analysis (Garvin, 1993).

This kind of employee engagement has been found to be effective in sustaining quality improvement efforts in leading organizations. In a study of four high-value hospitals, the most efficient organizations translated the tools of systems-based problem solving beyond their quality improvement departments, training their clinical and nonclinical staff in process improvement methods (Edwards et al., 2011). Such training yields a staff that is more engaged in problem solving and that, in solving problems, gains a sense of accomplishment and enthusiasm and generates forward momentum for further efforts (Edwards et al., 2011; Lukas et al., 2007). To encourage a spirit of continuous learning and improvement among health care employees, systems tools such as organizational management, human factors engineering, and process improvement could be incorporated into professional education and continuing education curricula (IOM and NAE, 2005; Spear, 2006).

Numerous examples of effective uses of systems-based problem solving show how engineering principles can be applied to embed quality, safety, and patient-centeredness into care delivery. A variety of such methods are available for achieving improvement in health care, including Total Quality Management, Six Sigma, Lean, Plan-Do-Study-Act cycles, and hybrid approaches, their success depending on various contextual factors (Chassin and Loeb, 2011; Kaplan et al., 2010). One application of systems engineering principles is for standardizing care protocols. Through multiple iterations of problem-solving cycles, learning organizations have been able to elucidate standard protocols and guidelines for a variety of clinical conditions and processes. In so doing, they have streamlined patient care while allowing for the variation in practice required to tailor treatment to each patient's unique circumstances.

For example, a team at Intermountain's LDS Hospital created a clinical practice guideline for managing ventilator settings in the treatment of acute respiratory distress syndrome. The guideline underwent multiple iterations, with 125 changes being made within the first 4 months of use, now down to 1-2 changes per month. Implementing this guideline has increased patient survival from 9.5 to 44 percent while saving physicians time and the hospital money (James and Savitz, 2011). Standard protocols for clinical processes also can improve safety. In 2009, Kaiser Permanente's Sepsis Care Performance Initiative established protocols for early intervention and treatment for sepsis; the result was a more than 50 percent decrease in sepsis mortality (Cosgrove et al., 2012). Additionally, in response to variations in practice and failures to follow evidence-based protocols, checklists have been developed to improve care for ventilated patients, for central venous catheterized intensive care unit patients, for surgical patients, and for patients with catheter-related blood stream infections (Berenholtz et al., 2004a,b; Hales and Pronovost, 2006; Haynes et al., 2009; Pronovost et al., 2006a). Such interventions are prime examples of system redesign to prevent human error in complex systems—errors that can cause downstream effects such as patient harm, poorer outcomes, and potential malpractice claims (Gawande, 2007; Hales and Pronovost, 2006; IOM, 2001; Kohn et al., 2000; Winters et al., 2011). Systems-based problem solving also has been applied off the front lines, as illustrated in Box 9-3.

Systems engineering methods have been used as well to reduce variability in hospital admissions. In response to mismatches between available resources and patient demand that result in long wait times for patients and empty beds for hospitals, learning organizations have implemented methods for decreasing the variability in patient admissions from emergency departments and elective procedures. Not only does the smoothing of peaks and

---

BOX 9-3
Application of Systems-Based Problem
Solving to Improve Medication Delivery

The principles of systems-based problem solving have been applied off the front lines to improve the efficiency of clinical support services, including pharmacy, imaging, and patient handoffs. For example, after discovering that medication orders often were not ready when nurses came to retrieve them, the pharmacy staff of University of Pittsburgh Medical Center South Side used systems engineering principles to improve the efficiency and timeliness of medication delivery. By analyzing the problem, they learned that physician orders for medications were handled in batches that were entered throughout the day, filled the next morning, and delivered the next afternoon. That method meant prescriptions were delivered 12-24 hours after being written, at which point patients' medication needs often had changed. This, in turn, led to time wasted in restocking old orders and workarounds to get patients the medications they needed.

To address the problem, the pharmacy staff worked as a team to determine what needs their unit was expected to meet and simulated their work to investigate the factors that were preventing them from meeting these needs. By addressing the identified problems, including the way drugs were stored, the delivery routes technicians took through the hospital, and the timing of medication processing, the pharmacy staff reduced the incidence of missing medications by 88 percent, the time spent looking for medications by 60 percent, the incidence of out-of-stock medications by 85 percent, and medication processing from once every 24 hours to once every 2 hours.

SOURCE: Spear, 2005.

---

valleys in patient flow improve both patients' experience and hospitals' financial position, but it also has the potential to reduce staff stress, which can lead to burnout, errors, and diminished safety and quality (Litvak and Bisognano, 2011; Litvak et al., 2005). Improvements in patient flow at Cincinnati Children's Hospital Medical Center, for example, enabled savings of $100 million in avoided capital expenses that would have gone to the purchase of 100 new beds. Improved patient flow also led to greater work satisfaction among staff and reduced wait times for patients (IOM, 2010; Joint Commission, 2009).

Continuous Feedback and Improvement

Beyond systems-based problem solving, systems that continuously learn and improve need to be adept at transferring the knowledge they gain throughout the organization. However, several barriers prevent such diffusion of new knowledge. As noted in Chapter 6, some types of knowledge are easier or more difficult to disseminate broadly than others, and environmental factors, such as health care payment policies and regulations, can further promote or inhibit knowledge uptake (Berwick, 2003; Greenhalgh et al., 2004; Rogers, 2003). One common challenge to the diffusion of knowledge throughout an organization is a lack of awareness that the knowledge exists; for example, one unit of a hospital may have the potential to benefit from knowledge produced by another but may not be aware of that unit's activities. As relationships among individuals in different units and departments are critical to meeting this challenge, the social dynamics of the organization come into play and influence the diffusion and uptake of new insights (Ford and Angermeier, 2008). Another potential barrier relates to whether the recipient is willing to receive new knowledge or recognizes how the knowledge might be applied in a new context. For example, a common challenge is resistance from leaders or workers who are accustomed to doing things in a particular way and would prefer to continue those practices.

Several methods—including reports, staff rotations, education and training programs, and adoption of new policies and standards that align with organizational goals—can be used to overcome these barriers and encourage knowledge transfer (Garvin, 1993; Lukas et al., 2007). These barriers also can be overcome by a strong organizational culture that values continuous improvement focused on patient-centered goals and by leadership that highlights the innovative work of front-line workers and unit leaders. One strategy for increased knowledge dissemination—the Framework for Spread—is described in Box 9-4.

Also essential to the development of a continuously learning health care system is learning from others. To this end, organizations need to seek out new perspectives from similarly situated institutions (Garvin, 1993). As is characteristic of dissemination in other industries, some health care organizations will be innovators and early adopters of new innovations, while others may be more hesitant to adopt the lessons of field leaders (Berwick, 2003; Rogers, 2003). Still other organizations may resist the adoption of interventions proven to improve quality, citing local conditions that make adoption unworkable. Finally, some organizations may adopt a new innovation enthusiastically only to find that their staff reject it because the organization lacks the business model, leadership, or cultural elements that make adoption sustainable. One means of supporting organizations that continually learn from others may be through the accreditation, certification, and licensure processes for health care organizations provided by the Joint Commission and state agencies.

While the importance of building a learning organization—one that has staff buy-in and adapts to local conditions—from within cannot be

---

BOX 9-4
The Framework for Spread

The Framework for Spread, developed by the Veterans Health Administration (VHA) in partnership with the Institute for Healthcare Improvement (IHI), describes six focus areas to consider when attempting to spread an innovation across a system: leadership, identification of better ideas, communication, social systems, measurement and feedback, and knowledge management. These components were put into practice with the goal of expanding the use of innovations that improve access to care. First, leaders set a systemwide goal of expanding access and communicated that goal broadly. They showed their support by allocating funding and staff time to the initiative, aligned other ongoing projects with the new goal, and established points of contact and steering committees to lead and manage the effort. To communicate the initiative and its advantages, the organization developed a booklet and used its website to explain and communicate the ideas, including examples of success with the initiative in other settings. Next, the VHA identified a target group of clinics that would serve as early adopters of the initiative and would influence their peers to promote further spread. These learning initiatives were undertaken in waves to raise awareness and transfer technical knowledge to early adopters, with extra education being provided when needed. Finally, the VHA monitored its success in spreading the access-to-care initiative by measuring clinic wait times and the percentage of clinics that had implemented the initiative and by using the VHA website to share tips and successes. As a result of these efforts, wait times for primary care appointments decreased from 60.4 days to 28.4 days in 2 years.

SOURCE: Nolan et al., 2005.

---

overstated, positive deviance is an approach that organizations can use to encourage learning from those that are farther along. The premise of positive deviance is that certain members of a community possess wisdom about the solution to a problem and that other community members can generalize this wisdom to their own institutions to improve performance (Bradley et al., 2009). The approach calls for in-depth analysis of the processes and workflows that improve quality in learning organizations that face risks similar to those faced by the potential adopting organization. With incentives to adopt new practices in place, the adopting organization then tests innovations by taking advantage of existing organizational resources to increase buy-in and the sustainability of the change. Finally, implementation of the innovation is monitored, and the results are communicated to stakeholders and other potential adopters (Bradley et al., 2009; Marsh et al., 2004). Box 9-5 presents an example of the use of the positive deviance approach to improvement.

Despite the potential of the positive deviance approach to improve quality and promote continuous learning, some caveats should be noted. First, the approach depends on the ability to clearly identify leading organizations on key performance measures, which requires rankings and applies only to processes that can be measured quantitatively. In addition, the approach requires that leading organizations be willing to share their methods and be open about their work, which may not always be the case (Bradley et al., 2009). Moreover, using positive deviance may have the unintended consequence of organizations adopting individual innovations in a piecemeal fashion instead of developing sustainable strategies for continuous learning and improvement. For this reason, de novo quality improvement research may better drive an institution toward continuous learning and improvement. Finally, undertaking large-scale quality-improvement projects under a positive deviance framework requires resources that many organizations cannot commit. In the case study in Box 9-5, for example, a grant

---

BOX 9-5
Positive Deviance Approach to Improvement at Cincinnati Children's Hospital Medical Center's Cystic Fibrosis Center

As part of a Robert Wood Johnson Foundation/Institute for Healthcare Improvement (IHI) Pursuing Perfection grant, Cincinnati Children's Hospital Medical Center undertook a project to improve the performance of its Cystic Fibrosis Center. The Medical Center worked with the Cystic Fibrosis Foundation to analyze the Cystic Fibrosis Center's performance. The evaluation results were surprising to the Medical Center, because it ranked in the 20th percentile for cystic fibrosis patient outcomes for lung function. In response to these findings, the organization formed a multidisciplinary group of parents and clinicians who decided to take a positive deviance approach to improving the Cystic Fibrosis Center's performance. They studied the top five cystic fibrosis centers, identified by the Cystic Fibrosis Foundation, and worked with those centers to learn how they were able to achieve consistently high performance. As a result, a number of process changes were made. To improve patients' lung function, the Cystic Fibrosis Center focused on daily airway clearance, teaching parents and patients more effective clearance techniques. To ensure that patients saw the appropriate caregivers and received well-coordinated care, the Center reviewed patients' charts before they came to clinic, developed coordinated care plans for each patient, determined which specialists should see the patients during each visit, and created a caregiver visit checklist. As a result of these efforts, by 2008 the Center's lung function outcomes had moved from the 20th to the 95th percentile.

SOURCE: Tucker and Edmondson, 2010.

from the Robert Wood Johnson Foundation was integral to the redesign of the treatment protocols of Cincinnati Children's Hospital Medical Center's Cystic Fibrosis Center.

Transparency as a Transformational Tool

One critical tool for promoting improvement is broad transparency. By linking provider performance to patient outcomes and measuring providers' utilization rates and performance against internal and external benchmarks, organizations can improve the quality and value of care provided and become better stewards of limited resources. Because most clinicians and organizations lack important data on their own performance and how it relates to that of their peers, such transparency empowers them to improve their performance and helps them improve care processes, reduce variations in practice, and reduce waste. Highly efficient organizations have been able to sustain transformational change by using internal performance information beyond administrative data to drive improvement efforts (Edwards et al., 2011; James and Savitz, 2011); an example is presented in Box 9-6. External transparency may also help organizations improve performance.

BOX 9-6
Transparency on Primary Care Performance
Yields Improvements at Denver Health

To improve performance and reduce variation in practice among primary care providers in 2006 Denver Health began developing preventive health and chronic disease patient registries for the 100,000 users of its community health center network. By using a single patient identifier to link care from multiple sites to each patient and focusing on high-impact, high-opportunity areas such as diabetes care, hypertension care, and cancer screening, Denver Health developed a system for monitoring provider performance, tracking service utilization, and supporting clinicians in managing patients between visits. To help clinicians understand their own performance, Denver Health created performance report cards with information aggregated across patients and time and populated by nearly real-time data. The report cards included transparent, unblinded data on clinicians' performance by site and by provider, and reduced variation and improved overall performance. Since their inception, Denver Health's report cards have led to a nearly twofold increase in colorectal cancer screening rates, a 20 percent increase in breast cancer screening rates, and an increase in hypertension control rates from 60 to 72 percent.

SOURCE: Cosgrove et al., 2012.

A study of the responses of 17 large, multispecialty physician groups to public reporting on the quality of the diabetes care they provided found that the reporting prompted increased implementation of diabetes improvement interventions (Smith et al., 2012).

ALIGNMENT OF INCENTIVES WITHIN AND ACROSS ORGANIZATIONS

While each of the factors discussed above is important, it is the organization's operational model—the way it aligns goals, resources, and incentives—that makes learning actionable. An organization's operational model can incentivize continuous learning, help eliminate variability and waste that do not contribute to quality care, enable savings that can be invested in improving care processes and patient health, and make improvement sustainable.

The concept of using an organization's operational model to drive sustainable improvement has gained traction in manufacturing and high-reliability industries. With the exception of a few standout institutions, however, continuous learning rarely is built into the operational model of health care organizations. Yet, doing so is critical as leaders need a plan to direct the allocation of resources to support continuous improvement, as well as strategies for what to measure, incentivize, and reward to actively embed a culture of improvement (Bagian, 2005; Schein, 2004). Several strategies have been developed for aligning an organization's operational model with continuous learning. New methods, such as value stream and cost mapping, that can be used to examine the benefits and waste at each step in the delivery of health care services have allowed organizations to learn from their own processes and eliminate waste and harmful variability. The cost savings achieved through these processes can then be allocated to investments that add value, such as information technology and analytic capabilities and staff time devoted to quality improvement projects (IOM, 2008; James and Savitz, 2011; Kaplan and Porter, 2011).

In addition to quality improvement gains, health care institutions' alignment of business practices with continuous learning may provide a competitive advantage. A learning organizational culture has been shown to be predictive of successful financial performance, and studies have found that financially successful organizations score highly on organizational health metrics, including training and development, communication, flexibility and openness to change, job satisfaction, managers facilitating and recognizing staff performance, and customer satisfaction (Barney, 1986; Boan and Funderburk, 2003; Fisher and Alford, 2000; Gordon and Ditomaso, 1992; Keller and Price, 2011; Rotemborg and Saloner, 1993; Senge, 1990). In addition, several health care organizations have found that embracing business practices that promote continuous learning and improvement enhances quality and reduces costs (Cosgrove et al., 2012). However, the health care reimbursement system traditionally has not rewarded learning, making it difficult for organizations to establish operational models that are advantageous from both a financial and a continuous improvement perspective. Current reimbursement systems may even penalize health care organizations that implement best practices by failing to pay for crucial steps in those evidence-based workflows (Toussaint, 2009). New payment models, several of which are outlined in the Patient Protection and Affordable Care Act, are emerging that may change the value proposition in favor of organizations with operational models that promote continuous learning and improvement. Chapter 8 explores the value proposition for creating a learning health care system in greater depth.

Conclusion 9-1: Realizing the potential of a continuously learning health care system will require a sustained commitment to improvement, optimized operations, concomitant culture change, aligned incentives, and strong leadership within and across organizations.

Related findings:

- *Systematic designs, processes, and problem solving improve productivity and outcomes.* Denver Health introduced Lean process improvement across the organization in 2006, and by 2012 had realized $151 million in financial benefits, as well as the lowest expected-to-observed hospital mortality rate in a consortium of academic medical centers and affiliated hospitals.
- *Organizational culture influences quality and outcomes over time.* One intervention that focused on teamwork training, coaching, and communication skills saw an 18 percent reduction in annual mortality, with adverse events continuing to decrease, versus only a 7 percent reduction in facilities not participating in the intervention.
- *Leadership matters in health care improvement.* One study found that hospitals that ranked in the top 5 percent for heart attack outcomes had strong leadership and a governance commitment to improvement, good communication and coordination, shared values and culture, and experience with problem solving and learning.
- *Board engagement guides quality improvement.* One survey found that hospitals governed by boards with a committee dedicated to quality were associated with more than 25 percent lower risk-adjusted mortality rates for three common medical conditions.

FRAMEWORK FOR ACHIEVING THE VISION[1]

Transitioning to a health care system characterized by continuous learning and improvement requires commitment on the part of the organizations that deliver care. One important goal of this transition is to optimize care delivery operations, continually improving the value achieved by care and streamlining processes to provide the best patient health outcomes. As described in Recommendation 7, organizations can use a variety of tools to meet this goal, and opportunities exist to share best practices in optimizing operations.

Recommendation 7: Optimized Operations

Continuously improve health care operations to reduce waste, streamline care delivery, and focus on activities that improve patient health. Care delivery organizations should apply systems engineering tools and process improvement methods to improve operations and care delivery processes.

Strategies for progress toward this goal:

- *Health care delivery organizations* should utilize systems engineering tools and process improvement methods to eliminate inefficiencies, remove unnecessary burdens on clinicians and staff, enhance patient experience, and improve patient health outcomes.
- The *Centers for Medicare & Medicaid Services,* the *Agency for Healthcare Research and Quality,* the *Patient-Centered Outcomes Research Institute, quality improvement organizations,* and *process improvement leaders* should develop a learning consortium aimed at accelerating training, technical assistance, and the collection and validation of lessons learned about ways to transform the effectiveness and efficiency of care through continuous improvement programs and initiatives.

A variety of factors, including an organization's culture, teamwork and partnership among its staff, its ability to analyze and improve upon care delivery processes, and its alignment of rewards and incentives, are crucial in driving and sustaining the transition to a system that continuously learns and improves. In addition to leadership, the governing bodies of health care organizations play a key role in promoting and sustaining

---

[1]Note that in Chapters 6-9, the committee's recommendations are numbered according to their sequence in the taxonomy in Chapter 10.

continuous learning and improvement. As fiduciaries with responsibility for the organizations' clinical and financial performance, governing bodies are accountable for the value of care delivered, and in turn can hold organizational leaders accountable for achieving that aim. Recommendation 10 outlines the commitments that leaders and governing boards of health care delivery organizations, as well as others, need to make to promote continuous learning and improvement.

Recommendation 10: Broad Leadership

Expand commitment to the goals of a continuously learning health care system. Continuous learning and improvement should be a core and constant priority for all participants in health care—patients, families, clinicians, care leaders, and those involved in supporting their work.

Strategies for progress toward this goal:

- *Health care delivery organizations* should develop organizational cultures that support and encourage continuous improvement, the use of best practices, transparency, open communication, staff empowerment, coordination, teamwork, and mutual respect and align rewards accordingly.
- *Leaders* of these organizations should define, disseminate, support, and commit to a vision of continuous improvement; focus attention, training, and resources on continuous learning; and build an operational model that incentivizes continuous improvement and ensures its sustainability.
- *Governing boards of health care delivery organizations* should support and actively participate in fostering a culture of continuous improvement, request continuous feedback on the progress being made toward the adoption of such a culture, and align leadership incentive structures accordingly.
- *Clinical professional specialty societies, health professional education programs, health professions specialty boards, licensing boards,* and *accreditation organizations* should incorporate basic concepts and specialized applications of continuous learning and improvement into health professions education; continuing education; and licensing, certification, and accreditation requirements.

As health care organizations continuously learn and improve, they can adapt to changes in the practice of medicine and developments in science and technology. Furthermore, increasing the learning capacity of health care organizations will improve the ability of the overall system to learn, as well as the ability of these organizations to deliver high-quality, high-value care to their patients.

REFERENCES

AHRQ (Agency for Healthcare Research and Quality). 2010. *Hospital survey on patient safety culture*. http://www.ahrq.gov/qual/patientsafetyculture/hospsurvindex.htm#Toolkit (accessed December 21, 2011).

Bagian, J. P. 2005. Patient safety: What is really at issue? *Frontiers of Health Services Management* 22(1):3-16.

Barnas, K. 2011. ThedaCare's business performance system: Sustaining continuous daily improvement through hospital management in a lean environment. *Joint Commission Journal on Quality and Patient Safety* 37(9):387-399.

Barney, J. B. 1986. Organizational culture: Can it be a source of sustained competitive advantage? *Academy of Management Review* 11(3):656-665.

Belmont, E., C. C. Haltom, D. A. Hastings, R. G. Homchick, L. Morris, J. Taitsman, B. M. Peters, R. L. Nagele, B. Schermer, and K. C. Peisert. 2011. A new quality compass: Hospital boards' increased role under the Affordable Care Act. *Health Affairs (Millwood)* 30(7):1282-1289.

Berenholtz, S. M., S. Milanovich, A. Faircloth, D. T. Prow, K. Earsing, P. Lipsett, T. Dorman, and P. J. Pronovost. 2004a. Improving care for the ventilated patient. *Joint Commission Journal on Quality Safety* 30(4):195-204.

Berenholtz, S. M., P. J. Pronovost, P. A. Lipsett, D. Hobson, K. Earsing, J. E. Farley, S. Milanovich, E. Garrett-Mayer, B. D. Winters, H. R. Rubin, T. Dorman, and T. M. Perl. 2004b. Eliminating catheter-related bloodstream infections in the intensive care unit. *Critical Care Medicine* 32(10):2014-2020.

Berwick, D. M. 2003. Disseminating innovations in health care. *Journal of the American Medical Association* 289(15):1969-1975.

Boan, D., and F. Funderburk. 2003. *Healthcare quality improvement and organizational culture*. Easton, MD: Delmarva Foundation.

Bradley, E. H., L. A. Curry, S. Ramanadhan, L. Rowe, I. M. Nembhard, and H. M. Krumholz. 2009. Research in action: Using positive deviance to improve quality of health care. *Implementation Science* 4:25.

Carroll, J. S., and A. C. Edmondson. 2002. Leading organisational learning in health care. *Quality & Safety in Health Care* 11(1):51-56.

Chassin, M. R., and J. M. Loeb. 2011. The ongoing quality improvement journey: Next stop, high reliability. *Health Affairs (Millwood)* 30(4):559-568.

Cleary, P. D. 2003. A hospitalization from hell: A patient's perspective on quality. *Annals of Internal Medicine* 138(1):33.

Colla, J. B., A. C. Bracken, L. M. Kinney, and W. B. Weeks. 2005. Measuring patient safety climate: A review of surveys. *Quality & Safety in Health Care* 14(5):364-366.

Connor, M., D. Duncombe, E. Barclay, S. Bartel, C. Borden, E. Gross, C. Miller, and P. R. Ponte. 2007. Creating a fair and just culture: One institution's path toward organizational change. *Joint Commission Journal on Quality and Patient Safety Joint Commission Resources* 33(10):617-624.

Conway, J. 2008. Getting boards on board: Engaging governing boards in quality and safety. *Joint Commission Journal on Quality and Patient Safety* 34(4):214-220.

Conway, J., F. Federico, K. Stewart, and M. Campbell. 2011. *Respectful management of serious clinical adverse events*. Cambridge, MA: Institute for Healthcare Improvement.

Cosgrove, D., M. Fisher, P. Gabow, G. Gottlieb, G. C. Halvorson, B. James, G. Kaplan, J. Perlin, R. Petzel, G. Steele, and J. Toussaint. 2012. *A CEO checklist for high-value health care.* Discussion Paper, Institute of Medicine, Washington, DC. http://www.iom.edu/~/media/Files/Perspectives-Files/2012/Discussion-Papers/CEOHighValueChecklist.pdf (accessed August 31, 2012).

Curry, L. A., E. Spatz, E. Cherlin, J. W. Thompson, D. Berg, H. H. Ting, C. Decker, H. M. Krumholz, and E. H. Bradley. 2011. What distinguishes top-performing hospitals in acute myocardial infarction mortality rates? A qualitative study. *Annals of Internal Medicine* 154(6):384-390.

Denison, D., and A. Mishrah. 1995. Toward a theory of organizational science. *Organization Science* 6(2):204-223.

Edmondson, A., R. Bohmer, and G. Pisano. 2001. Speeding up team learning. *Harvard Business Review* 79(9):125.

Edwards, J. N., S. Silow-Carroll, and A. Lashbrook. 2011. *Achieving efficiency: Lessons from four top-performing hospitals.* New York: The Commonwealth Fund.

Federico, F., and D. Bonacum. 2010. Strengthening the core. Middle managers play a vital role in improving safety. *Healthcare Executive* 25(1):68-70.

Fisher, C., and R. Alford. 2000. Consulting on culture. *Consulting Psychology: Research and Practice* 52(3).

Ford, R., and I. Angermeier. 2008. Creating a learning health care organization for participatory management: A case analysis. *Journal of Health Organization and Management* 22(3):269-293.

Furman, C., and R. Caplan. 2007. Applying the Toyota production system: Using a patient safety alert system to reduce error. *Joint Commission Journal on Quality and Patient Safety* 33(7):376-386.

Garvin, D. A. 1993. Building a learning organization. *Harvard Business Review* 71(4):78-91.

Garvin, D. A., A. C. Edmondson, and F. Gino. 2008. Is yours a learning organization? *Harvard Business Review* 86(3):109.

Gawande, A. 2007. The checklist: If something so simple can transform intensive care, what else can it do? *New Yorker* 86-101.

Gordon, G. G., and N. Ditomaso. 1992. Predicting corporate performance from organizational culture. *Journal of Management Studies* 29(6):783-798.

Government Accountability Office. 2011. *Value in health care: Key information for policymakers to assess efforts to improve quality while reducing costs.* Washington, DC: Government Accountability Office.

Greenhalgh, T., G. Robert, F. Macfarlane, P. Bate, and O. Kyriakidou. 2004. Diffusion of innovations in service organizations: Systematic review and recommendations. *Milbank Quarterly* 82(4):581-629.

Hales, B. M., and P. J. Pronovost. 2006. The checklist: A tool for error management and performance improvement. *Journal of Critical Care* 21(3):231-235.

Halvorson, G. C. 2009. *Health care will not reform itself: A user's guide to refocusing and reforming American health care.* New York: CRC Press.

Haynes, A. B., T. G. Weiser, W. R. Berry, S. R. Lipsitz, A. H. Breizat, E. P. Dellinger, T. Herbosa, S. Joseph, P. L. Kibatala, M. C. Lapitan, A. F. Merry, K. Moorthy, R. K. Reznick, B. Taylor, A. A. Gawande, and Safe Surgery Saves Lives Study Group. 2009. A surgical safety checklist to reduce morbidity and mortality in a global population. *New England Journal of Medicine* 360(5):491-499.

Heifetz, R. A., and D. L. Laurie. 2001. The work of leadership. *Harvard Business Review* 79(11):131.

IHI (Institute for Healthcare Improvement). 2006. *A framework for leadership of improvement.* Cambridge, MA: IHI.

IHI. 2007. *Protecting 5 million lives from harm. Getting started kit: Governance leadership "boards on board."* http://www.longwoods.com/product/download/code/19364 (accessed August 31, 2012).

IOM (Institute of Medicine). 2001. *Crossing the quality chasm: A new health system for the 21st century.* Washington, DC: National Academy Press.

IOM. 2008. *Creating a business case for quality improvement research: Expert views, workshop summary.* Washington, DC: The National Academies Press.

IOM. 2010. *The healthcare imperative: Lowering costs and improving outcomes: Workshop series summary.* Washington, DC: The National Academies Press.

IOM and NAE (National Academy of Engineering). 2005. *Building a better delivery system: A new engineering/health care partnership.* Washington, DC: The National Academies Press.

James, B. C., and L. A. Savitz. 2011. How Intermountain trimmed health care costs through robust quality improvement efforts. *Health Affairs (Millwood)* 30(6):1185-1191.

Jiang, H. J., C. Lockee, K. Bass, and I. Fraser. 2008. Board engagement in quality: Findings of a survey of hospital and system leaders. *Journal of Healthcare Management American College of Healthcare Executives* 53(2):121-134; discussion 135.

Jiang, H. J., C. Lockee, K. Bass, and I. Fraser. 2009. Board oversight of quality: Any differences in process of care and mortality? *Journal of Healthcare Management* 54(1):15-29.

Joint Commission. 2009. *Managing patient flow in hospitals: Strategies and solutions.* 2nd ed., edited by E. Litvak. Oak Brook, IL: Joint Commission Resources, Inc.

Kaplan, H. C., P. W. Brady, M. C. Dritz, D. K. Hooper, W. M. Linam, C. M. Froehle, and P. Margolis. 2010. The influence of context on quality improvement success in health care: A systematic review of the literature. *Milbank Quarterly* 88(4):500-559.

Kaplan, R. S., and M. E. Porter. 2011. How to solve the cost crisis in health care. *Harvard Business Review* 47-64.

Keller, S., and C. Price. 2011. Organizational health: The ultimate competitive advantage. *McKinsey Quarterly,* June. http://www.mckinseyquarterly.com/Organizational_health_The_ultimate_competitive_advantage_2820 (accessed August 31, 2012).

Klein, K. J., and J. S. Sorra. 1996. The challenge of innovation implementation. *Academy of Management Review* 21(4):1055-1080.

Kohn, L. T., J. Corrigan, and M. S. Donaldson. 2000. *To err is human: Building a safer health system.* Washington, DC: National Academy Press.

Leape, L. L., and D. M. Berwick. 2005. Five years after To Err Is Human: What have we learned? *Journal of the American Medical Association* 293(19):2384-2390.

Litvak, E., and M. Bisognano. 2011. More patients, less payment. Increasing hospital efficiency in the aftermath of health reform. *Health Affairs (Millwood)* 30(1):76-80.

Litvak, E., P. I. Buerhaus, F. Davidoff, M. C. Long, M. L. McManus, and D. M. Berwick. 2005. Managing unnecessary variability in patient demand to reduce nursing stress and improve patient safety. *Joint Commission Journal on Quality and Patient Safety* 31(6):330-338.

Lukas, C. V., S. K. Holmes, A. B. Cohen, J. Restuccia, I. E. Cramer, M. Shwartz, and M. P. Charns. 2007. Transformational change in health care systems: An organizational model. *Health Care Management Review* 32(4):309-320.

Mardon, R. E., K. Khanna, J. Sorra, N. Dyer, and T. Famolaro. 2010. Exploring relationships between hospital patient safety culture and adverse events. *Journal of Patient Safety* 6(4):226-232.

Marsh, D. R., D. G. Schroeder, K. A. Dearden, J. Sternin, and M. Sternin. 2004. The power of positive deviance. *British Medical Journal* 329(7475):1177-1179.

Maxfield, D., J. Grenny, R. Lavandero, and L. Groah. 2005. *The silent treatment: Why safety tools and checklists aren't enough to save lives.* http://www.silenttreatmentstudy.com/ (accessed May 16, 2012).

Menkes, J. 2011. Three traits every CEO needs. *The Conversation*, May 11. http://blogs.hbr.org/cs/2011/05/three_traits_every_ceo_needs.html (accessed August 31, 2012).

Nasca, T. J., I. Philibert, T. Brigham, and T. C. Flynn. 2012. The next GME accreditation system—rationale and benefits. *New England Journal of Medicine* 366(11):1051-1056.

Neily, J., P. D. Mills, Y. Young-Xu, B. T. Carney, P. West, D. H. Berger, L. M. Mazzia, D. E. Paull, and J. P. Bagian. 2010. Association between implementation of a medical team training program and surgical mortality. *Journal of the American Medical Association* 304(15):1693-1700.

Neily, J., P. D. Mills, N. Eldridge, B. T. Carney, D. Pfeffer, J. R. Turner, Y. Young-Xu, W. Gunnar, and J. P. Bagian. 2011. Incorrect surgical procedures within and outside of the operating room: A follow-up report. *Archives of Surgery* 146(11):1235-1239.

Nolan, K., M. W. Schall, F. Erb, and T. Nolan. 2005. Using a framework for spread: The case of patient access in the Veterans Health Administration. *Joint Commission Journal on Quality and Patient Safety* 31(6):339-347.

Parmelli, E., G. Flodgren, F. Beyer, N. Baillie, M. E. Schaafsma, and M. P. Eccles. 2011. The effectiveness of strategies to change organisational culture to improve healthcare performance: A systematic review. *Implementation Science* 6:33.

Pfeffer, J., and R. I. Sutton. 2006. Evidence-based management. *Harvard Business Review* 84(1):62.

Pisano, G. P., R. M. J. Bohmer, and A. C. Edmondson. 2001. Organizational differences in rates of learning: Evidence from the adoption of minimally invasive cardiac surgery. *Management Science* 47(6):752-768.

Pronovost, P., D. Needham, S. Berenholtz, D. Sinopoli, H. Chu, S. Cosgrove, B. Sexton, R. Hyzy, R. Welsh, G. Roth, J. Bander, J. Kepros, and C. Goeschel. 2006a. An intervention to decrease catheter-related bloodstream infections in the ICU. *New England Journal of Medicine* 355(26):2725-2732.

Pronovost, P. J., S. M. Berenholtz, C. A. Goeschel, D. M. Needham, J. B. Sexton, D. A. Thompson, L. H. Lubomski, J. A. Marsteller, M. A. Makary, and E. Hunt. 2006b. Creating high reliability in health care organizations. *Health Services Research* 41(4, Pt. 2):1599-1617.

Reinertsen, J. L., and K. M. Johnson. 2010. Rounding to influence. Leadership method helps executives answer the "hows" in patient safety initiatives. *Healthcare Executive* 25(5):72-75.

Rogers, E. M. 2003. *Diffusion of innovations.* 5th ed. New York: Free Press.

Rotemborg, J. J., and G. Saloner. 1993. Leadership style and incentives. *Management Science* 39(11).

Schein, E. H. 2004. *Organizational culture and leadership.* San Francisco, CA: Jossey-Bass.

Scott, T., R. Mannion, H. Davies, and M. Marshall. 2003. The quantitative measurement of organizational culture in health care: A review of the available instruments. *Health Services Research* 38(3):923-945.

Senge, P. M. 1990. *The leader's new work: Building learning organizations.* Cambridge, MA: Sloan Management Review.

Silversin, J., and M. J. Kornacki. 2000. Creating a physician compact that drives group success. *Medical Group Management Journal* 47(3):54-58, 60, 62.

Sinkowitz-Cochran, R. L., K. H. Burkitt, T. Cuerdon, C. Harrison, S. Gao, D. Scott Obrosky, R. Jain, M. J. Fine, and J. A. Jernigan. 2011. The associations between organizational culture and knowledge, attitudes, and practices in a multicenter Veterans Affairs quality improvement initiative to prevent methicillin-resistant Staphylococcus aureus. *American Journal of Infection Control* 40(2):138-143.

Smith, M. A., A. Wright, C. Queram, and G. C. Lamb. 2012. Public reporting helped drive quality improvement in outpatient diabetes care among Wisconsin physician groups. *Health Affairs* 31(3):570-577.

Spear, S. J. 2005. Fixing health care from the inside, today. *Harvard Business Review* 83(9):78.

Spear, S. J. 2006. Fixing healthcare from the inside: Teaching residents to heal broken delivery processes as they heal sick patients. *Academic Medicine* 81(Suppl. 10):S144-S149.

Spear, S. J., and M. Schmidhofer. 2005. Ambiguity and workarounds as contributors to medical error. *Annals of Internal Medicine* 142(8):627-630.

Toussaint, J. 2009. Writing the new playbook for U.S. health care: Lessons from Wisconsin. *Health Affairs (Millwood)* 28(5):1343-1350.

Tucker, A., and A. Edmondson. 2010. Cincinnati Children's Hospital Medical Center. *Harvard Business School*, June 28. http://hbswk.hbs.edu/item/6441.html (accessed August 31, 2012).

Vaughn, T., M. Koepke, E. Kroch, W. Lehrman, S. Sinha, and S. Levey. 2006. Engagement of leadership in quality improvement initiatives: Executive quality improvement survey results. *Journal of Patient Safety* 2(1).

Vigorito, M. C., L. McNicoll, L. Adams, and B. Sexton. 2011. Improving safety culture results in Rhode Island ICUs: Lessons learned from the development of action-oriented plans. *Joint Commission Journal on Quality and Patient Safety* 37(11):509-514.

Wachter, R. M. 2010. Patient safety at ten: Unmistakable progress, troubling gaps. *Health Affairs (Millwood)* 29(1):165-173.

Weiner, B. J., J. A. Alexander, and S. M. Shortell. 1996. Leadership for quality improvement in health care; empirical evidence on hospital boards, managers, and physicians. *Medical Care Research and Review* 53(4):397-416.

Weiner, B. J., S. M. Shortell, and J. Alexander. 1997. Promoting clinical involvement in hospital quality improvement efforts: The effects of top management, board, and physician leadership. *Health Services Research* 32(4):491-510.

Winters, B. D., M. S. Aswani, and P. J. Pronovost. 2011. Commentary: Reducing diagnostic errors: Another role for checklists? *Academic Medicine* 86(3):279-281.

Young, T., S. Brailsford, C. Connell, R. Davies, P. Harper, and J. H. Klein. 2004. Using industrial processes to improve patient care. *British Medical Journal* 328(7432):162-164.

10

Actions for Continuous Learning, Best Care, and Lower Costs

Implementing the actions delineated in Chapters 6-9 and achieving the vision of continuous learning and improvement for the health care system will depend on broad leadership by the complex network of decentralized and loosely associated individuals and organizations that make up the current system. Given the complexity of the system and the interconnectedness of its various sectors, no one sector acting alone can bring about the scope and scale of transformative change necessary to develop a system that continuously learns and improves. Each stakeholder brings different strengths, skills, needs, and expertise to the task of improving the system; faces unique challenges; and is accountable for different aspects of the system's success. Hence, collaboration among individuals and organizations in a given stakeholder group, as well as between stakeholders, will be necessary to produce effective and sustainable change. This chapter summarizes the recommendations presented in Chapters 6 through 9 and then describes the roles of the various stakeholders in the system in implementing these recommendations.

ACHIEVING THE VISION

Based on the findings and conclusions identified in the course of its work, the committee recommends specific actions, supported by the material presented in Chapters 6-9, that will accelerate progress toward continuous learning, best care, and lower costs. The committee's recommendations are collected below, grouped into three categories as summarized in Box 10-1: foundational elements, care improvement targets, and a supportive

---

BOX 10-1
Categories of the Committee's Recommendations

Foundational Elements

Recommendation 1: *The digital infrastructure.* Improve the capacity to capture clinical, care delivery process, and financial data for better care, system improvement, and the generation of new knowledge.
Recommendation 2: *The data utility.* Streamline and revise research regulations to improve care, promote the capture of clinical data, and generate knowledge.

Care Improvement Targets

Recommendation 3: *Clinical decision support.* Accelerate integration of the best clinical knowledge into care decisions.
Recommendation 4: *Patient-centered care.* Involve patients and families in decisions regarding health and health care, tailored to fit their preferences.
Recommendation 5: *Community links.* Promote community-clinical partnerships and services aimed at managing and improving health at the community level.
Recommendation 6: *Care continuity.* Improve coordination and communication within and across organizations.
Recommendation 7: *Optimized operations.* Continuously improve health care operations to reduce waste, streamline care delivery, and focus on activities that improve patient health.

Supportive Policy Environment

Recommendation 8: *Financial incentives.* Structure payment to reward continuous learning and improvement in the provision of best care at lower cost.
Recommendation 9: *Performance transparency.* Increase transparency on health care system performance.
Recommendation 10: *Broad leadership.* Expand commitment to the goals of a continuously learning health care system.

---

policy environment. Also identified are the stakeholders whose engagement is necessary for the implementation of each recommendation. Each recommendation describes the core improvement aim for the area, followed by specific strategies representing initial steps stakeholders should take in acting on the recommendation. Additional activities will have to be undertaken by numerous stakeholder groups to sustain and advance the continuous improvement required.

Foundational Elements

Recommendation 1: The Digital Infrastructure

Improve the capacity to capture clinical, care delivery process, and financial data for better care, system improvement, and the generation of new knowledge. Data generated in the course of care delivery should be digitally collected, compiled, and protected as a reliable and accessible resource for care management, process improvement, public health, and the generation of new knowledge.

Strategies for progress toward this goal:

- *Health care delivery organizations* and *clinicians* should fully and effectively employ digital systems that capture patient care experiences reliably and consistently, and implement standards and practices that advance the interoperability of data systems.
- *The National Coordinator for Health Information Technology, digital technology developers,* and *standards organizations* should ensure that the digital infrastructure captures and delivers the core data elements and interoperability needed to support better care, system improvement, and the generation of new knowledge.
- *Payers, health care delivery organizations,* and *medical product companies* should contribute data to research and analytic consortia to support expanded use of care data to generate new insights.
- *Patients* should participate in the development of a robust data utility; use new clinical communication tools, such as personal portals, for self-management and care activities; and be involved in building new knowledge, such as through patient-reported outcomes and other knowledge processes.
- The *Secretary of Health and Human Services* should encourage the development of distributed data research networks and expand the availability of departmental health data resources for translation into accessible knowledge that can be used for improving care, lowering costs, and enhancing public health.
- *Research funding agencies and organizations,* such as the *National Institutes of Health,* the *Agency for Healthcare Research and Quality,* the *Veterans Health Administration,* the *Department of Defense,* and the *Patient-Centered Outcomes Research Institute,* should promote research designs and methods that draw naturally on existing care processes and that also support ongoing quality improvement efforts.

Recommendation 2: The Data Utility

Streamline and revise research regulations to improve care, promote the capture of clinical data, and generate knowledge. Regulatory agencies should clarify and improve regulations governing the collection and use of clinical data to ensure patient privacy but also the seamless use of clinical data for better care coordination and management, improved care, and knowledge enhancement.

Strategies for progress toward this goal:

- The *Secretary of Health and Human Services* should accelerate and expand the review of the Health Insurance Portability and Accountability Act (HIPAA) and institutional review board (IRB) policies with respect to actual or perceived regulatory impediments to the protected use of clinical data, and clarify regulations and their interpretation to support the use of clinical data as a resource for advancing science and care improvement.
- *Patient and consumer groups, clinicians, professional specialty societies, health care delivery organizations, voluntary organizations, researchers,* and *grantmakers* should develop strategies and outreach to improve understanding of the benefits and importance of accelerating the use of clinical data to improve care and health outcomes.

Care Improvement Targets

Recommendation 3: Clinical Decision Support

Accelerate integration of the best clinical knowledge into care decisions. Decision support tools and knowledge management systems should be routine features of health care delivery to ensure that decisions made by clinicians and patients are informed by current best evidence.

Strategies for progress toward this goal:

- *Clinicians and health care organizations* should adopt tools that deliver reliable, current clinical knowledge to the point of care, and organizations should adopt incentives that encourage the use of these tools.
- *Research organizations, advocacy organizations, professional specialty societies,* and *care delivery organizations* should facilitate the

development, accessibility, and use of evidence-based and harmonized clinical practice guidelines.

- *Public and private payers* should promote the adoption of decision support tools, knowledge management systems, and evidence-based clinical practice guidelines by structuring payment and contracting policies to reward effective, evidence-based care that improves patient health.
- *Health professional education programs* should teach new methods for accessing, managing, and applying evidence; engaging in lifelong learning; understanding human behavior and social science; and delivering safe care in an interdisciplinary environment.
- *Research funding agencies and organizations* should promote research into the barriers and systematic challenges to the dissemination and use of evidence at the point of care, and support research to develop strategies and methods that can improve the usefulness and accessibility of patient outcome data and scientific evidence for clinicians and patients.

Recommendation 4: Patient-Centered Care

Involve patients and families in decisions regarding health and health care, tailored to fit their preferences. Patients and families should be given the opportunity to be fully engaged participants at all levels, including individual care decisions, health system learning and improvement activities, and community-based interventions to promote health.

Strategies for progress toward this goal:

- *Patients and families* should expect to be offered full participation in their own care and health and encouraged to partner, according to their preference, with clinicians in fulfilling those expectations.
- *Clinicians* should employ high-quality, reliable tools and skills for informed shared decision making with patients and families, tailored to clinical needs, patient goals, social circumstances, and the degree of control patients prefer.
- *Health care delivery organizations,* including programs operated by the *Department of Defense,* the *Veterans Health Administration,* and *Health Resources and Services Administration,* should monitor and assess patient perspectives and use the insights thus gained to improve care processes; establish patient portals to facilitate data sharing and communication among clinicians, patients, and families; and make high-quality, reliable tools available for shared decision making with patients at different levels of health literacy.

- The *Agency for Healthcare Research and Quality,* partnering with the *Centers for Medicare & Medicaid Services, other payers,* and *stakeholder organizations,* should support the development and testing of an accurate and reliable core set of measures of patient-centeredness for consistent use across the health care system.
- The *Centers for Medicare & Medicaid Services* and *other public and private payers* should promote and measure patient-centered care through payment models, contracting policies, and public reporting programs.
- *Digital technology developers* and *health product innovators* should develop tools to assist individuals in managing their health and health care, in addition to providing patient supports in new forms of communities.

Recommendation 5: Community Links

Promote community-clinical partnerships and services aimed at managing and improving health at the community level. Care delivery and community-based organizations and agencies should partner with each other to develop cooperative strategies for the design, implementation, and accountability of services aimed at improving individual and population health.

Strategies for progress toward this goal:

- *Health care delivery organizations* and *clinicians* should partner with *community-based organizations* and *public health agencies* to leverage and coordinate prevention, health promotion, and community-based interventions to improve health outcomes, including strategies related to the assessment and use of web-based tools.
- *Public and private payers* should incorporate population health improvement into their health care payment and contracting policies and accountability measures.
- *Health economists, health service researchers, professional specialty societies,* and *measure development organizations* should continue to improve measures that can readily be applied to assess performance on both individual and population health.

Recommendation 6: Care Continuity

Improve coordination and communication within and across organizations. Payers should structure payment and contracting to reward effective communication and coordination between and among members of a patient's care team.

Strategies for progress toward this goal:

- *Health care delivery organizations* and *clinicians,* partnering with *patients, families,* and *community organizations,* should develop coordination and transition processes, data sharing capabilities, and communication tools to ensure safe, seamless patient care.
- *Health economists, health service researchers, professional specialty societies,* and *measure development organizations* should develop and test metrics with which to monitor and evaluate the effectiveness of care transitions in improving patient health outcomes.
- *Public and private payers* should promote effective care transitions that improve patient health through their payment and contracting policies.

Recommendation 7: Optimized Operations

Continuously improve health care operations to reduce waste, streamline care delivery, and focus on activities that improve patient health. Care delivery organizations should apply systems engineering tools and process improvement methods to improve operations and care delivery processes.

Strategies for progress toward this goal:

- *Health care delivery organizations* should utilize systems engineering tools and process improvement methods to eliminate inefficiencies, remove unnecessary burdens on clinicians and staff, enhance patient experience, and improve patient health outcomes.
- The *Centers for Medicare & Medicaid Services,* the *Agency for Healthcare Research and Quality,* the *Patient-Centered Outcomes Research Institute, quality improvement organizations,* and *process improvement leaders* should develop a learning consortium aimed at accelerating training, technical assistance, and the collection and validation of lessons learned about ways to transform the effectiveness and efficiency of care through continuous improvement programs and initiatives.

Supportive Policy Environment

Recommendation 8: Financial Incentives

Structure payment to reward continuous learning and improvement in the provision of best care at lower cost. Payers should structure payment models, contracting policies, and benefit designs to reward care that is effective and efficient and continuously learns and improves.

Strategies for progress toward this goal:

- *Public and private payers* should reward continuous learning and improvement through outcome- and value-oriented payment models, contracting policies, and benefit designs. Payment models should adequately incentivize and support high-quality team-based care focused on the needs and goals of patients and families.
- *Health care delivery organizations* should reward continuous learning and improvement through the use of internal practice incentives.
- *Health economists, health service researchers, professional specialty societies,* and *measure development organizations* should partner with *public and private payers* to develop and evaluate metrics, payment models, contracting policies, and benefit designs that reward high-value care that improves health outcomes.

Recommendation 9: Performance Transparency

Increase transparency on health care system performance. Health care delivery organizations, clinicians, and payers should increase the availability of information on the quality, prices and cost, and outcomes of care to help inform care decisions and guide improvement efforts.

Strategies for progress toward this goal:

- *Health care delivery organizations* should collect and expand the availability of information on the safety, quality, prices and cost, and health outcomes of care.
- *Professional specialty societies* should encourage transparency on the quality, value, and outcomes of the care provided by their members.
- *Public and private payers* should promote transparency in quality, value, and outcomes to aid plan members in their care decision making.

- *Consumer and patient organizations* should disseminate this information to facilitate discussion, informed decision making, and care improvement.

Recommendation 10: Broad Leadership

Expand commitment to the goals of a continuously learning health care system. Continuous learning and improvement should be a core and constant priority for all participants in health care—patients, families, clinicians, care leaders, and those involved in supporting their work.

Strategies for progress toward this goal:

- *Health care delivery organizations* should develop organizational cultures that support and encourage continuous improvement, the use of best practices, transparency, open communication, staff empowerment, coordination, teamwork, and mutual respect and align rewards accordingly.
- *Leaders* of these organizations should define, disseminate, support, and commit to a vision of continuous improvement; focus attention, training, and resources on continuous learning; and build an operational model that incentivizes continuous improvement and ensures its sustainability.
- *Governing boards of health care delivery organizations* should support and actively participate in fostering a culture of continuous improvement, request continuous feedback on the progress being made toward the adoption of such a culture, and align leadership incentive structures accordingly.
- *Clinical professional specialty societies, health professional education programs, health professions specialty boards, licensing boards,* and *accreditation organizations* should incorporate basic concepts and specialized applications of continuous learning and improvement into health professions education; continuing education; and licensing, certification, and accreditation requirements.

Given the interconnected nature of the problems to be solved, it will be important to take the actions identified above in concert. To elevate the quantity of evidence available to inform clinical decisions, for example, it is necessary to increase the supply of evidence by expanding the clinical research base; make the evidence easily accessible by embedding it in clinical technological tools, such as clinical decision support; encourage use of the evidence through appropriate payment, contracting, and regulatory policies and cultural factors; and assess progress toward the goal using reliable metrics and appropriate transparency. The absence of any one of these factors will substantially limit overall improvement. To guide success, progress on the recommendations in this report should be monitored continuously.

Implementing the actions detailed above and achieving the vision of continuous learning and improvement will depend on the exercise of broad leadership by the complex network of decentralized and loosely associated individuals and organizations that make up the health care system. Given the complexity of the system and the interconnectedness of its different actors and sectors, no one actor or sector alone can bring about the scope and scale of transformative change necessary to develop a system that continuously learns and improves. Each stakeholder brings different strengths, skills, needs, and expertise to the task of improving the system, faces unique challenges, and is accountable for different aspects of the system's success. There is a distinct need for collaboration between and among stakeholders to produce effective and sustainable change.

PATIENTS, CONSUMERS, CAREGIVERS, COMMUNITIES, AND THE PUBLIC

Roles in Learning

As the focus of health care, patients are central to the success of improvement initiatives. Any large-scale change will require the participation of patients as partners, with the system building trust on every dimension. Patients can motivate continuous improvement by setting high expectations for their care in terms of quality, value, and use of scientific evidence and by selecting health care services, clinicians, health care organizations, and plans that meet those expectations. Patients also can promote learning and improvement by engaging in their own care; sharing decision making with their clinicians; and, with the help of their caregivers, directly applying evidence to their self-care and self-management on an ongoing basis. As their needs progress, patients can seek effective and efficient services that align most closely with their goals.

Challenges to Learning

There are several impediments to patients and the broader public playing a central role in improving the health care system. Notably, the culture of health care often does not encourage or support shared decision making. Even when patients are encouraged to play a role in decisions about their care, they often lack understandable, reliable information—from evidence on the efficacy of different treatment options to information on the quality of different providers and health care organizations—that is customized to their needs, preferences, and health goals. In addition, health care needs to be tailored to a patient's health literacy, as people have different abilities to obtain, comprehend, and use health information to make care decisions (Brach et al., 2012).

In addition, there are challenges to measuring patient empowerment and patient-centered care. Without accurate and reliable measures, it is difficult to determine whether initiatives aimed at achieving greater patient empowerment are successful or to reward clinicians and health care organizations that provide patient-centered care. Several organizations, such as the National Quality Forum (NQF) and the National Committee for Quality Assurance (NCQA), have begun to address this need with respect to defining and measuring aspects of health care performance that relate to patient-centered care. Once measurement has been accomplished, moreover, there are further challenges in communicating this information to patients in an understandable and relevant format such that it can easily be applied to care decisions. These challenges are beginning to be addressed by several public reporting initiatives, including national initiatives such as Hospital Compare and regional initiatives such as Minnesota Community Measurement and the Wisconsin Collaborative for Healthcare Quality, which have begun to incorporate patient experience metrics into their public reporting efforts.

Opportunities

While the challenges described above are considerable, several opportunities exist for increasing patient involvement in the health care system. Organizations have implemented new methods for gathering patient feedback, from patient advisory councils to surveys; clinicians have introduced new communication and shared decision-making processes; and insurers have begun to account for patient-centeredness in payment. Further, health information technology offers new ways for patients and providers to communicate, and new mobile devices and sensors allow patients to monitor their conditions continuously. Leveraging these opportunities will increase patient involvement in improving health care.

Next Steps

To help achieve a learning health care system, patients will need to play the following roles:

- Engage actively in their own care and health and, where appropriate, that of family members and loved ones through approaches that include questioning, education and lifelong learning, the use of information and technology, shared decision making, and self-management of their health and conditions.

- Partner with all stakeholders to ensure that health care meets their needs, as well as those of their community and the public overall.
- Contribute to continuous learning by providing feedback at every level of their care experience.
- Participate in the development of a robust data utility and the use of digital tools for care management and coordination.
- Take advantage of access to information, knowledge, and educational opportunities to become more actively involved in their health.

CLINICIANS AND THEIR TEACHERS

Roles in Learning

The health care professionals who deliver care are cornerstones of any effort to improve health care. These professionals—including more than 800,000-870,000 active physicians, 2.7 million registered nurses, 250,000 pharmacists, and many additional health professionals practicing in the United States during 2010—represent the front lines of health care delivery and the primary interface for patients and consumers (HRSA, 2008; Staiger et al., 2009; U.S. Bureau of Labor Statistics, 2011). Engaging this sector is essential to progress in health care, from expanding the supply of clinical information, to promoting the use of evidence, to involving patients in their care and health.

The roles and responsibilities of clinicians are changing over time. Health care is evolving from a profession in which solo practitioners provided all aspects of care for a patient to one in which a team of clinicians is involved in meeting a patient's health needs. For example, Medicare patients see an average of seven physicians, including five specialists, split among four different practices (Pham et al., 2007). The changing landscape of medicine necessitates an increased focus on coordinating, sharing information, and working across specialty and professional lines. In this new team-based environment, clinicians across disciplinary lines need to work together to maintain and improve a patient's health, with different clinicians playing complementary roles based on their training and education (IOM, 2011b).

In addition, there is a trend toward greater transparency and accountability in health care, paralleling a similar trend occurring throughout society. New initiatives are focused on measuring and publicly reporting the quality of clinicians, the quality of hospitals, the prices for medical services, the costs of care episodes, and the health outcomes of different procedures and devices. These metrics are being applied to payment policies, from value-based insurance design to tiered networks, as an additional lever for accountability. This trend will change clinical practice as clinicians adapt and respond to these external factors.

Challenges to Learning

Although health care professionals strive to provide the best care to their patients, they face many challenges to the consistent delivery of efficient, high-quality care. Current practice experience falls short of this ideal in part because of inefficient workflows and support systems—which result in long delays for such straightforward tasks as patient follow-up and appointment scheduling—and because of the lack of adequate training and infrastructure to support the practice of high-quality care. The proliferation and fragmentation of information, expertise, and care delivery processes greatly compound the complex task faced by health care professionals when they try to deliver the right care at the right time. Moreover, the financial incentives for providers often are misaligned, rewarding volume of services over care quality and health outcomes. Overcoming these obstacles will depend increasingly on a team-based approach to care whereby clinicians coordinate care with each other and with community-based support services.

Opportunities

New methods of educating health care professionals and other health care workers, as well as new models for continuing to develop their competencies, will be needed to support a learning health care system. The current clinical training programs for each profession often operate independently from each other, which may limit an interprofessional view of care and teamwork (IOM, 2003). Education and continuing education need to focus on methods for using new evidence in clinical decision making, engaging in lifelong learning, understanding human behavior and social science, and delivering safe care in an interdisciplinary team environment (AAMC, 2011; Lucian Leape Institute Roundtable on Reforming Medical Education, 2010). To ensure that clinical leaders have the tools necessary to support large-scale improvement, additional opportunities are needed for educating health care workers in organizational management, systematic problem-solving techniques, and process improvement. Initiatives such as the Institute for Healthcare Improvement's (IHI's) Open School have been developed to address these needs, although additional projects will be needed to disseminate these tools widely. Additionally, given that effective communication with patients is crucial, clinical education needs to teach methods for communicating information to patients and engaging them actively in the clinical decision-making process.

New technologies and payment policies will assist health care professionals seeking to move toward continuous learning and improvement. The development of a robust information technology infrastructure will enable universal access to electronic health records; allow access to large databases for quality improvement; and enable broader access to decision support tools and knowledge repositories containing updated medical evidence, as well as evidence-based guidelines. Further, new incentives—financial, regulatory, and others—are being tested that would reward providers for applying evidence to patient care, delivering high-quality services, and improving their patients' health (Bovbjerg and Berenson, 2012).

Next Steps

To help achieve a learning health care system, clinicians and their teachers need to play the following roles:

- Embrace a culture of continuous improvement, with a focus on sharing and learning within and across systems.
- Optimize current educational programs to meet the knowledge and team-based needs of today and tomorrow for clinical care, management, and leadership.
- Optimize the care continuum with careful process design and robust technology.
- Partner with patients and families to set goals and make decisions based on clinical needs, social circumstances, and the degree of control patients prefer in their care, as well as acquire tools and skill sets for explaining clinical concepts, risks, and benefits to patients and their families.
- Collaborate with stakeholders on important health policy questions, such as payment reform and the application of clinical data to improving outcomes.
- Utilize digital health record systems in meaningful ways to capture patient experience and apply decision support at every level of their practice.

PROFESSIONAL SPECIALTY SOCIETIES

Roles in Learning

Bringing together clinicians and providing a forum for action, professional specialty societies play important roles in promoting learning. Many societies create regularly reviewed guidelines that summarize the current state of the science for a specific specialty, with some developing performance measures that build on those guidelines. Other societies have developed advanced data infrastructures for assessing performance with specific procedures or conditions, such as the registries created by the American College of Cardiology and The Society of Thoracic Surgeons. Still others have developed quality improvement initiatives for improving safety and quality, such as the American College of Surgeons' National Surgical Quality Improvement Program.

Challenges to Learning

Professional specialty societies seeking to play a greater role in learning face cultural, resource, and technical challenges (Ferris et al., 2007). On the cultural front, there are outstanding questions about the evolving nature of professionalism and the interest in self-regulation. With regard to resource and technical challenges, developing the data infrastructure for registries and quality improvement programs requires substantial investments in resources and significant technical expertise.

Opportunities

Several recent clinician led initiatives are aimed at improving the value achieved from health care. Some, such as the Choosing Wisely campaign spearheaded by the American Board of Internal Medicine (ABIM) Foundation and nine medical specialty groups, focus on identifying treatments or interventions that may provide little benefit to the general patient population (Cassel and Guest, 2012). The purpose of the campaign is to encourage discussions between patients and clinicians about the benefits and risks of different treatments and diagnostic technologies. This work, building on the Good Stewardship project (Good Stewardship Working Group, 2011), is intended to expand to additional specialty areas over time.

Next Steps

To help achieve a learning health care system, professional specialty societies need to play the following roles:

- Collaborate with other stakeholders to consider the necessary common core data elements and measures for managing high-impact conditions.
- Facilitate, along with other relevant organizations, the development, accessibility, and use of evidence-based clinical practice guidelines.

- Develop measures that can be applied to manage health on both the individual and population levels, assess performance and value, and evaluate the effectiveness of care transitions.
- Collect and make available information on the quality and outcomes of care.

DELIVERY SYSTEM LEADERS

Roles in Learning

Because of their size and care capacities, health care delivery organizations play a critical role in driving improvement in the health care system by using new practice methods, setting standards, and sharing resources and information with other care delivery organizations. In addition, many of these organizations have made significant investments in health information technology and in building their research capacity, which has allowed them to become leaders in generating and using evidence to improve patient care; many academic health centers and health systems have developed substantial research infrastructures for deepening clinical and biomedical understanding. Further, changes in health care have elevated the role of health care organizations in the delivery of care. Whereas many physicians traditionally practiced in small independent practices, physicians have increasingly joined large health care delivery systems over the past several years. As a result, the number of physician practices owned by hospitals increased from 20 percent in 2002 to 55 percent in 2008 (Kocher and Sahni, 2011). Although many physicians continue to work in small practices, the growth in physician employment by health care delivery organizations has made these institutions even more central stakeholders.

Challenges to Learning

Many institutions still struggle to implement sustainable, transformational system changes. They face both external obstacles, such as financial incentives that emphasize quantity of services over quality, and internal challenges in efforts to achieve improvement. To overcome these obstacles and become organizations that continuously learn and improve, they must adopt systematic problem-solving techniques and operational models that encourage and reward sustained quality and improved patient outcomes, and foster leadership and a culture that provide a strong foundation for improvement efforts. The accreditation, certification, and licensure processes for health care organizations provided by the Joint Commission and state agencies may support these efforts. Finally, the lessons learned by pioneer organizations need to be disseminated more broadly so that the entire system can benefit from the knowledge gained through the initiatives of individual organizations.

Opportunities

Opportunities exist to learn from the many industries that have developed new methods for improving safety, reliability, quality, and value. Organizations have learned how to manage and analyze large volumes of information; how to coordinate large numbers of workers to provide products or services with consistent quality; and how to ensure reliable performance, even under conditions of high risk. A number of these methods could potentially be adapted to health care to improve performance. In doing so, it will be important to consider several factors specific to health care, such as patient diversity and the technical complexity of modern medicine, as well as local factors that could affect implementation.

Next Steps

To help achieve a learning health care system, leaders of health care delivery organizations need to play the following roles:

- Set bold, mission-driven aims for clinical, financial, service, and experience outcomes against a frank assessment of the current reality, and implement those aims with a prioritized, aligned approach.
- Embrace a culture of continuous improvement, with a focus on sharing and learning within and across systems.
- Partner with patients, the public, communities, clinicians, and other stakeholders to, for example, achieve progress on the use of clinical data and patient perspectives to improve care.
- Promote transparency of process and performance.
- Collaborate with organizations within and beyond the traditional health care system to leverage prevention, health promotion, and community-based interventions to expand coordination and improve health.
- Optimize the care continuum with careful, systematic process design and robust technology.
- Develop and adopt tools that deliver clinical knowledge to the point of care.

HEALTH INSURERS

Roles in Learning

In 2010, private health insurance plans provided health benefits for 64 percent of the total U.S. population, and public payers, including Medicare, Medicaid, the Children's Health Insurance Program, the Department of Defense, and Department of Veterans Affairs health benefits programs, provided coverage to 31 percent (with some individuals receiving coverage from a mix of public and private sources) (DeNavas-Walt et al., 2011). As organizations that interact directly with patients, insurers have the ability to support patients as they seek to maintain healthy behaviors and access quality health care services. Further, insurance company policies determine the financial realities for health care providers and have a strong influence on how providers practice. While traditional reimbursement schedules have rewarded volume of services, recent insurer initiatives tie incentives to care quality or patient health outcomes to reward high performance.

Challenges to Learning

The insurance industry is operating in an environment of rising costs (Auerbach and Kellermann, 2011). In the employer-sponsored insurance market, health care premiums for family coverage have increased by 113 percent over the past decade (Kaiser Family Foundation and Health Research & Educational Trust, 2011). As a result, more families are unable to afford coverage; the number of uninsured Americans rose to 50 million in 2010 (DeNavas-Walt et al., 2011). In addition to the general challenges related to rising costs and waste, insurers face challenges related to new treatments and technologies, the aging of the population, and the increase in chronic conditions. Some insurers have developed new systems for applying evidence to their payment models, contracting policies, and benefit design. Yet these organizations often lack access to sufficient evidence on the efficacy of different treatments and interventions.

Opportunities

Private and public payers have undertaken multiple initiatives to improve value and promote the application of scientific evidence. These initiatives range from value-based purchasing, to medical homes, to accountable care organizations, to value-based insurance design. One notable example is policies on coverage with evidence development, which allow the coverage of new treatments and technologies while an evidence base for their effectiveness is being built. Other initiatives include multipayer claims databases, such as the Wisconsin Health Information Organization and the Health Care Cost Institute, that support the development of new insights regarding cost and value. These initiatives, many of which have shown success, provide new opportunities to deepen the knowledge base with respect to which payment models work under different circumstances, as well as encourage further innovation in the development of value initiatives.

Recent initiatives to expand the research infrastructure on clinical effectiveness, such as the Patient-Centered Outcomes Research Institute (PCORI), will help address the current gaps in evidence. To this end, PCORI has been allocated funding of $210 million for the first 3 years, rising to $500 million annually from 2014 to 2019 (Washington and Lipstein, 2011). Although it is premature to judge PCORI's work, increasing the level of knowledge on comparative effectiveness is critical to building a learning health care system.

One noteworthy new body is the Center for Medicare & Medicaid Innovation, which is charged with testing and evaluating innovative payment and delivery system models that could improve care quality while slowing cost growth in Medicare, Medicaid, and the Children's Health Insurance Program. Although the Patient Protection and Affordable Care Act outlines approximately 20 areas that the Innovation Center could consider at the outset, the legislation provides substantial flexibility for the exploration of different models. Successful models may be diffused to a larger patient population upon approval by the Secretary of Health and Human Services. The Innovation Center's ultimate goal is to promote the rapid development and diffusion of innovative payment and delivery models that are successful in improving quality and value. Through a number of ongoing initiatives, such as the Partnership for Patients, the Innovation Center will play an important role in improving care delivery and payment policies in Medicare and Medicaid and ensuring that payment policies support continuous learning by clinicians and health care organizations—a critical goal for a learning health care system. Although it is too soon to judge the effectiveness of the Center's work, the goal of improving payment policies is a critical one.

Next Steps

To help achieve a learning health care system, health insurers need to play the following roles:

- Seek to align incentives in support of high-quality, high-value, evidence-based care, including alignment among multiple payers and across the care continuum.

- Continually improve the value achieved by payment models, contracting policies, and benefit design while minimizing administrative burdens and expanding knowledge about the results of different payment and contracting models.
- Support increased research in clinical effectiveness and cross-industry application of the research results.
- Make longitudinal datasets available for research and public health purposes.
- Promote transparency to support care decisions and improvement efforts.
- Ensure a balanced focus on all outcomes (clinical, financial, service, and experience) and at multiple levels (individual, population).

EMPLOYERS

Roles in Learning

Given that employer-sponsored health insurance covers 55 percent of the population, employers and their employees bear a substantial proportion of health care costs (DeNavas-Walt et al., 2011). In return, they depend on the health care system to ensure that their employees remain healthy and productive. To this end, employers have increasingly supported efforts to improve quality and value by using their purchasing power to drive improvement efforts through contracts with providers and insurers, the design of benefit plans, and the provision of incentives and information for employees. Using such tools, employers can promote the application of evidence to care; encourage the use of high-quality, high-value providers and health care organizations; support positive changes in health behaviors; and expand the use of scientific evidence when employees make care decisions. Many employers have indicated their willingness to support continuous learning and improvement by introducing payment and contracting policies that reward safe, high-quality, high-value care that improves health.

Challenges to Learning

Rising health care costs have eroded employer-sponsored health care coverage and its generosity. Currently, 60 percent of employers offer coverage to their employees. In 2011, employer contributions to health insurance for family coverage averaged more than $4,100, up 230 percent in a decade (Kaiser Family Foundation and Health Research & Educational Trust, 2011). Health care costs have become a major expense for employers, threatening their competitiveness in a global economy. Costs, however, are only part of the problem; employers also consider the return (in terms of employee health) that they receive from this investment. Yet, recent statistics suggest that substantial waste and inefficiency result in expenditures that do not improve care quality or patient health.

Opportunities

The tools available to employers to improve health care quality and value are limited by a lack of clinical evidence. New efforts to increase the clinical knowledge base, such as PCORI, will help address this challenge.

Next Steps

To help achieve a learning health care system, employers need to play the following roles:

- Use their purchasing power to drive high-quality, high-value health care.
- Actively engage their employees in health and wellness through workplace wellness programs, partnerships, educational resources, and the design of benefit plans.
- Engage with employees to understand their unique values, needs, and expectations.
- Incentivize employees to use high-quality, high value providers as measured by clinical, financial, service, and experience outcomes.
- Share industry-specific business practices and systematic approaches to process improvement with the health care community in the spirit of learning within and across community partners.

HEALTH RESEARCHERS

Roles in Learning

Health researchers are critical to building the evidence base for care effectiveness and value. These investigators consider both individual treatments and interventions and broader delivery system initiatives, conducting quantitative and qualitative evaluations, cost-benefit analyses, and organizational studies. Given this broad charge, the health researcher community includes those involved in the design and operation of clinical trials, the development of clinical registries and clinical databases, the creation of standards and metrics, modeling and simulation studies, studies of health services and care delivery processes, and the aggregation of study results into systematic reviews and clinical guidelines. This work has been supported by a number of agencies and organizations, including the Agency for Healthcare Research and Quality (AHRQ), the National Institutes of Health (NIH), and PCORI.

Challenges to Learning

This stakeholder group faces several challenges as it works to build knowledge. The financial resources for research and development are limited as a result of economic and budgetary constraints. Further, public awareness of and participation in the clinical research enterprise has recently decreased, with fewer individuals expressing interest in participating in clinical trials (Woolley and Propst, 2005). Investigators also have expressed concern about the ability to share data and glean insights from clinical data because of the current regulatory framework (IOM, 2009a). Results of previous surveys of health researchers suggest that the current formulation and interpretation of privacy rules have increased the cost and time to conduct research, that different institutional interpretations of the Health Insurance Portability and Accountability Act (HIPAA) and associated regulations have impeded collaboration, and that the rules have made it difficult to recruit subjects (Association of Academic Health Centers, 2008; Greene et al., 2006; IOM, 2009a; Ness, 2007).

Transforming the research enterprise will require new efforts to build trust among patients and the public. Building this trust will in turn require increasing confidence in the results of clinical research, being open and honest about the risks and benefits of this type of research, and ensuring confidence in the privacy and security safeguards for health data. Technically, new approaches are needed to reduce the expense and effort of conducting the research, to improve the applicability of its results to clinical decisions, and to identify smaller effects and effects on different populations.

Finally, this sector will need to consider how to accelerate the translation of evidence into practice using technological and nontechnological tools, accounting for the factors that affect the dissemination of initiatives in the health care system. The products of the nation's clinical data utility and research enterprise are useless unless they are disseminated and put into practice. Yet current systems that generate new clinical knowledge and those that implement such knowledge are largely disconnected and poorly coordinated. Although many effective, evidence-based practices, therapeutics, and interventions are developed every year, only some become widely used in a meaningful way. Overcoming this obstacle will require a focus on the dissemination and translation of research, new partnerships between clinical and health service researchers and clinicians in implementing research results, and additional research into the dissemination and diffusion of scientific evidence in the system.

Opportunities

New efforts to increase the knowledge base on clinical effectiveness, such as PCORI, along with the work of existing research agencies, such as NIH and AHRQ, will help broaden the scope of the clinical research that is undertaken. Further, many research organizations have initiated high-profile efforts to improve the quality and efficiency of clinical trials, including initiatives at NIH and the Food and Drug Administration's Clinical Trials Transformation Initiative. Based on these efforts and the work of academic research leaders, new types of research trials have been developed, such as pragmatic clinical trials, delayed design trials, and cluster randomized controlled trials (see Chapter 6 for a description of these types of trials) (Campbell et al., 2007; Eldridge et al., 2008; Tunis et al., 2003, 2010). Advanced statistical methods, including Bayesian analysis, allow for adaptive research designs that can learn as a research study advances, making studies more flexible (Chow and Chang, 2008). These new methods are designed to reduce the expense and effort of conducting research, to improve the applicability of research results to clinical decisions, to improve the ability to identify smaller effects, and to offer an alternative when traditional methods are not feasible.

In addition to new research methods, advances in statistical analysis, simulation, and modeling now supplement traditional methods for conducting trials. Given that even the most tightly controlled trials show a distribution of patient responses to a given treatment or intervention, new statistical techniques can help segment results for different populations. Further, new Bayesian techniques for data analysis can disentangle the effects of different clinical interventions on overall population health (Berry et al., 2006). With the growth in computational power, newly developed models can replicate physiological pathways and disease states (Eddy and Schlessinger, 2003; Stern et al., 2008). These models can then be used to simulate clinical trials and individualize clinical guidelines according to a patient's particular situation and biology, which can improve health status while reducing costs (Eddy et al., 2011). As computational power increases, the potential applications of these simulation and modeling tools will continue to advance.

In addition, novel technologies allow for new means of collecting health care data directly from patients. Enabled by advances in mobile technologies and informatics, patients and consumers now have the ability to be involved in collecting and sharing data on their personal condition. This vision is being realized through biobanks operated by disease-specific organizations, in addition to social networking sites. Examples of social networking sites that aim to promote patient participation in research include PatientsLikeMe®, Love/Avon Army of Women, and Facebook health groups. While these patient-initiated approaches face challenges, especially related to bias in self-reporting, data quality, and protection against discrimination, their prevalence can only be expected to increase.

Next Steps

To help achieve a learning health care system, health researchers need to play the following roles:

- Actively engage with care communities to advance understanding of clinical research and clinical trials and thereby enhance balanced consideration of and enrollment in clinical trials.
- Develop and implement new methods for conducting clinical research that overcome the limitations of the traditional research enterprise.
- Partner with patients to build trust in the clinical research enterprise.
- Optimize, through formal and informal structures, the linkages among basic research, clinical research, public health, and care delivery through such means as technology, communities of learning, and cross-industry collaboration.
- Engage in efforts to advance publication and learning as a result of quality improvement efforts.
- Advance the science of dissemination and implementation, with a focus on practical strategies for expanding the diffusion of clinical research.

DIGITAL TECHNOLOGY DEVELOPERS

Roles in Learning

Digital technology developers have emerged to meet the growing demand to capture, store, retrieve, and share information in virtually every aspect of health care. The range of newly digitalized services is remarkable, encompassing products that assist in scheduling and billing, claims processing and payment, supply and equipment inventory maintenance, individual patient records, medication prescribing and tracking, decision support systems, postmarket product monitoring, and disease and treatment registries. Fundamentally, the work of this sector focuses on improving the access of patients and health care providers to reliable, high-quality evidence; enhancing patient-provider communication and interaction; seamlessly and continuously capturing measures of patient health at ever finer levels of granularity; promoting operational effectiveness and efficiency; improving the ability to manage and analyze large quantities of data; and improving research on clinical effectiveness and quality of care.

Challenges to Learning

Digital technology developers face multiple challenges to increasing the digital resources for health care. One of the greatest challenges is the need to develop standards that foster data sharing and data quality. For example, sharing of electronic health records is impeded by the fact that a variety of such systems are in use, each of which stores data using different methods and in different formats. Overcoming these challenges will require technological solutions, such as interoperability strategies; methods for highlighting the quality of the data; and ways to identify the data's source, context, and provenance. In addition, given the complex and demanding nature of modern health care practice, it is necessary to ensure that these tools can be seamlessly integrated into providers' daily workflow without causing disruptions in their clinical routine.

Opportunities

An opportunity to promote the adoption of health information technologies was recently provided by the Health Information Technology for Economic and Clinical Health (HITECH) Act, part of the American Recovery and Reinvestment Act. This legislation formalized the Office of the National Coordinator for Health Information Technology in the Department of Health and Human Services and provided substantial financial incentives for health care providers and hospitals to adopt and use electronic health records. Resources devoted to those programs include $2 billion for programs by the National Coordinator, as well as almost $30 billion in Medicare and Medicaid incentive payments to physicians and hospitals (Blumenthal, 2009; Buntin et al., 2010). Notably, the act encourages not only the adoption but also the meaningful use of such record systems. The criteria for incentive eligibility in the first stage of meaningful use were released by CMS on July 13, 2010. The aim of this stage was to capture clinical data in a standardized format within electronic health records and make the data accessible to authorized users (Blumenthal and Tavenner, 2010). Subsequent stages of meaningful use are currently under development. They will focus on the secure exchange of health information for care coordination and will drive more advanced uses of health information technology systems (Buntin et al., 2010).

Next Steps

To help achieve a learning health care system, digital technology developers need to play the following roles:

- Ensure that electronic health record systems and other digital technologies capture and deliver the core data elements needed to support knowledge generation.
- Partner with patients, the delivery system, insurers, researchers, innovators, regulators, and other stakeholders.
- Collaborate in the development of core datasets for different diseases and conditions to support clinical care, improvement, and research.
- Develop tools that assist individuals in managing their health and health care and that provide opportunities for building communities to support patient efforts.
- Consider interoperability and integration in clinical workflows in designing digital health systems.

HEALTH PRODUCT INNOVATORS AND REGULATORS

Roles in Learning

By conducting clinical research and developing innovative new treatments and interventions, health product innovators play a pivotal role in a learning health care system. In 2010, the biopharmaceutical segment of the market conducted research and development for more than 3,000 products in development (Pharmaceutical Research and Manufacturers of America, 2011). Regulators, including the Food and Drug Administration, play an important role as well in several aspects of the health care system, from the introduction of medical products to surveillance of existing products.

Challenges to Learning

As with other research sectors, these stakeholders face challenges in generating new clinical evidence. The current research paradigm often requires substantial investments of money and time to answer important questions, limiting the amount of research that can be conducted to answer important questions and develop new products. The research enterprise is especially challenged in understanding how different treatments affect patients in everyday settings and in distinguishing the effects of a treatment in different population groups. Regulators similarly face challenges in providing a regulatory framework that ensures safety and effectiveness throughout a product's life cycle (IOM, 2009b, 2011a,c).

Opportunities

Health product innovators and regulators will be affected by new developments in the design of health plan benefits, such as the coverage with evidence development designs noted above that provide payment for interventions while evidence on their efficacy continues to be generated. Further, the digital infrastructure will provide new opportunities to gather postmarket surveillance data and identify potential adverse reactions, as well as unexpected indications for a therapy. Finally, the development of new research methods will allow for more granular assessments of a product's effectiveness, including the patient populations that benefit (or do not), allowing for more effective use of the product. The industry has an opportunity to build on its productive partnerships in clinical effectiveness research to further advance the capacities of the field.

Developments in digital technology allow for new linkages between health product innovators and regulators. Given their interest in the safety and effectiveness of pharmaceuticals, devices, and other products, regulators collect and analyze substantial amounts of data to evaluate whether a product is safe and effective for its indicated use. For the health care system to continuously learn and improve, health care knowledge must continuously be generated. On the regulatory level, evidence on a product's effectiveness needs to be updated after the product's introduction. One initiative aimed at addressing this concern is the Food and Drug Administration's Sentinel Initiative, which is focused on building a national electronic system to monitor the safety of drugs. A related pilot initiative is the Mini-Sentinel network, whose mission is to learn about the barriers and challenges to establishing this type of large-scale product safety monitoring system.

Next Steps

To help achieve a learning health care system, health product innovators and regulators need to play the following roles:

- Build a learning system across the industry, anchored in ethical practice, that allows for the most effective public-private partnerships, learning, and diffusion of innovation.
- Probe the unique systems, processes, and needs of high-quality, high-value health care, and conduct applied research on innovative approaches to meeting those needs.

- Partner with the health care organizations in the communities in which they and their employees live to address identified opportunities for improvement.
- Develop tools that assist individuals in managing their health and health care.

GOVERNANCE

Roles in Learning

All governance groups, from boards of health care organizations to governmental bodies, need to be actively involved in promoting a learning health care system. The leadership of these groups, often in collaborative forms, will be necessary to motivate the actions required to create a learning health care system.

Hospital and health care delivery system boards have a crucial role in guiding their organizations toward continuous learning and improvement. Boards are responsible for the quality of care provided, the financial health and reputation of the organization, oversight of the organization's executives, and formulation of the organization's mission (Belmont et al., 2011; Conway, 2008). Better outcomes are associated with organizations in which the board spends time on health care quality concepts, sets a quality agenda, formally monitors quality performance metrics, interacts with staff on strategy, and rewards executive leadership based on measured quality and safety goals (IHI, 2007; Jiang et al., 2009; Vaughn et al., 2006).

Challenges to Learning

As stated earlier, many institutions still struggle to implement sustainable, transformational system changes. The challenges range from health care payment incentives that encourage greater use of health care services to an organizational culture opposed to large-scale change. There also is a need to diffuse the lessons learned by pioneer organizations more broadly, so that the whole system can benefit from the knowledge gained through the initiatives of individual organizations.

Opportunities

As noted earlier, many industries have developed new methods for improving safety, reliability, quality, and value. These methods hold great promise. Encouraging and rewarding their application in health care organizations is an important task of governing bodies.

Furthermore, health care organizations have the opportunity to incorporate and promote learning throughout their governance structures, from governing boards to professional governance bodies. The professional governance bodies, such as a hospital's medical committee, generally monitor clinical practice patterns and review professional standards, allowing for an opportunity to promote evidence-based practices and highlighting areas within the organization that achieve high performance. Other committees and governance structures in the organization have similar opportunities to encourage continuous improvement from all the organization's employees.

Next Steps

To help achieve a learning health care system, governing bodies need to play the following roles:

- Embrace a culture of continuous improvement, with a focus on sharing and learning within and across systems.
- Set bold mission-driven aims for clinical, financial, service, and experience outcomes against a frank assessment of the current reality.
- Affirm the primary role of health care organizations in serving their communities by working to improve the care experience, population health, and the value of care.
- Establish vibrant collaboratives, with clear aims and expectations for improvement across the care continuum, connecting community, health care delivery, public health, regulatory, employer, insurer, education, and other key stakeholders.

THE CHALLENGE

Missed opportunities for better health care have real human and economic impacts. If the care in every state were of the quality delivered by the highest-performing state, an estimated 75,000 fewer deaths would have occurred across the country in 2005 (McCarthy et al., 2009; Schoenbaum et al., 2011). Current waste in health care diverts resources from productive uses—estimates suggest almost $750 billion in opportunity costs in 2009 that could be used for improving care on many dimensions (IOM, 2010). It is only through shared commitments, in alignment with a supportive policy environment, that the opportunities offered by science and information technology can be captured. The nation's health and economic futures—best care at lower cost—depend on the ability to steward the evolution of a continuously learning health care system.

REFERENCES

AAMC (Association of American Medical Colleges). 2011. *Behavioral and social science foundations for future physicians*. Washington, DC: AAMC.

Association of Academic Health Centers. 2008. *HIPAA creating barriers to research and discovery: HIPAA problems widespread and unresolved since 2003*. http://www.aahcdc.org/policy/reddot/AAHC_HIPAA_Creating_Barriers.pdf (accessed June 9, 2011).

Auerbach, D. I., and A. L. Kellermann. 2011. A decade of health care cost growth has wiped out real income gains for an average US family. *Health Affairs* 30(9):1630-1636.

Belmont, E., C. C. Haltom, D. A. Hastings, R. G. Homchick, L. Morris, J. Taitsman, B. M. Peters, R. L. Nagele, B. Schermer, and K. C. Peisert. 2011. A new quality compass: Hospital boards' increased role under the Affordable Care Act. *Health Affairs (Millwood)* 30(7):1282-1289.

Berry, D. A., L. Inoue, Y. Shen, J. Venier, D. Cohen, M. Bondy, R. Theriault, and M. F. Munsell. 2006. Modeling the impact of treatment and screening on U.S. breast cancer mortality: A Bayesian approach. *Journal of the National Cancer Institute Monographs* (36):30-36.

Blumenthal, D. 2009. Stimulating the adoption of health information technology. *New England Journal of Medicine* 360(15):1477-1479.

Blumenthal, D., and M. Tavenner. 2010. The "meaningful use" regulation for electronic health records. *New England Journal of Medicine* 363(6):501-504.

Bovbjerg, R. R., and R. A. Berenson. 2012. *The value of clinical practice guidelines as malpractice "safe harbors."* Washington, DC: Urban Institute.

Brach, C., B. Dreyer, P. Schyve, L. M. Hernandez, C. Baur, A. J. Lemerise, and R. Parker. 2012. *Attributes of a health literate organization*. Discussion Paper, Institute of Medicine, Washington, DC. http://iom.edu/~/media/Files/Perspectives-Files/2012/Discussion-Papers/BPH_Ten_HLit_Attributes.pdf (accessed August 31, 2012).

Buntin, M. B., S. H. Jain, and D. Blumenthal. 2010. Health information technology: Laying the infrastructure for national health reform. *Health Affairs (Millwood)* 29(6):1214-1219.

Campbell, M. J., A. Donner, and N. Klar. 2007. Developments in cluster randomized trials and statistics in medicine. *Statistics in Medicine* 26(1):2-19.

Cassel, C. K., and J. A. Guest. 2012. Choosing wisely: Helping physicians and patients make smart decisions about their care. *Journal of the American Medical Association* 307(17):1801-1802.

Chow, S. C., and M. Chang. 2008. Adaptive design methods in clinical trials—a review. *Orphanet Journal of Rare Diseases* 3:11.

Conway, J. 2008. Getting boards on board: Engaging governing boards in quality and safety. *Joint Commission Journal on Quality and Patient Safety* 34(4):214-220.

DeNavas-Walt, C., B. D. Proctor, and J. C. Smith. 2011. *Income, poverty, and health insurance coverage in the United States: 2010*. Washington, DC: U.S. Census Bureau.

Eddy, D. M., and L. Schlessinger. 2003. Archimedes: A trial-validated model of diabetes. *Diabetes Care* 26(11):3093-3101.

Eddy, D. M., J. Adler, B. Patterson, D. Lucas, K. A. Smith, and M. Morris. 2011. Individualized guidelines: The potential for increasing quality and reducing costs. *Annals of Internal Medicine* 154(9):627-634.

Eldridge, S., D. Ashby, C. Bennett, M. Wakelin, and G. Feder. 2008. Internal and external validity of cluster randomised trials: Systematic review of recent trials. *British Medical Journal* 336(7649):876-880.

Ferris, T. G., C. Vogeli, J. Marder, C. S. Sennett, and E. G. Campbell. 2007. Physician specialty societies and the development of physician performance measures. *Health Affairs (Millwood)* 26(6):1712-1719.

Good Stewardship Working Group. 2011. The "top 5" lists in primary care: Meeting the responsibility of professionalism. *Archives of Internal Medicine* 171(15):1385-1390.

Greene, S. M., A. M. Geiger, E. L. Harris, A. Altschuler, L. Nekhlyudov, M. B. Barton, S. J. Rolnick, J. G. Elmore, and S. Fletcher. 2006. Impact of IRB requirements on a multicenter survey of prophylactic mastectomy outcomes. *Annals of Epidemiology* 16(4):275-278.

HRSA (Health Resources and Services Administration). 2008. *The physician workforce: Projections and research into current issues affecting supply and demand.* Washington, DC: U.S. Department of Health and Human Services.

IHI (Institute for Healthcare Improvement). 2007. *Protecting 5 million lives from harm. Getting started kit: Governance leadership "boards on board."* http://www.longwoods.com/product/download/code/19364 (accessed August 31, 2012).

IOM (Institute of Medicine). 2003. *Health professions education: A bridge to quality.* Washington, DC: The National Academies Press.

IOM. 2009a. *Beyond the HIPAA privacy rule: Enhancing privacy, improving health through research.* Washington, DC: The National Academies Press.

IOM. 2009b. *Leadership commitments to improve value in health care: Finding common ground: Workshop summary.* Washington, DC: The National Academies Press.

IOM. 2010. *The healthcare imperative: Lowering costs and improving outcomes: Workshop series summary.* Washington, DC: The National Academies Press.

IOM. 2011a. *Building a national framework for the establishment of regulatory science for drug development: Workshop summary.* Washington, DC: The National Academies Press.

IOM. 2011b. *The future of nursing: Leading change, advancing health.* Washington, DC: The National Academies Press.

IOM. 2011c. *Medical devices and the public's health: The FDA 510(k) clearance process at 35 years.* Washington, DC: The National Academies Press.

Jiang, H. J., C. Lockee, K. Bass, and I. Fraser. 2009. Board oversight of quality: Any differences in process of care and mortality? *Journal of Healthcare Management* 54(1):15-29.

Kaiser Family Foundation and Health Research & Educational Trust. 2011. *Employer health benefits: 2011 annual survey.* Menlo Park, CA: Kaiser Family Foundation and Health Research & Educational Trust.

Kocher, R., and N. R. Sahni. 2011. Hospitals' race to employ physicians—the logic behind a money-losing proposition. *New England Journal of Medicine* 364(19):1790-1793.

Lucian Leape Institute Roundtable on Reforming Medical Education. 2010. *Unmet needs: Teaching physicians to provide safe patient care.* Boston, MA: National Patient Safety Foundation.

McCarthy, D., S. How, C. Schoen, J. Cantor, and D. Belloff. 2009. *Aiming higher. Results from a state scorecard on health system performance.* New York: Commonwealth Fund Commission on a High Performance Health System.

Ness, R. B. 2007. Influence of the HIPAA privacy rule on health research. *Journal of the American Medical Association* 298(18):2164-2170.

Pham, H. H., D. Schrag, A. S. O'Malley, B. Wu, and P. B. Bach. 2007. Care patterns in Medicare and their implications for pay for performance. *New England Journal of Medicine* 356(11):1130-1139.

Pharmaceutical Research and Manufacturers of America. 2011. *Pharmaceutical industry profile 2011.* Washington, DC: Pharmaceutical Research and Manufacturers of America.

Schoenbaum, S. C., C. Schoen, J. L. Nicholson, and J. C. Cantor. 2011. Mortality amenable to health care in the United States: The roles of demographics and health systems performance. *Journal of Public Health Policy* 32(4):407-429.

Staiger, D. O., D. I. Auerbach, and P. I. Buerhaus. 2009. Comparison of physician workforce estimates and supply projections. *Journal of the American Medical Association* 302(15):1674-1680.

Stern, M., K. Williams, D. Eddy, and R. Kahn. 2008. Validation of prediction of diabetes by the Archimedes model and comparison with other predicting models. *Diabetes Care* 31(8):1670-1671.

Tunis, S. R., D. B. Stryer, and C. M. Clancy. 2003. Practical clinical trials: Increasing the value of clinical research for decision making in clinical and health policy. *Journal of the American Medical Association* 290(12):1624-1632.

Tunis, S. R., J. Benner, and M. McClellan. 2010. Comparative effectiveness research: Policy context, methods development and research infrastructure. *Statistics in Medicine* 29(19):1963-1976.

U.S. Bureau of Labor Statistics. 2011. *Occupational employment statistics: Occupational profiles (May 2011 estimates)*. http://www.bls.gov/oes/current/oes_stru.htm#29-0000 (accessed May 15, 2012).

Vaughn, T., M. Koepke, E. Kroch, W. Lehrman, S. Sinha, and S. Levey. 2006. Engagement of leadership in quality improvement initiatives: Executive quality improvement survey results. *Journal of Patient Safety* 2(1).

Washington, A. E., and S. H. Lipstein. 2011. The Patient-Centered Outcomes Research Institute—promoting better information, decisions, and health. *New England Journal of Medicine* 365(15):e31.

Woolley, M., and S. M. Propst. 2005. Public attitudes and perceptions about health-related research. *Journal of the American Medical Association* 294(11):1380-1384.

Appendix A

Glossary

Community—Groups of people defined in many ways, such as by geography, culture, disease or condition, occupation, and workplace.

Complexity—A property of a system that consists of multiple interrelated components and is also difficult to analyze and understand because of its complicated nature.

Continuous learning and improvement—The process of ongoing measurement and analysis to inform changes in the delivery of care. Continuous learning occurs both intra- and interinstitutionally and relies on the real-time capture and use of data on patient experience, outcomes, and process measures.

Cost—Price multiplied by the volume of services or products used, or the total sum of money spent at a given level (patients, organizations, state, national).

Evidence—Information from clinical experience that has met some established test of validity, with the appropriate standard determined according to the requirements of the intervention and clinical circumstance. (IOM Roundtable on Value & Science-Driven Health Care Charter)

Evidence-based—Being based on reliable evidence while accounting appropriately for individual variation in patient needs. (IOM Roundtable on Value & Science-Driven Health Care Charter)

Genomics—A field of study concerned with hereditary information of organisms.

High-value—A characteristic achieved through maximizing value by improving outcomes, lowering costs, or both.

Informatics—A field of study concerned with the effective use of information to answer scientific questions.

Learning health care system—A health care system in which science, informatics, incentives, and culture are aligned for continuous improvement and innovation, with best practices seamlessly embedded in the care process, patients and families active participants in all elements, and new knowledge captured as an integral by-product of the care experience (Charter, IOM Roundtable on Value & Science-Driven Health Care).

Patient-centered outcomes—Outcomes of clinical care that are most important to patients.

Price—The amount charged for a given health care service or product. It is important to note that there are frequently multiple prices for the same service or product, depending on the patient's insurance status and payer, as other factors.

Proteomics—A field of study that examines the structure and function of proteins.

Systems engineering—An interdisciplinary approach to the design, management, and analysis of complex systems to achieve objectives such as efficiency, quality, and safety.

Value—Assessed using the following heuristic: $\text{Value} = \dfrac{\text{Outcomes}}{\text{Cost}}$

Appendix B

A CEO Checklist for High-Value Health Care

The following IOM Discussion Paper, "A CEO Checklist for High-Value Health Care," was released in June 2012 by the IOM Roundtable on Value & Science-Driven Health Care. The document can also be found online at http://www.iom.edu/CEOChecklist.

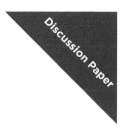

A CEO Checklist for High-Value Health Care

Delos Cosgrove, Michael Fisher, Patricia Gabow, Gary Gottlieb,
George Halvorson, Brent James, Gary Kaplan, Jonathan Perlin,
Robert Petzel, Glenn Steele, and John Toussaint*

June 2012

*Participants in the IOM Roundtable on Value & Science-Driven Health Care

*The views expressed in this discussion paper are those of the authors and not
necessarily of the authors' organizations or of the Institute of Medicine. The paper
is intended to help inform and stimulate discussion. It has not been subjected to the
review procedures of the Institute of Medicine and is not a report of the Institute of
Medicine or of the National Research Council.*

INSTITUTE OF MEDICINE
OF THE NATIONAL ACADEMIES
Advising the nation • Improving health

AUTHORS

Delos Cosgrove, MD
President and CEO
Cleveland Clinic

Michael Fisher
President and CEO
Cincinnati Children's Hospital
  Medical Center

Patricia Gabow, MD
Chief Executive Officer
Denver Health and Hospital Authority

Gary Gottlieb, MD, MBA
President and CEO
Partners HealthCare System, Inc.

George Halvorson
Chairman and CEO
Kaiser Permanente

Brent James, MD, MStat
Executive Director
Intermountain Institute for Care
  Delivery Research

Gary Kaplan, MD
Chairman and CEO
Virginia Mason Health System

Jonathan Perlin, MD, PhD
President, Clinical and Physician Services
HCA, Inc.

Robert Petzel, MD
Undersecretary for Health
Department of Veterans Affairs

Glenn Steele, MD, PhD
President and CEO
Geisinger Health System

John Toussaint, MD
Chief Executive Officer
ThedaCare Center for Healthcare Value

The authors were assisted by the following individuals:

Albert Bothe, MD
Geisinger Health System

Jonathan Darer, MD, MPH
Geisinger Health System

Duane Davis, MD
Geisinger Health System

Tejal Gandhi, MD
Partners HealthCare System, Inc.

Uma Kotagal, MBBS, MSc
Cincinnati Children's Hospital

Tom Lee, MD
Partners HealthCare System, Inc.

Peter Markell
Partners HealthCare System, Inc.

J. Michael McGinnis, MD, MPP
Institute of Medicine

Geraldine McGlynn, MEd
Veterans Health Administration

E. Lynn Miller
Geisinger Health System

Kathleen Paul
Virginia Mason Health System

Brian Powers
Institute of Medicine

Lucy Savitz, PhD
Intermountain Healthcare

Pat Schrepf
Virginia Mason Health System

Earl Steinberg, MD
Geisinger Health System

Leigh Stuckhardt, JD
Institute of Medicine

Jed Weissberg, MD
Kaiser Permanente

Robert Wyllie, MD
Cleveland Clinic

As leaders of health care organizations, we are acutely aware of the pressures that rising health care costs place on individuals, employers, and the government, as we are of unacceptable shortfalls in the quality and efficiency of care. But we have also learned, through experiences in our own institutions and through communication and collaboration with colleagues in others, that better outcomes at lower costs can be achieved through care transformation initiatives that yield improved results, more satisfied patients, and cultures of continuous learning. These transformation efforts have generated certain foundational lessons relevant to every CEO and Board member, and the health care delivery organizations they lead. We have assembled these lessons here as a *A CEO Checklist for High-Value Health Care* to describe touchstone principles, illustrated with case examples, central not only to our work to date, but to sustaining and reinforcing the system-wide transformation necessary for continuous improvement in the face of rapidly increasing pressures, demands, and market changes.

This *Checklist* is intended to be a living and dynamic document, and we invite both suggestions to improve its utility and reach, and co-signing by our CEO colleagues who wish to support these strategies for effective, efficient, and continuously improving health care for all Americans.

NEEDS AND OPPORTUNITIES

Health care in the United States is at a critical point. Excessive costs are no longer tenable and mediocre outcomes are no longer tolerable. For 32 of the past 40 years, health care costs have grown faster than the rest of the U.S. economy.[1] Federal health care costs—expected to reach $950 billion in 2012—will become the largest contributor to the national debt.[2] States, too, are being crippled by health care costs. Medicaid now consumes almost a quarter of state budgets, crowding out investments in education and infrastructure.[3] In the private sector, escalating costs have eroded the bottom line for employers who purchase health care for their employees and have eliminated any appreciable gains in income for American families during the past decade.[4,5] Purchasers simply cannot afford the status quo.

Despite these expenditures, outcome shortfalls are pervasive. Population health measures such as life expectancy and preterm birth lag behind those of almost every other developed nation. Patients are still harmed by medical errors. Recent assessments indicate that 10 years after the IOM report *To Err Is Human* estimated that medical errors cause up to 98,000 deaths in hospitals each year,[6] roughly 15 percent of hospital patients are still being harmed during their stays.[7] Poor care coordination places further strain on patients and the system, with roughly 20 percent of discharged elderly patients returning to the hospital within 30 days.[8] Faced with concerns about the cost and quality of health care, purchasers are developing concrete plans to leverage their buying power to reduce expenditures and demand high-value care—care that achieves better outcomes at lower costs.

These are the realities for health care executives today. As demand for high-value health care builds, care delivery leaders face the near-term imperative to transform the way their organizations operate. We know the potential for improvement exists. The amount of waste in the system—estimated to be at least 30 percent[9]—provides both the opportunity and the mandate for transformation. Replacing wasteful practices and procedures with those marked by effectiveness and efficiency can improve health outcomes and bottom lines at a time when pressures are growing on both counts.

> The Checklist's 10 items reflect the strategies that, in our experiences and those of others, have proven effective and essential to improving quality and reducing costs.

Given the urgency at hand, each of us, with the assistance of farsighted staff and in cooperation with many of you in other institutional leadership positions, has been engaged in these kinds of efforts. To aid and accelerate the system-wide transformation necessary, we have assembled what we are calling "A CEO Checklist for High-Value Care" (the Checklist). The Checklist's 10 items reflect the strategies that, in our experiences and those of others, have proven effective and essential to improving quality and reducing costs. They describe the foundational, infrastructure, care delivery, and feedback components of a system oriented around value, and represent basic opportunities—indeed obligations—for hospital and health care delivery system CEOs and Boards to improve the value of health care in their institutions.

The strategies in this Checklist are not, of course, of the "one-and-done" variety. Rather, the items we present here are elements that must become core components of an organization's DNA. In some ways, they represent more a credo of commitment than a simple checklist, but each Checklist item is every bit as vital as the items on the checklists routinely used by pilots taking complicated aircraft into quickly changing conditions. Taken together, the Checklist provides a blueprint for improving quality and reducing cost amid a changing landscape.

We realize that while the elements on the Checklist are necessary to achieve high-value health care within an institution, they are not sufficient to reach full potential across the system. Forces outside the control of any single institution—economic incentives that reward volume over value, inequitable access to needed services, poor linkage of community and clinical services, and unnecessary regulatory requirements—can all serve as barriers to the transformation required. However pervasive, we cannot allow these issues to obscure the substantial gains that can be achieved from the steps well within our control as leaders of our institutions.

What follows is an item-by-item review of the basic issues, opportunities, and expectations for the 10 items on the Checklist, along with case material that briefly describes a sample of our experiences. To improve readability and access, we have been deliberately brief in the case descriptions, but more details may be found in the material in Appendix I, where follow-up contact information is also provided for additional conversations. Because this paper addresses the system-level issues that are central to achieving high-value health care, we do not discuss or spotlight some important work that has been developed around individual services that are often overused, unnecessary, or otherwise wasteful. In recognition of the utility of such analyses and inventories, we have included summaries of some of that work in Appendix II.

Ultimately, the transition to high-value care will be led and championed by executives who recognize high quality and lower cost as institutional aims, and will be sustained by a system-wide culture of continuous improvement. When successfully implemented, these systematic improvements that reduce waste and improve outcomes will maximize the value of health care delivered in the United States.

A CHECKLIST
FOR HIGH-VALUE HEALTH CARE

Just as we offer an invitation to each staff and Board member of our respective institutions to hold us accountable for fully engaging, implementing, and sustaining attention to every Checklist item, we invite you to be in touch as we work together to build the field of health care transformation and better health for all Americans.

Foundational elements

✓ **Governance priority**—visible and determined leadership by CEO and Board

✓ **Culture of continuous improvement**—commitment to ongoing, real-time learning

Infrastructure fundamentals

✓ **IT best practices**—automated, reliable information to and from the point of care

✓ **Evidence protocols**—effective, efficient, and consistent care

✓ **Resource utilization**—optimized use of personnel, physical space, and other resources

Care delivery priorities

✓ **Integrated care**—right care, right setting, right providers, right teamwork

✓ **Shared decision making**—patient–clinician collaboration on care plans

✓ **Targeted services**—tailored community and clinic interventions for resource-intensive patients

Reliability and feedback

✓ **Embedded safeguards**—supports and prompts to reduce injury and infection

✓ **Internal transparency**—visible progress in performance, outcomes, and costs

FOUNDATIONAL ELEMENTS

To create lasting, sustainable change, the pursuit of continuous improvement and better value for patients must define an organization's culture, mission, and leadership. It is a pursuit that is never complete, but with a relentless operational ethos of continuous improvement and assessment, we can achieve the value potential for the care within our institutions and the health of the populations we serve.

✓ **Governance priority**—visible and determined leadership by CEO and Board

✓ **Culture of continuous improvement**—commitment to ongoing, real-time learning

✓ Governance Priority
Visible and determined leadership by CEO and Board

Senior executive leaders and Board members are the central stewards of high-value care. Responsible for both our institutions' financial health and the quality of care provided, we are inherently the most visible champions for a culture of continuous improvement in quality and high-value care. Our steadfast engagement with front-line staff, management, and other organizational leaders to evaluate performance and explore opportunities for improvement is the key ingredient to achieving high-value care. Similarly, engaging our Boards as fully informed and visible partners in our quality and value innovations will foster stronger attention to and appreciation of the rewards from related staff efforts, engender more dynamic and productive meetings on the issues, and improve the reward structure to focus on reinforcing the culture of continuous improvement.

QUESTIONS WE ASK OURSELVES, OUR SENIOR LEADERS, AND OUR BOARDS TO ASSESS PROGRESS:

- What is our strategy for continuous improvement in the effectiveness and efficiency of care, and are we reinforcing it with every member of our organization?

- What else can our Board and its members do to emphasize and help drive our continuous improvement efforts?

✓ Culture of Continuous Improvement

Commitment to ongoing, real-time learning

The sustainability of efforts to improve the quality and value of care is contingent on an institutional culture of continuous improvement. Evaluating tasks and processes to identify better approaches allows hospitals to reduce waste, improve outcomes, and yield significant savings. Rather than prescribing behavior, managers and executives who teach problem solving, develop standard work, and remove barriers to improvement help their employees excel. This requires a management system built on the tenants of respect for all people in the organization, in which leadership behavior is focused on humility, facilitation, and mentorship. Front-line staff are taught to

1. analyze processes to identify waste and inefficiency,

2. propose changes to eliminate wasted resources and effort,

3. test proposed solutions on a small scale, and

4. if successful, scale the improvements to the entire organization. This process is never complete. Existing workflows must be continually refined and new opportunities for improvement continually sought.

A culture of continuous improvement demands that all workers apply this method to their tasks to drive iterative improvements in the efficiency of hospital operations.

QUESTIONS WE ASK OURSELVES AND OUR SENIOR LEADERS TO ASSESS PROGRESS:

- In what ways are our employees at every level supported and empowered to improve effectiveness, efficiency, and outcomes in their daily work?

- What tools have we built into our processes for continuous feedback and action to improve care delivery?

OUR EXPERIENCES { Culture of Continuous Improvement }

Denver Health adopted Lean as the philosophy and toolset to use in redesigning care. Lean is built on respect for people and continuous improvement, and focuses on reducing waste from the customer perspective.

- **Better care:** Achieved lowest observed-to-expected hospital mortality (among University Healthsystem Consortium)
- **Lower costs:** Since 2006, $158 million in financial benefit realized despite a 60 percent increase in uncompensated care

Virginia Mason adapted elements of the Toyota Production System to develop the Virginia Mason Production System (VMPS), aimed at identifying and eliminating waste and inefficiency in the many processes of health care delivery.

- **Better care:** Patients spend more value-added time with providers and experience fewer errors
- **Lower costs:** Multiple years of 4 to 5 percent margins

ThedaCare implemented the Business Performance System, a management process that supports front-line workers to solve problems every day. This moves away from a project mentality for improvement to a system transformation that builds a continuous improvement culture.

- **Better care:** 88 percent of safety and quality indicators improved; 85 percent of customer satisfaction indicators improved; 83 percent of staff engagement indicators improved
- **Lower costs:** Days cash on hand increased from 180 to 202 ($36 million improvement); cash-flow margin improved from 10.5 percent to almost 12.5 percent

INFRASTRUCTURE FUNDAMENTALS

Infrastructure components serve as foundation stones that enable the delivery of high-value care. As fundamental as governance and culture, certain technical capabilities promote the delivery of best practices and enable quality-improvement processes and assessment. These infrastructure elements are often critical first steps to transitioning to a system of high-value health care. Many of the specific care delivery and reliability strategies discussed below rely on a robust internal infrastructure.

✓ **IT best practices**—automated, reliable information to and from the point of care

✓ **Evidence protocols**—effective, efficient, and consistent care

✓ **Resource utilization**—optimized use of personnel, physical space, and other resources

✓ IT Best Practices

Automated, reliable information to and from the point of care

Reliable information systems are critical not just to ensure care quality, but also to improve efficiency in administrative and other process measures. Implementing EHRs and other technologies to enhance connectivity and efficiency can achieve cost savings and improve quality. These systems aid hospitals in automating order entry and reducing paperwork; optimizing staffing levels and scheduling; managing equipment and resources; defining care protocols and providing clinical decision support; managing billing and revenue cycles; reducing adverse drug events and duplicate tests; and improving care coordination.

QUESTIONS WE ASK OURSELVES AND OUR SENIOR LEADERS TO ASSESS PROGRESS:

- How well is our IT system used to help providers streamline administrative tasks and improve the care experience and patient outcomes?

- How well is our EHR aligned with Meaningful Use requirements?

OUR EXPERIENCES { IT Best Practices }

Geisinger implemented a series of health IT initiatives to improve quality and enhance efficiency, such as electronic health records; a health information exchange; ePrescribing modules; a data warehouse; and comprehensive document management.

- **Lower costs:** During the past 5 years, savings of $1.7 million from reduced chart pulls; more than $600,000 from reduced printing and faxing; more than $500,000 per year from reduced nursing staff time through ePrescribing; and more than $1 million from reduced transcription

HCA implemented Barcode Medication Administration (BCMA) in all of its hospitals. BCMA combines an electronic medication administration record of the specific medications ordered for the patient with barcode verification of the patient's identity (armband) and medication (label).

- **Better care:** Fewer adverse drug events; reduced length of stay
- **Lower costs:** 58.5 percent reduction in the total number of liability claims related to medication errors

Veterans Health Administration's Adverse Drug Event Reporting System (VA ADERS) was created to streamline and improve ADE monitoring. VA ADERS is an integrated web-based application that fully automates the ADE reporting process (including direct submission to FDA MedWatch) through a single portal for all facilities. VA ADERS allows for a wide range of pharmacovigilance functions as well as an improved ability to make pharmacy-benefit and formulary-management decisions.

- **Better care:** Seven-fold increase in ADE reporting; standardized reports on ADEs available to all VA medical centers, with breakdowns by facility and region

Kaiser Permanente's electronic medical library helps give caregivers access to the information they need when they need it, even in the exam room at the point of care, in order to best treat Kaiser's members and patients. The system contains data from thousands of medical texts and journals, and includes a full array of recommended best practices, proven care protocols, and advice.

- **Better care:** More than 10,000 uses per day of the electronic medical library by Kaiser clinicians; single site of contact for all clinical content for faster dissemination of best practices, new medical information, and new medical science

Cleveland Clinic has integrated a "hard stop" function into their computerized physician order entry system to reduce medically unnecessary same-day duplicate tests. Providers are able to override the stop through a call to the clinical pathology group.

- **Lower costs:** 13 percent reduction in blood gas determinations; $10,000 in monthly savings for laboratory tests (excluding blood gas); $117,000 in first-month savings for molecular testing

✓ Evidence Protocols
Effective, efficient, and consistent care

The delivery of high-value care is contingent on having the best information on what treatment works best for whom, and under what circumstances. Evidence-based protocols for managing the diagnosis and treatment of various conditions improve the reproducibility and standardization of care while allowing for tailoring to the unique needs of individual patients. Evidence-based protocols go beyond guidelines. Integrated within an EHR, they automatically provide clinicians with the best evidence about a particular condition as well as a decision pathway for diagnosis and treatment. Experience suggests that evidence-based care protocols may be most effective when developed and refined within institutions, blending protocols developed elsewhere with local issues and circumstances.

QUESTIONS WE ASK OURSELVES AND OUR SENIOR LEADERS TO ASSESS PROGRESS:

- For which of our most common and highest-cost conditions and procedures do we not yet have evidence-based care protocols? What is our strategy for filling these gaps and keeping others current?

- Which of our care protocols are not yet integrated into provider workflows via our EHR and what is our plan to fully integrate them?

OUR EXPERIENCES { Evidence Protocols }

Geisinger cardiac surgeons identified evidence- or consensus-based best practices from nationally published guidelines for patients undergoing elective coronary artery bypass. A variety of standardized order sets, decision-support tools, and reminders were created in the EHR, with tracking and reporting of adherence to the provision of each element of care.

- **Better care:** 67 percent reduction in operative morality; 1.3-day decrease in length of stay
- **Lower costs:** Revenue minus expense improved by more than $1,900 per case; cost per case for the Geisinger Health Plan decreased by 4.8 percent

HCA developed a "bundle" of standardized, evidence-based care practices related to high-risk obstetrical conditions in order to improve patient outcomes and reduce the costs of perinatal services.

- **Better care:** Maternal death rate of ~6.5 per 100,000 births (compared to national average of 13)
- **Lower costs:** $68 million in system-wide annual savings; 75 percent reduction in malpractice claim costs

Virginia Mason embedded pre-established evidence-based decision rules into the existing workflow of providers at the point of ordering an advanced imaging test to reduce variability. If the provider cannot specify an appropriate evidence-based decision rule, the test cannot be ordered.

- **Better care:** Reduced delays for necessary imaging; no unnecessary tests
- **Lower costs:** Substantial decrease in imaging utilization: MRI rate for headache by 23.2 percent; lumbar MRI rate by 23.4 percent; and sinus CT rate by 26.8 percent

Intermountain Healthcare applied rigorous evidence protocols and process improvement methodology to more than 60 clinical processes that constitute roughly 80 percent of care delivered. One example is the elective induction of labor. When women arrive at an Intermountain labor and delivery facility, nurses, through the EMR, must demonstrate that all criteria for elective delivery are met. If the criteria are not met, approval/consultation is required to proceed.

- **Better care:** Inappropriate elective induction rate fell from 28 percent to less than 2 percent; women spend 750 fewer hours in delivery per year
- **Lower costs:** Over c-section rate ~40 percent lower than national average, producing overall cost savings of $50 million; $10 million reduction in maternal and newborn variable costs per year

Kaiser Permanente's Healthy Bones Program, conceived by KP orthopedists, is a set of measures to identify and proactively treat patients at risk for osteoporosis and hip fractures. Physicians participating in the program implemented a number of initiatives, including increasing the use of bone density tests (DXA scans) and anti-osteoporosis medications, adding osteoporosis education and home health programs, and standardizing practice guidelines for osteoporosis management.

- **Better care:** During the course of 5 years, the Healthy Bones Program reduced hip fracture rates for at-risk patients by nearly 50 percent

✓ Resource Utilization
Optimized use of personnel,
physical space, and other resources

Providing high-value care requires the
efficient use of finite resources, yet much
of health care today is suboptimal on
both counts. Operations-management
tools can help improve returns on fixed-
capital investments. Variability in the flow
of patients into a hospital unit results in
overcrowding, worse health outcomes due to
fluctuations in staffing levels, increased staff
stress, lower patient and staff satisfaction,
reduced access to care, and higher costs.[10]
Strategies such as Queuing Theory and
Variability Methodology can be used to
eliminate sources of artificial variability,
improving occupancy without increasing
staffing or capacity or reducing lengths
of stay. Furthermore, systematic process-
improvement efforts such as Lean can be
used to make more efficient use of personnel
and other resources. Structured analysis
of daily work can eliminate inefficiencies,
increase value-added time spent with
patients, reduce staff stress, and optimize
the use of supplies and other resources.

QUESTIONS WE ASK OURSELVES AND
OUR SENIOR LEADERS TO ASSESS
PROGRESS:

- What procedures have we put in place for
  continuous monitoring of patient flow,
  occupancy, and staffing levels for each
  major service line?

- What indices do we use to identify and
  eliminate unnecessary and wasteful
  fluctuations, variation, and inefficiencies
  in each element?

OUR EXPERIENCES { Resource Utilization }

Cincinnati Children's implemented a series of operations-management interventions to smooth patient flow through the intensive care unit to reduce daily artificial variation and make bed occupancy more predictable.

- **Better care:** Fewer delays in/cancelling of elective surgeries due to bed availability
- **Lower costs:** $100 million in capital costs (75 new beds) avoided due to improved patient flow

Virginia Mason used the tools and methods of the Virginia Mason Production System to reduce inefficiencies in the workflow of nurses. Using 5-day workshops (Rapid Process Improvement), nursing teams analyzed their work and implemented methods to improve efficiency. For example, instead of the usual method of caring for patients throughout a unit, nurses now work as a team with a patient-care technician in "cells" (groups of rooms located near each other).

- **Better care:** Nurses spend 90 percent of time in direct patient care (compared to 35 percent); nurses can more easily monitor patients and quickly attend to needs; enhanced communication among team members; improved skill–task alignment

Intermountain Healthcare actively addressed inefficiencies in the supply chain using an evidence-based approach. Internal supply chain experts work with Intermountain's clinical staff to develop effective processes and strategies that remove the supply burden from caregivers. These teams analyze supply chains to identify the practices and products that drive the best outcomes.

- **Better care:** 2.3 percent reduction in catheter-associated bloodstream infections
- **Lower costs:** More than $200 million in savings during the past 5 years

CARE DELIVERY PRIORITIES

The core motivation for any hospital or health system is to deliver care that is safe, effective, patient-centered, timely, efficient, and equitable.[11] Certain strategies can help care-delivery organizations reengineer care around these principles. Often, this involves changing the existing construct of care delivery to one of open collaboration with patients, team-based care, delivery of care within and outside the hospital, and more active management of the health of the patient population by allocating resources based on severity of need.

✓ **Integrated care**—right care, right setting, right providers, right teamwork

✓ **Shared decision making**—patient–clinician collaboration on care plans

✓ **Targeted services**—tailored community and clinic interventions for resource-intensive patients

✓ Integrated Care

Right care, right setting, right providers, right teamwork

In response to financial pressures and patient preferences, hospitals and health systems must find new ways to deliver care in the most appropriate and cost-efficient setting. Targeted clinics, home care programs, and other models aimed at ensuring that care is delivered in the most appropriate setting can help reduce costs and improve outcomes. This sort of integration promotes patients' participation in their care, allows for monitoring of key chronic disease indicators, and reduces hospital readmissions that are stressful for patients and costly for health systems. Results improve when these efforts are supplemented by teaming and partnership strategies that promote care integration, as well as staffing patterns that optimize skill–task alignment.

QUESTIONS WE ASK OURSELVES AND OUR SENIOR LEADERS TO ASSESS PROGRESS:

- What procedures ensure optimal care transitions, both within units of the hospital and between the hospital and the community?

- How do we assess which care setting is most cost-effective and appropriate to the patient experience and outcome?

- How do we define the patient's care team and ensure that each care step is delivered by the most appropriate team member?

OUR EXPERIENCES ⟨ Integrated Care ⟩

Partners HealthCare's Connected Cardiac Care Program (CCCP) is a home monitoring program for heart failure (HF) patients at risk for hospitalization. CCCP's core components are care coordination, education, and development of self-management skills through the use of telemonitoring. Patients use home monitoring equipment to submit weight, blood pressure, heart rate, and symptoms on a daily basis.

- **Better care:** 51 percent reduction in HF hospital readmission; 44 percent reduction in non-HF hospital readmission
- **Lower costs:** More than $10 million in savings to date ($8,155 per patient)

Geisinger leveraged two key components of its integrated health system structure—Geisinger Clinic and Geisinger Health Plan—to develop an advanced medical home model, named ProvenHealth Navigator® (PHN). The PHN model has five core elements: (1) re-engineered patient-centered primary care, (2) integrated population management, (3) 360° care systems to form a medical neighborhood, (4) measurement of quality of care, and (5) a value-based reimbursement model.

- **Better care:** 18.2 percent decrease in acute admissions; 20 percent decrease in readmissions
- **Lower costs:** 7.1 percent reduction in the total cost of care during the past 5 years

Veterans Health Administration's Patient-Aligned Care Teams (PACT) improved veterans' access to high-quality primary care. PACTs, the VHA's version of the Patient-Centered Medical Home, deliver evidence-based, value-oriented, patient-centered team-based care with a focus on prevention and population health. To facilitate and improve access to care, PACTs employ multiple modalities, such as telephone clinics, home telehealth, secure messaging, and mobile apps.

- **Better care:** 15 percent increase in same-day access to primary care physicians
- **Lower costs:** 8 percent reduction in urgent care visits; 4 percent reduction in admission rates

✓ Shared Decision Making

Patient–clinician collaboration on care plans

Patient-centered care hinges on shared decisions. Shared decision processes help hospital staff inform patients about the risks and benefits of various treatment options and give patients the opportunity to consider how these options align with their goals for care and communicate these goals with their care providers. These processes encourage open communication among patients and ensure the development of an evidence-based care plan free of duplication and waste. Once properly informed about their care options, patients often reveal preferences for lower-cost and less-intensive treatments, which can reduce costs associated with overuse.

QUESTIONS WE ASK OURSELVES AND OUR SENIOR LEADERS TO ASSESS PROGRESS:

- What tools are being provided to our clinicians to aid in the communication of complex medical information to patients and their families?

- How do we require and facilitate the routine engagement of patients and their families as fully-informed, active decision makers in the planning and execution of their care?

OUR EXPERIENCES { Shared Decision Making }

ThedaCare's Collaborative Care Units are a redesign of inpatient care that focuses on those elements of care that add value to the patient experience. The basic unit of collaborative care is the interdisciplinary team with the patient at the center. On admission, a physician, nurse, discharge planner, and pharmacist jointly meet the patient and, with the patient's input, develop a single plan of care.

- **Better care:** Average length of stay dropped 10 to 15 percent; medication reconciliation errors were eliminated and compliance with care protocols improved; patient satisfaction scores rose to 95 percent (from 68 percent)
- **Lower costs:** 25 percent reduction in direct and indirect costs of inpatient care

Cleveland Clinic initiated a care-enhancement process for patients undergoing lung transplants to improve patient and family engagement with clinicians and care plans. Daily "huddles" with the patient and all caregivers were initiated to inform the patient and family of expected progress and develop a consistent plan among caregivers.

- **Better care:** 1.5-day reduction in average length of stay; 3 percent improvement in 30-day survival; 28 percent improvement in patient satisfaction with clinician communication
- **Lower costs:** 6 percent reduction in total cost of care

✓ Targeted Services

Tailored community and clinic interventions for resource-intensive patients

Patients who visit emergency rooms more frequently than others, whose illnesses require extensive inpatient care, and whose health care costs are among the highest in the community are a key cost-driver for health care institutions. A recent report from the Agency for Healthcare Research and Quality found that 5 percent of the American population is responsible for roughly half of the nation's health expenditures.[12] To better target care for these highest-risk patients, health care systems can employ patient-stratification techniques to identify these patients, ensure timely and appropriate access to care, and customize their treatment. Current inadequacies in the safety net and reimbursement hurdles for nontraditional models of care make this challenging, but we have found several viable strategies for targeting services to those who need them most. Care coordination, case management, and improved transitions can all enhance the care experience while reducing the costs associated with readmissions and visits to the emergency department (ED).

QUESTIONS WE ASK OURSELVES AND OUR SENIOR LEADERS TO ASSESS PROGRESS:

- What is our procedure for identifying, engaging, and tailoring the management of high-risk, resource-intensive patients?

- What resources are we dedicating to the targeting and intensive management of the health of these patients, here and in the community?

OUR EXPERIENCES { Targeted Services }

Cincinnati Children's, partnering with local physician practices, launched a large-scale asthma-improvement initiative across 38 community-based pediatric practices. This comprehensive initiative uses population segmentation to specifically target the "high-risk" cohort, and helps enable the delivery of best care through components such as multidisciplinary-practice quality-improvement teams; real-time patient-, practice-, and network-level data/reporting; and automated routing of ED/urgent care visit and admission alerts to primary care practices.

- **Better care:** 92 percent adherence to best practices for care management; 93 percent of parents rate their child's asthma as under control
- **Lower costs:** In the past year, 92 avoided admissions ($322,000 in savings) and 266 avoided ED/urgent care visits

Partners HealthCare System participated in a 3-year demonstration project to test strategies to improve the coordination of high-cost Medicare patients. To help primary care physicians manage these patients, case managers were integrated into primary care practices. Case managers developed personal relationships with enrolled patients and worked closely with physicians to help identify gaps in patient care, coordinate providers and services, facilitate communication (especially during transitions), and help educate patients and providers.

- **Better care:** 20 percent reduction in admissions; 13 percent reduction in ED visits
- **Lower costs:** $2.65 saved for every $1 spent; 7 percent net savings for each patient in the program

Virginia Mason worked with Boeing to launch the Intensive Outpatient Care Program (IOCP) to improve quality of care and reduce costs for Boeing's most expensive employees and their adult dependents. IOCP participants were enrolled in an intensified chronic care model centered on intensive in-person, telephonic, and email contacts. Services include frequent proactive outreach by an RN, education in self-management of chronic conditions, rapid access to and care coordination by the IOCP team, and direct involvement of specialists in primary care contacts, including behavioral health when feasible.

- **Better care:** 14.8 percent improvement in physical function; 17.6 percent improvement in timeliness of care
- **Lower costs:** 33 percent reduction in per capita claims; 56.5 percent reduction in work days missed

Kaiser Permanente, in conjunction with the President's Advisory Council on HIV/AIDS, the VA, and NCQA, developed and piloted a series of performance measures to improve care and reduce disparities among its 20,000 patients with HIV. Kaiser Permanente's best practices for HIV/AIDS care include quality-improvement programs that measure gaps in care; testing, prevention, and treatment guidelines; multidisciplinary care team models that emphasize the "medical home"; and education for both providers and patients.

- **Better care:** 94 percent median treatment adherence among patients regularly in care and on antiretroviral therapy; HIV mortality rates that are half the national average; 69 percent of all HIV-positive patients have maximal viral control (compared to 19-35 percent nationally)

RELIABILITY AND FEEDBACK

No single action, project, or program can drive transformation. Continuous improvement on the delivery of high-value care requires health care institutions to continually monitor and improve reliability and performance. Building safeguards into clinical workflows helps prevent adverse events, and providing decision support for providers ensures that the right care is delivered. Equally important are the collection and analysis of feedback data on cost, quality, and outcomes. Transparency in internal metrics helps organizations encourage a culture of high-value care through good stewardship of resources and improved performance on outcomes indicators.

✓ **Embedded safeguards**—supports and prompts to reduce injury and infection

✓ **Internal transparency**—visible progress in performance, outcomes, and costs

✓ Embedded Safeguards

Supports and prompts to reduce injury and infection

Reducing preventable patient harm is a fundamental aspect of high-value care. System-level factors such as procedures to guide the delivery of care, checklists, and care protocols can be embedded to create an environment that guards against human error. Such interventions support front-line workers in their tasks and promote a culture of consistent, reliable, high-quality care.

QUESTIONS WE ASK OURSELVES AND OUR SENIOR LEADERS TO ASSESS PROGRESS:

- For which of the most common injuries and errors have we developed or adapted specific protocols to reduce their incidence, and what are the priorities ahead?

- How are these protocols fully integrated into existing workflows, such as through prompts in our EHR?

OUR EXPERIENCES { Embedded Safeguards }

Cincinnati Children's implemented a bundle of interventions—a robust detection system to accomplish real-time awareness and analysis of all failures, microsystem-level process and outcome data, and standardized pediatric process bundles—to reduce rates of specific hospital-acquired conditions.

- **Better care:** 85 percent reduction in ventilator-associated pneumonia; >50 percent reduction in catheter-associated bloodstream infections; 43 percent reduction in class I and II surgical site infections
- **Lower costs:** $5.6 million saved per year

HCA conducted a multi-year effort to reduce central line–associated bloodstream infections (CLABSIs). This program incorporates the latest evidence-based recommendations, including insertion and maintenance practices, supply standardization of central-line kits, and competency training for all HCA physicians as part of their biannual credentialing.

- **Better care:** Up to 200 lives saved; 57.4 percent decrease in hospital-acquired bloodstream infections within the ICU since 2006; 80 HCA facilities with zero hospital-acquired bloodstream infections
- **Lower costs:** $17.5 million saved system-wide annually ($44,000 per case)

Kaiser Permanente established early-intervention protocols for diagnosing and treating community-acquired sepsis. Nursing, physician, informatics, and quality leaders translated existing guidelines into specific competencies, practices, and roles for the care delivery staff. Patient care protocols in the ED and ICU were changed to provide early-recognition and treatment-intervention opportunities.

- **Better care:** Sepsis mortality reduced by over half; 3.5-day reduction in the length of stay for patients with a principal diagnosis of sepsis; ~3-fold increase in the number of sepsis cases diagnosed

Partners HealthCare implemented pharmacy barcoding at Brigham and Women's Hospital to reduce serious medication errors. Pharmacists barcode-scan all medications dispensed from the pharmacy to ensure that the medications match the physicians' orders. Nurses at the bedside then scan the medications prior to administration to patients, and are alerted about possible errors.

- **Better care:** 31 percent reduction in serious medication-administration errors; increased on-time medication availability on nursing units
- **Lower costs:** $3.3 million in cumulative 5-year savings (costs recouped within first year)

Veterans Health Administration's Methicillin-Resistant Staphylococcus Aureus (MRSA) Prevention Initiative was implemented in 2007 to decrease MRSA infections acquired at acute care facilities nationwide. The program focused on a bundle of evidence-based best practices known to prevent MRSAs and the leadership of a MRSA Prevention Coordinator (MPC) charged with overseeing implementation at each medical center.

- **Better care:** 1,000 prevented MRSA infections and a 62 percent reduction in ICU MRSA rates nationwide from October 2007 to June 2010; currently, more than 70 percent of VHA facilities have zero MRSAs monthly

✓ Internal Transparency

Visible progress in performance, outcomes, and costs

Variability in clinician practices is inevitable—even within high-performing organizations. By making providers aware of variations in practice, their utilization rates, and their performance against internal and external benchmarks, institutions can guide providers' behavior toward improved value. Additionally, making health care providers aware of the costs associated with procedures encourages better stewardship of limited resources.

QUESTIONS WE ASK OURSELVES AND OUR SENIOR LEADERS TO ASSESS PROGRESS:

- How do we measure and benchmark adherence to evidence protocols, service utilization rates, and performance on quality, costs, and outcomes?

- What are our procedures for using performance data to improve outcomes and reduce variability, costs, and waste?

- How do we communicate clinician-specific performance data back to clinicians, and how can we improve that communication?

OUR EXPERIENCES { Internal Transparency }

Denver Health developed preventive-health and chronic-disease patient registries for users of their community health center network. One aspect of this system is the creation of performance report cards aggregated across patients and time and populated by nearly real-time data. An essential feature of the report cards has been non-blinded display of performance by site of primary care and by primary care provider, which drove reduced variation and improved overall performance.

- **Better care:** During the past 3 years, colorectal cancer screening rates nearly doubled; breast cancer screening rates increased by 20 percent; hypertension control rates increased from 60 percent to 72 percent

Cleveland Clinic implemented web-based business intelligence tools to collect and display provider performance data for a wide variety of metrics in order to engage providers in quality improvement and waste reduction. By giving providers transparent access to metrics that identify variations in practice, utilization rates, and performance against internal and external benchmarks, Cleveland Clinic has seen dramatic reductions in waste, improved quality, and a sustained change in culture.

- **Better care:** >40 percent reduction in central-line infections; 50 percent reduction in urinary-tract infections (UTIs)
- **Lower costs:** Cost avoidance of $30,000 for each central-line infection and $5,000 for each UTI

THE YIELD

Estimates vary, but several assessments concluded that at least 30 percent of our nation's health expenditures—roughly $750 billion—do not improve health.[13] We believe that the type of system-level improvements outlined in the Checklist hold the key to capturing this lost value. It is difficult to attribute dollars saved to the various items in the Checklist, because each is interrelated and, as discussed, some are fundamental enablers of more targeted strategies. However, when taken as part of a broad strategy to improve quality, our experiences have yielded promising results. To help give a sense of the possible yield of operationalizing a commitment to high-value care, displayed below are selected examples of better care and lower costs achieved within each of our institutions. If these results could be scaled nationally, the effect would be truly transformational.

BETTER CARE			
LIVES SAVED	67% decrease in elective CABG mortality at Geisinger	HIV mortality rate half the national average at Kaiser Permanente	Up to 200 lives saved at HCA from reduced CLABSIs
HEALTH GAINED	50% reduction in heart failure readmissions at Partners	~60% reduction in ICU MRSA rates at VHA	~20% reduction in admissions and readmissions for medical-home patients at Geisinger
PEOPLE SATISFIED	95% percent of patients at ThedaCare's Collaborative Care Unit rate it 5 out of 5	More than 90% satisfaction with Geisinger's medical home	~18% improvement in timeliness of care at the Virginia Mason IOCP program

LOWER COSTS			
THE RIGHT CARE	$10 million saved ($8,000 per patient) with Partners heart failure home monitoring	$17.5 million saved system-wide at HCA from decreased CLABSIs	$6.3 million saved from reduced surgical site infections at Cincinnati Children's
AT REDUCED COST	7.1% reduction in total cost of care for medical-home patients at Geisinger	25% reduction in direct and indirect costs of patient care in ThedaCare Collaborative Care Unit	35% reduction in indirect cost of inpatient care for high-cost Medicare beneficiaries at Partners
EFFICIENTLY DELIVERED	$100 million in capital costs avoided at Cincinnati Children's	$158 million in financial benefit at Denver Health since 2006	$200 million saved in 5 years through supply chain improvement at Intermountain

OPPORTUNITIES
TO ADVANCE HIGH-VALUE CARE

The items in this Checklist reflect core elements for the health care transformation needed to deliver high-value care—better outcomes at lower costs. On the other hand, many of the levers for true transformation lie outside the control of institutional leaders and in the domain of broader, system-wide policies and incentives. In many ways, we are operating in a time of turbulent optimism. Recent legislation and changes in the health care marketplace afford numerous opportunities for change, but systemic barriers to successful transformation remain.

Reference has already been made to the challenges faced by each of us at the individual and institutional levels, and the challenges to the efficient operation of the system as a whole. In addition, prevailing system-wide payment models have placed an economic disincentive on adopting some of the cost-containment strategies outlined above. In a system that rewards volume over value, many health care delivery organizations have invested in expensive technologies and equipment, hired unnecessary personnel, and expanded their brick-and-mortar operations. This kind of overcapitalization creates an economic incentive to maximize revenue from capital that has already been invested, rather than seek out opportunities to reduce costs and improve quality. Few institutions have been spared the consequences of this phenomenon, including our own, but working to address it is a very real mandate, and a core motivator

of our interest in sharing experiences on ways to improve. Most fundamental to enabling the transition envisioned is the alignment of incentives and operations to reflect the principles of high-value care. Patients, and employers who share in paying for their care, should be provided information and incentives to seek out institutions that provide high-value care, and delivery sites should be reimbursed in accordance with the value of care delivered.

Faced with the extreme consequences of growing costs, many purchasers are beginning to leverage their power to demand high-value care. Employers are attempting to rein in health care costs by contracting with providers and insurers, redesigning benefit plans, and providing incentives and information to employees. Individuals, too, are increasingly looking to contain health care expenditures. Mounting costs for individual coverage as well as cost-sharing/shifting in group plans have increased consumer discretion. While this shift is already under way in some markets, considerable progress is still needed. Accelerating this progress revolves around increasing transparency on cost and outcomes. Only with the knowledge of which delivery sites provide the best care for the lowest cost can employers and other purchasers drive volume to institutions that provide high-value care.

Reimbursement models that favor high-value care also create an imperative

> Patients, and employers who share in paying for their care, should be provided information and incentives to seek out institutions that provide high-value care, and delivery sites should be reimbursed in accordance with the value of care delivered.

for health care delivery system transformation. Here, too, progress is under way. In the private market, Blue Cross Blue Shield of Massachusetts' Alternative Quality Contract and Geisinger's ProvenCare® are models of bundled, value-based reimbursement that are receiving increasing attention. Several pilot initiatives are also under way in the private sector. UnitedHealth Group began an episode-based reimbursement plan for oncology practices, and the Integrated Healthcare Association launched a Bundled Episode Payment Pilot Program involving several of the nation's largest private insurers. The shift toward value-based reimbursement is also occurring at the state level. In the face of acute budget pressures, more and more states are shifting Medicaid enrollees to managed-care plans. For example, New York and Florida—two of the states with the largest Medicaid populations—plan to enroll all beneficiaries in managed-care plans within the next several years.[14]

A fundamental opportunity for transitioning toward value-based reimbursement lies with the federal government and in the implementation of certain provisions in recent health reform legislation. The Centers for Medicare & Medicaid Services has been experimenting with value-based reimbursement pilots for years, but elements of the Affordable Care Act (ACA) have the potential to accelerate this transition. Provisions in the ACA establish programs for bundled payments, value-based purchasing, and for reducing Medicare payments to hospitals for errors and avoidable readmissions. One particularly relevant provision is the Medicare Shared Savings

> Further progress is necessary, but the demand for high-value care is clearly growing. Employers, individuals, private insurers, and public payers are all facing pressure to contain costs, and are seeking health care delivery organizations that can do so while maintaining quality.

Program, designed to spur the development of Accountable Care Organizations (ACOs). Under this program, ACOs are responsible for providing high-quality care and, if they reduce costs for Medicare patients, share in the savings.

The ACA also created the Center for Medicare & Medicaid Innovation, which is charged with investing a budget of $10 billion over the next 10 years to accelerate the development and implementation of innovative payment and delivery models for Medicare, Medicaid, and the Children's Health Insurance Program (CHIP). The Innovation Center already launched programs for the development of ACOs and Patient-Centered Medical Homes, as well as bundled payment initiatives for acute care. While the initial target of the Innovation Center is cost reduction in federal programs, its ultimate goal is to develop scalable models for all payer arrangements.

Further progress is necessary, but the demand for high-value care is clearly growing. Employers, individuals, private insurers, and public payers are all facing pressure to contain costs, and are seeking health care delivery organizations that can do so while maintaining quality. Current and forthcoming initiatives provide considerable incentives to implement the strategies for high-value care described in this Checklist.

IMPLEMENTATION AGENDA

The items in the Checklist describe the foundational, infrastructure, care delivery, and feedback components of a system oriented around value. They are our best approximation of the interventions key to improving health care while lowering costs, and to weathering impending regulatory and reporting changes and shifting purchaser demands. The business case for their adoption is compelling. For leaders using this Checklist as a resource to improve the value of care provided in their institutions, particular attention should be paid to the phasing and sequencing of adoption. We have found that early successes are affirming and will pave the way for continued improvement. Ultimately, the cadence for implementation will be derived from the particular culture of the institution and the needs of its patient population.

Successful implementation of the items on this Checklist is dependent on close partnerships between executives and their Boards. Responsibility rests with hospital health system leaders to embrace higher quality and lower costs as institutional aims, to foster a culture that prioritizes high-value care, to determine a path forward, and to steward and sustain the transformation. While executives oversee the day-to-day operations of the institution, the Board is ultimately accountable for the organization's clinical and financial success, for its reputation in and commitment to the community, and for partnering with executives to shape the organization's mission. In turn, Boards bear responsibility for holding the organization and its executives accountable for the outcomes achieved and for fostering high-value care as an institutional priority.

Partnerships with insurers and employers are also fundamentally important in building demand for and enabling the transition to high-value care. This has been a critical step for many of us as we have attempted to improve the value of care delivered in our institutions. Our experiences with these initiatives have brought to light the advantages of direct, transparent communication with purchasers, payers, and consumers. Such partnerships can help accelerate the shift to reimbursement models that favor high-value care and ensure that adhering to the strategies in this Checklist is fiscally sustainable.

Ultimately, it is our responsibility to improve care delivery in our institutions. More broadly, as health care community leaders, responsibility rests with us for eliminating waste from the system and reinvesting it to maximize the quality and efficiency of health care in the United States. It is our utmost desire that all of us, together, rise to the challenges of a changing health care landscape and transform our organizations into engines of sustainable, efficient, high-quality care for all Americans. We invite your partnership in this effort.

Join us in the Checklist

Please contact us at CEOChecklist@nas.edu to become a co-signatory.

REFERENCES

1. Centers for Medicare and Medicaid Services. 2012. *National health expenditure data*. Available at: http://www.cms.gov/Research-Statistics-Data-and-Systems/Statistics-Trends-and-Reports/NationalHealthExpendData/index.html (accessed May 22, 2012).

2. Keehan, S. P., A. M. Sisko, C. J. Truffer, J. A. Poisal, G. A. Cuckler, A. J. Madison, J. M. Lizonitz, and S. D. Smith. 2011. National health spending projections through 2020: Economic recovery and reform drive faster spending growth. *Health Affairs* 30(8):1-12.

3. The quarter of state budgets figure used includes both federal and state Medicaid contributions, as well as all federal contributions to the total budget. National Association of State Budget Officers. 2011. *State Expenditure Report 2010 (Fiscal 2009-2011 Data)*. Available at http://www.nasbo.org/sites/default/files/Summary%20-%20State%20Expenditure%20Report.pdf (accessed April 25, 2012); Kaiser Family Foundation. 2011. *Moving ahead amid fiscal challenges: A look at Medicaid spending, coverage and policy trends results from a 50-state Medicaid budget survey for state fiscal years 2011 and 2012*. Available at http://www.kff.org/medicaid/upload/8248.pdf (accessed January 23, 2012).

4. Kaiser Family Foundation. 2011. *Employer Health Benefits Survey*. Available at http://ehbs.kff.org/pdf/2011/8225.pdf (accessed November 4, 2011).

5. Auerbach, D., and A. L. Kellermann. 2011. A decade of health care cost growth has wiped out real income gains for an average US family. *Health Affairs* 30(9):1630-1636.

6. Institute of Medicine. 1999. *To err is human: Building a safer health system*. Washington, DC: National Academy Press.

7. Landrigan, C. P., G. J. Parry, C. B. Bones, A. D. Hackbarth, D. A. Goldmann, and P. J. Sharek. 2010. Temporal trends in rates of patient harm resulting from medical care. *New England Journal of Medicine* 363(22):2124-2134; U.S. Department of Health and Human Services. Office of Inspector General. 2010. *Adverse events in hospitals: National incidence among Medicare beneficiaries*. Washington, DC: Department of Health and Human Services.

8. Jencks, S. F., M. V. Williams, and E. A. Coleman. 2009. Rehospitalizations among patients in the medicare fee for-service program. *New England Journal of Medicine* 360(14):1418-1428.

9. Institute of Medicine. 2010. *The healthcare imperative: Lowering costs and improving outcomes*. Washington, DC: The National Academies Press.

10. Litvak, E., and M. Bisognano. 2011. More patients, less payment: Increasing hospital efficiency in the aftermath of health reform. *Health Affairs* 30(1):76-80.

11. Institute of Medicine. 2001. *Crossing the quality chasm: A new health system for the 21st century*. Washington, DC: National Academy Press.

12. Cohen, S. B., and W. Yu. 2011. *The concentration and persistence in the level of health expenditures over time: Estimates for the U.S. population, 2008-2009*. Available at http://meps.ahrq.gov/mepsweb/data_files/publications/st354/stat354.pdf (accessed January 17, 2012).

13. James, B., and K. B. Bayley. 2006. *Cost of poor quality or waste in integrated delivery system settings. Final report*. Rockville, MD: Agency for Healthcare Research and Quality; Fisher, et al. 2003. The implications of regional variations in medicare spending. *Annals of Internal Medicine* 138(4):273-298; Institute of Medicine. 2010. *The healthcare imperative: Lowering costs and improving outcomes*. Washington, DC: The National Academies Press.

14. Iglehart, J.K. 2011. Desperately seeking savings: States shift more Medicaid enrollees to managed care. *Health Affairs* 30(9):1627-1629.

Case Material Supporting Checklist Items

The cases presented here are more detailed descriptions of our institutions' experiences implementing the 10 Checklist items, along with follow-up contact information for additional conversations.

Foundational elements

✓ **Governance priority**—visible and determined leadership by CEO and Board

CASE Leading Commitment to Value at Virginia Mason Health System

In order to better orient its leaders toward quality, Virginia Mason (VM) Health System leadership and the Board of Directors developed a new strategic plan that adopted the business case for quality as a key strategy with an unequivocal focus on the patient. Responsible governance is a foundational element of VM's strategic plan. VM's board, comprised of a wide range of community members, is ultimately responsible and accountable for the organization's success. Responsible governance means a Board that is committed to doing everything necessary to ensure a clinically superb, fiscally healthy, and innovative environment. At VM, this means that:

- The Board receives regular education about health care quality issues
- The Board is structured to emphasize quality
- The Board spends significant time at each of its meetings attending to quality
- Executive review and compensation are tied to specific quality metrics
- The organization can demonstrate improvements in quality and outcomes during the last 3 years
- Focus on quality is evidenced in the Board's approach to finance—both in terms of capital allocation and operating priorities

RESULTS

Virginia Mason received the inaugural Leapfrog Governance for Quality Award (an award given to one hospital or health system in the country annually) for the work its Board has done to mobilize the organization to improve the quality of patient care.

FOR MORE INFORMATION

Please contact: Lynne Chafetz, JD (lynne.chafetz@vmmc.org)

CASE   Board Governance and Engagement at Kaiser Permanente

To increase Board attention to quality and continuous improvement, Kaiser Permanente (KP) initiated a Quality Systems Assessment (QSA), supplemented by surveys of front-line staff, managers, and organizational leaders about our Quality strategy, visibility to the Board, and performance. As a result, a series of recommendations were made, including the use of whole-system performance measures; establishment of direct communication between the regions and the Board; evaluation of performance through multiple reporting methods; and differentiation of hospital versus health plan actions. KP developed the Big Q Performance Metrics Dashboard—a comprehensive and integrated view of KP's quality and service performance in six key domains: clinical effectiveness, safety, service, resource stewardship, risk management, and equitable care. KP caregivers and Board members use the Big Q dashboard to track KP's performance relative to national benchmarks, as well as trends over time.

RESULTS

As a result of the QSA process and ongoing Board engagement and leadership, Kaiser Permanente has been able to:

- Improve patient satisfaction
- Achieve nation-leading performance in quality of care
- Identify the gaps between the perspectives of leaders and the front line
- Improve awareness of quality and accountability throughout the organization
- Develop a culture of patient- and family-focused care

FOR MORE INFORMATION

Please contact: Jed Weissberg, MD (jed.weissberg@kp.org)

FOUNDATIONAL ELEMENTS

✓ **Culture of Continuous Improvement**—commitment to ongoing, real-time learning

CASE Lean Improvement Efforts at Denver Health

In order to reduce waste from the customer perspective, and to build respect for people and continuous improvement into its operations, in 2005, Denver Health adopted Lean—a strategy for reducing waste and improving continuously—as the philosophy and toolset to use in redesigning care. Denver Health utilized a two-pronged approach to implement Lean: (1) organizational leaders (Black Belts) trained in Lean used Lean in their day-to-day work to identify and eliminate waste and (2) week-long rapid-improvement events were derived from 16 areas of focus or "value streams." The areas of focus spanned the entire integrated system of care, from paramedics to obstetrics and from back-office functions to clinical care.

RESULTS

- Since August 2006, $158 million in financial benefit realized despite a 60 percent increase in uncompensated care
- Achieved lowest observed-to-expected hospital mortality (among University Healthsystem Consortium)
- Widespread employee acceptance of Lean philosophy—78 percent of employees understand how Lean enables Denver Health to meet its mission

FOR MORE INFORMATION

Please contact: Phil Goodman (philip.goodman@dhha.org)

CASE   The Virginia Mason Production System

To identify and eliminate waste and inefficiency in the main processes of health care delivery, in 2002, Virginia Mason (VM) Health System adapted elements of the Toyota Production System to develop the Virginia Mason Production System (VMPS). VMPS is a daily part of work at VM and is integral to the organization's success. All leaders attend mandatory VMPS leadership training, are required to lead at least one formal improvement event each year, and are expected to routinely coach and train staff in how to improve their work using VMPS tools and methods. Managers from all areas routinely serve periods in the Kaizen Promotion Office, the team that guides improvement work. VMPS strategies range from small-scale ideas tested and implemented immediately to long-range planning that redesigns new spaces and processes. VM has completed 1,280 continuous-improvement activities involving staff, patients, and guests.

RESULTS

- Steadily improved financial health—multiple years of 4 to 5 percent margins
- Patients spend more value-added time with providers
- Better patient safety, less delay in seeing physicians for care and more timely results and treatments
- Reduction of waste in administrative processes

FOR MORE INFORMATION

Please contact: Diane Miller (diane.miller@vmmc.org)

FOUNDATIONAL ELEMENTS
CULTURE OF CONTINUOUS IMPROVEMENT—COMMITMENT TO ONGOING, REAL-TIME LEARNING

CASE Business Performance System at ThedaCare

To ensure the sustainability of its system-improvement efforts, in 2008, ThedaCare implemented the Business Performance System, a management system to deliver and sustain improvement-management processes and to support front-line workers in solving problems every day. Sustainable improvement results require moving away from a project mentality for improvement to a system transformation that builds a continuous-improvement culture. This, in turn, requires standard work for management, which means managers and executives have a new playbook for their behaviors and actions. The system starts with an 8:00 to 10:00 a.m. meeting-free zone each day. During this time, all managers and executives attend "gemba," which means they go to where the "real work" is done or where value is added to the customer. They spend this time in the ED, ICU, or clinic, etc. They go with a specific set of questions concerning the quality, safety, people, delivery, and cost of delivering care that day. Problems are identified by staff, managers, and executives, which are then solved immediately by front-line staff, who are given the tools, training, and encouragement they need to tackle almost any problem. The 10 components of the Business Performance System are taught in a 16-week mandatory course for managers and executives. This learning occurs not in a classroom but in the workplace, supported by knowledgeable coaches. The students must prove competency through observation to be installed as a permanent manager.

RESULTS

- 88 percent of safety and quality indicators improved; 85 percent of customer satisfaction indicators improved
- 83 percent of staff-engagement indicators improved
- 50 percent of financial indicators improved
- Days cash on hand increased from 180 to 202 (a $36 million improvement) from 2008-2011
- Cash-flow margin improved from 10.3 percent to almost 12.3 percent from 2008-2011
- 4 percent profit margin in 2011, despite a doubling of Medicaid volume

FOR MORE INFORMATION

Please contact: ThedaCare Center for Healthcare Value (info@createvalue.org)

INFRASTRUCTURE FUNDAMENTALS

✓ **IT Best Practices**—automated, reliable information to and from the point of care

CASE Streamlining Administrative Processes with Health IT at Geisinger

To improve quality and enhance efficiency at 40 outpatient centers and 3 hospitals, Geisinger implemented a series of health IT initiatives. The foundation of this effort was an electronic health record, but it has subsequently expanded to include a health information exchange, ePrescribing modules, a data warehouse and comprehensive document management.

RESULTS

During the past 5 years:

- $1.7 million saved from reduced chart pulls
- More than $600,000 saved from reduced printing and faxing
- $500,000 saved from reduced cost of management of outside documents
- More than $500,000 saved per year from reduced nursing-staff time through ePrescribing
- More than $1 million saved from reduced transcription

FOR MORE INFORMATION

Please contact: James M. Walker, MD, FACP (jmwalker@geisinger.edu)

CASE Barcode Medication Administration at HCA

To improve the efficiency of medication ordering and delivery practices, HCA implemented Barcode Medication Administration (BCMA) in all of its hospitals. BCMA combines an electronic medication-administration record of the specific medications ordered for a patient with barcode verification of patient identity (armband) and medication (label). The nurse or therapist uses this technology while administering medications to ensure general confirmation of the "Five Rights" of medication administration (right patient, right medication, right route, right dose, and right time). Full deployment of BCMA in all inpatient settings was completed in 2005.

RESULTS

- 58.5 percent reduction in the total number of liability claims related to medication errors
- Readiness for Stage 2 Meaningful Use requirement for secure bedside medication administration
- Improved data capture for billing on administration and accuracy of charges
- Improved inventory control

FOR MORE INFORMATION

Please contact: Karla Miller, PharmD (karla.miller@hcahealthcare.com)

CASE The VA Adverse Drug Event Reporting System

In order to streamline and improve adverse drug event (ADE) monitoring capabilities for pharmacovigilance, the VA created a national database known as the VA Adverse Drug Event Reporting System (VA ADERS). VA ADERS is an integrated web-based application that fully automates the ADE reporting process (including direct submission to FDA MedWatch) through a single portal for all VA facilities. VA ADERS allows for a wide range of pharmacovigilance functions, including building standardized reports, looking at preventability issues, and engaging in ad hoc evaluations of possible safety signals (case finding), which can then undergo further scrutiny and evaluation as deemed necessary. Compared to the VA's legacy database, VA ADERS has improved the efficiency of adverse drug reaction coding. Overall, VA ADERS' function is integral to the VA's contemporary pharmacovigilance efforts, and it plays an important role in many VA pharmacy benefits and formulary management decisions.

RESULTS

- Seven-fold increase in reported ADEs
- Ability to generate standardized reports on adverse drug reactions and events with breakdowns by region and by facility

FOR MORE INFORMATION

Please contact: Michael Valentino, RPh, MHSA (michael.valentino@va.gov)
Fran Cunningham, Pharm.D (fran.cunningham@va.gov)

INFRASTRUCTURE FUNDAMENTALS
IT BEST PRACTICES—AUTOMATED, RELIABLE INFORMATION TO AND FROM THE
POINT OF CARE

CASE   Enterprise Data Warehouse at Intermountain Healthcare

To improve the effectiveness and efficiency of clinical management, Intermountain Healthcare constructed an enterprise data warehouse (EDW) function that compliments the electronic medical record (EMR) system used across its 23 hospitals and 200-plus clinics. The Intermountain EDW consists of a number of "data marts" organized by high-priority clinical processes. The contents of a data mart are derived from the evidence-based best practice guideline that a series of condition-specific standing Intermountain teams generate to manage clinical care delivery. A data mart functions as a clinical registry, tracking all patients who experience a particular clinical process over time. It produces a full set of process-management reports, organized as a series of nested dashboards with increasing levels of detail. The EDW system draws together a series of parallel data flows into coordinated information. For example, the EDW combines financial data (case mix information, insurance claims submissions, and detailed information from Intermountain's activity-based costing systems); clinical data (data from laboratory, microbiology, blood bank, imaging, procedure room, and bedside charting EMR systems); and patient satisfaction information (CMS-mandated HCHAPS data and a more detailed internal survey).

RESULTS

Development of Intermountain's EDW has allowed for:

• The ability to track individual patient results in real time
• The ability to monitor patients across all of their concurrent conditions
• Full integration of clinical, financial, and care-process data

FOR MORE INFORMATION

Please contact: Lucy Savitz, PhD (lucy.savitz@imail.org)

CASE   Reducing Overuse Through Computerized Physician Order Entry (CPOE) at Cleveland Clinic

To reduce medically unnecessary same-day duplicate tests, Cleveland Clinic initiated a review of all computerized order sets and monitored the frequency of laboratory tests that show no significant variation during at least a 24-hour period of time. All standard order sets were updated, and after background collection of data, Cleveland Clinic initiated a same-day block or "hard stop" of eight laboratory tests. When duplicate orders were placed within the electronic medical record, providers were notified of the current day's result or that the test was pending. A provider override system was created via a call to the clinical pathology group. The "hard stop" preventing ordering was expanded to 100 and later to 1,241 individual tests. A second tier of screening was instituted for genetic testing. After collaboration with the relevant clinical providers, a series of molecular tests for 30 conditions were restricted to providers with appropriate training to independently order the tests. Others were required to consult a genetic counselor prior to ordering tests.

RESULTS

- 13 percent reduction in blood gas determinations
- $10,000 in monthly savings for laboratory tests (excluding blood gas)
- $117,000 in first-month savings for molecular testing
- Ability to target and educate providers found to most frequently order unnecessary tests

FOR MORE INFORMATION

Please contact: Robert Wyllie, MD (wyllier@ccf.org)

INFRASTRUCTURE FUNDAMENTALS
IT BEST PRACTICES—AUTOMATED, RELIABLE INFORMATION TO AND FROM THE
POINT OF CARE

CASE The Kaiser Permanente Electronic Medical Library

To give caregivers quick, comprehensive access to the latest practice protocols in real time, Kaiser Permanente (KP) built an electronic medical library, an online compendium of research-based guidelines, evidence-based care standards, and clinical material. The electronic medical library helps give KP caregivers access to the information they need when they need it, even in the exam room at the point of care, in order to best treat KP's members and patients. The system allows a single site of contact for all clinical content, leading to faster dissemination of best practices, new medical information, and new medical science across KP.

RESULTS

- Contains data from thousands of medical texts and journals, and includes a full array of recommended best practices, proven care protocols, and advice

- More than 10,000 uses per day of the electronic medical library by KP clinicians

FOR MORE INFORMATION

Please contact: Jed Weissberg, MD (jed.weissberg@kp.org)

INFRASTRUCTURE FUNDAMENTALS

✓ **Evidence Protocols**—effective, efficient, and consistent care

CASE Improving Coronary Artery Bypass Graft (CABG) Surgery at Geisinger

To improve care delivered to patients undergoing elective coronary artery bypass, Geisinger cardiac surgeons identified evidence-based or consensus-based best practices from nationally published guidelines. After 40 best practices were agreed on, workflow from initial evaluation to postoperative rehabilitation was redesigned by the entire surgical team of providers to ensure reliable performance of each desired element of care. A variety of standardized order sets, decision-support tools, and reminders were created in the electronic health record with tracking and reporting of adherence to the provision of each element of care.

RESULTS

- 67 percent reduction in operative mortality
- 1.3-day decrease in length of stay
- Revenue minus expense improved by more than $1,900 per case
- Cost per case for Geisinger Health Plan decreased by 4.8 percent
- 23 percent increase in contribution margin for the episode of care (decision to operate to 90 days post discharge)

FOR MORE INFORMATION

Please contact: Alfred Casale, MD (ascasale@geisinger.edu)

INFRASTRUCTURE FUNDAMENTALS
EVIDENCE PROTOCOLS—EFFECTIVE, EFFICIENT, AND CONSISTENT CARE

CASE Perinatal Services at HCA

HCA delivers a quarter-million babies yearly in 110 hospitals, representing nearly 6 percent of all U.S. babies born and reflecting a patient population more heterogeneous than the United States at large. To improve patient outcomes and reduce costs, HCA developed a "bundle" of standardized, evidence-based care practices related to high-risk obstetrical conditions. Standardized competencies were developed for fetal monitoring, requiring delivery nurses to prove ability in accurate monitoring and creating core requirements for physicians for credentialing and privileging. Guidelines were also developed for safe use of oxytocin and misoprostol and administration to appropriate patients. HCA also developed a variety of patient-safety protocols and programs designed to reduce the risk of maternal death. These included a novel policy that called for the universal use of pneumatic compression devices (for DVT prophylaxis) in all women undergoing C-sections.

RESULTS

- 75 percent reduction in malpractice-claim costs since 2010
- $68 million in system-wide annual savings
- Maternal death rate of ~6.5 per 100,000 births (compared to national average of 13)

FOR MORE INFORMATION

Please contact: Janet Meyers, RN, MBA (janet.meyers@hcahealthcare.com)

CASE Imaging Utilization at Virginia Mason Health System

Advanced imaging is a well-documented driver of high costs. At Virginia Mason (VM), review of medical records revealed substantial variation in provider use of advanced imaging. After an intensive program of provider education failed to result in improvement, VM began a plan to embed pre-established evidence-based decision rules into the existing workflow of providers at the point of ordering an advanced imaging test. Decision rules were installed in the software application used to schedule each of the advanced imaging studies. The format is that of a checklist, requiring the provider to click on the evidence-based indication for the imaging study to complete the electronic scheduling sequence. The same click needed to order the imaging study also specifies the evidence-based indication for the test. If the provider cannot specify an appropriate evidence-based decision rule, the test cannot be ordered.

RESULTS

- The MRI rate for headache decreased by 23.2 percent; the lumbar MRI rate decreased by 23.4 percent; and the sinus CT rate decreased by 26.8 percent
- No added provider time, no waits or delays to patient care, and minimal administrative cost

FOR MORE INFORMATION

Please contact: Robert Mecklenberg, MD (robert.mecklenburg@vmmc.org)

INFRASTRUCTURE FUNDAMENTALS
EVIDENCE PROTOCOLS—EFFECTIVE, EFFICIENT, AND CONSISTENT CARE

CASE Active Care Management at Intermountain Healthcare

To improve the efficiency and effectiveness of care, in 1996, Intermountain launched a long-term strategic initiative to extend full management oversight to high-priority clinical processes. Now, more than 60 such processes (which represent almost 80 percent of care delivered) are under active management. "Active management" means (1) an evidence-based best practice guideline, blended into clinical workflows; (2) an aligned data system, also embedded into clinical workflows, that tracks guideline variance in parallel with intermediate and final clinical, cost, and service outcomes; (3) full integration into Intermountain's electronic medical record system; and (4) a full set of educational materials for patients, family, and professional staff. An example of a clinical process under active management is elective induction of labor. It embeds into the clinical workflow at the point where a woman, referred by her obstetrician, first comes to an Intermountain labor and delivery facility for elective induction. Intermountain's nurses review the nine criteria established by the American College of Obstetrics and Gynecology (ACOG) for appropriate elective induction. If the woman meets all criteria, the induction and delivery proceeds. Otherwise, the nurses contact the referring obstetrician, as the guideline requires consultation from the department chair or a high-risk pregnancy specialist before induction can take place. Since its implementation in 2001, the guidelines and protocol continue to be refined.

RESULTS

- Inappropriate elective induction rate fell from 28 percent to less than 2 percent
- Over c-section rate approximately 40 percent lower than the national average; overall cost savings of $50 million
- $10 million reduction in maternal and newborn variable costs per year
- Women spend 750 fewer hours in delivery per year, freeing up resources for the delivery of an additional 1,500 infants

FOR MORE INFORMATION
Please contact: Lucy Savitz, PhD (lucy.savitz@imail.org)

CASE The Healthy Bones Program at Kaiser Permanente

To reduce the incidence of osteoporosis and hip fractures, Kaiser Permanente (KP) instituted the Healthy Bones Program—a set of measures to identify and proactively treat at-risk patients. Conceived by KP orthopedists, physicians participating in the program implemented a number of initiatives, including increasing the use of bone density tests (DXA scans) and anti-osteoporosis medications; adding osteoporosis education and home health programs; and standardizing practice guidelines for osteoporosis management.

RESULTS

During the course of 5 years, the Healthy Bones Program has:

- Tracked more than 625,000 male and female patients over the age of 50 in Southern California who had specific risk factors for osteoporosis and/or hip fractures
- Reduced hip fracture rates for at-risk patients by nearly 50 percent

FOR MORE INFORMATION

Please contact: Tadashi Funahasi, MD (tadashi.t.funahashi@kp.org)

INFRASTRUCTURE FUNDAMENTALS

✓ **Resource Utilization**—optimized use of personnel, physical space, and other resources

CASE Smoothing Patient Flow at Cincinnati Children's Hospital Medical Center

To smooth patient flow through the intensive care unit (ICU), Cincinnati Children's implemented a series of operations-management interventions, with the goal of reducing daily artificial variation to make bed occupancy more predictable. To do this, staff analyzed patient-flow dynamics, evaluating surgical providers' predicted need for intensive care and predicted length of stay (LOS). When a procedure was scheduled, surgical providers made initial LOS estimates on the basis of personal experience, the complexity of the case, patient co-morbidities, best-practice plans, and historical data. The electronic surgical scheduling system was revised so that the operative case and an ICU bed (if needed postoperatively) were scheduled (reserved) at the same time. In addition, the surgeon estimated a projected LOS when the case was initially scheduled. Reserved beds were continuously monitored, and the computerized scheduling system restricted operative-case scheduling if a bed was needed and the elective case limit for that day had been reached. An admission control model was used to limit the maximum allowable elective surgical cases requiring ICU access per day. A simulation model was developed for the ICU to predict bed occupancy for all medical and surgical (elective and emergent) patients. The information from this simulation was used to identify the appropriate admission-control limit (cap) for elective surgical cases that would allow maximum occupancy while minimizing the need to cancel elective cases. This cap was adjusted if available staffed beds increased or decreased due to construction or changes in capacity. Finally, a morning huddle was established. This 6:00 a.m. meeting, including the chief of staff, manager of patient services, and representatives from the operating room, pediatric ICUs, and anesthesia, was used to confirm ICU bed availability and anticipate needs for the next day. Over time, the morning huddle strategy broadened to include discharge prediction of outflow units. This allowed demand/capacity matching for patients transferring from the pediatric ICU to patient floors, reserving available open beds for predicted outgoing ICU patients and ensuring bed access for new elective surgical patients.

RESULTS

- $100 million in capital costs (75 new beds) avoided due to improved flow and patient placement
- Decrease in variability of new elective surgical admissions
- Decrease of diversion of patients to other units and delay/cancelation of surgical procedures
- Elimination of occasions in which beds in the pediatric ICU were not available when needed for urgent medical or surgical use

FOR MORE INFORMATION

Please contact: Uma Kotagal, MBBS, MSc (uma.kotagal@cchmc.org)

CASE Reducing Inefficiencies in Nurses' Workflow at Virginia Mason
Health System

In most hospitals, nurses spend only about 35 percent of their time on direct
patient care. Using the tools and methods of the Virginia Mason Production
System (VMPS), nursing teams increased that metric to 90 percent. They used
5-day workshops (Rapid Process Improvement) to evaluate their work and
make improvements. For example, instead of the usual method of caring for
patients throughout a unit, nurses work as a team with a patient-care technician
in "cells" (groups of rooms located near each other).

RESULTS

- Enhanced communication among team members and better
  skill–task alignment
- Allows nurses to more easily monitor patients and quickly attend to needs
- Most commonly used supplies for each unit were moved to patient rooms so
  that nurses reduced time spent walking back and forth to get supplies. Steps
  walked per day were reduced from 10,000 to approximately 1,200

FOR MORE INFORMATION

Please contact: Charleen Tachibana, RN (charleen.tachibana@vmmc.org)

INFRASTRUCTURE FUNDAMENTALS
RESOURCE UTILIZATION—OPTIMIZED USE OF PERSONNEL, PHYSICAL SPACE, AND
OTHER RESOURCES

CASE — Supply Chain Management at Intermountain Healthcare

In order to improve patient care and reduce costs, Intermountain Healthcare used an evidence-based approach to improve supply chain efficiency. Intermountain's supply chain organization (SCO) works with Intermountain's clinical programs to develop effective processes and strategies for supply chain management. Key to the SCO strategy is removing the supply burden from caregivers. When Intermountain found that a significant number of central line–associated bloodstream infections (CLABSIs)—which impact patient recovery and are non-reimbursable—were occurring in the bone marrow transplant unit, a committee consisting of clinicians and supply chain experts was formed to research the practices and products associated with superior outcomes.

RESULTS

- Overall: More than $200 million in savings during the past 5 years from supply chain improvements
- For CLABSI: 2.3 percent reduction in the rate of infections; 32 percent reduction in cost per line

FOR MORE INFORMATION

Please contact: Lucy Savitz, PhD (lucy.savitz@imail.org)

CARE DELIVERY PRIORITIES

✓ **Integrated Care**—right care, right setting, right provider, right teamwork

CASE Connected Cardiac Care Program at Partners

To better monitor patients' health outside the hospital setting, Partners introduced the Connected Cardiac Care Program (CCCP), a home monitoring program for heart failure (HF) patients at risk for hospitalization. CCCP's core components are care coordination, education, and development of self-management skills through the use of telemonitoring. Patients use equipment (a monitoring device and peripherals) in their home to submit weight, blood pressure, heart rate, and symptoms on a daily basis for 4 months. Telemonitoring nurses monitor these vitals, respond to out-of-parameter alerts, and guide patients through structured biweekly heart failure education.

RESULTS

- More than $10 million in savings to date ($8,155 per patient)
- 51 percent reduction in HF hospital readmission and 44 percent reduction in non-HF hospital readmission
- Improved patient understanding of heart failure and self-management skills
- High levels of clinician and patient receptivity and satisfaction

FOR MORE INFORMATION

Please contact: Joseph Kvedar, MD (jkvedar@partners.org)

CARE DELIVERY PRIORITIES
INTEGRATED CARE—RIGHT CARE, RIGHT SETTING, RIGHT PROVIDER, RIGHT TEAMWORK

CASE Geisinger's ProvenHealth Navigator®

To better integrate patient care, in 2006, Geisinger leveraged two key components of its integrated health system structure—Geisinger Clinic, which delivers primary care, and Geisinger Health Plan (GHP), which handles insurance risk and provides population health management services—to develop an advanced medical-home model named ProvenHealth Navigator® (PHN). The PHN model has five core elements: (1) re-engineered patient-centered primary care; (2) integrated population management; (3) 360° care systems to form a medical neighborhood; (4) measurement of quality of care; and (5) a value-based reimbursement model. The PHN model is in use at 42 primary care sites (plus 9 non-employed groups) that care for more than 300,000 lives.

RESULTS

Data from the past 5 years on 80,000 GHP members were analyzed and yielded:

- 7.1 percent reduction in the total cost of care during 5 years
- 91 percent of patients rate the quality of care as better than in the past
- 93 percent of physicians would recommend PHN as a model to other primary care physicians
- 18.2 percent decrease in risk-adjusted acute admissions
- 20 percent decrease in risk-adjusted re-admissions
- 99 percent of the patient population agrees that care management works with them effectively

FOR MORE INFORMATION

Please contact: Thomas Graf, MD (trgraf@geisinger.edu)

CASE   Patient-Aligned Care Teams (PACT) at the Veterans Health Administration

In order to improve the delivery of primary care, the Veterans Health Administration (VHA) developed and implemented Patient-Aligned Care Teams (PACT), the VHA's model of the patient-centered medical home. The PACT model is data-driven, evidence-based, and value-oriented, and strives to deliver patient-centered, team-based care with a focus on prevention and population health. To facilitate and improve access to primary care for veterans, the Department of Veterans Affairs (VA) has made multiple modalities available, such as telephone clinics, home telehealth, secure messaging, and mobile apps. Also, in order to give PACT the skills needed to deliver optimal care via this new model, intensive training was provided to the primary care workforce. To test this new model of care delivery, the VA simultaneously funded five regional "demonstration labs" designed to evaluate PACT innovations, and, in turn, improve and accelerate the quality and impact of system-wide PACT implementation.

RESULTS

- ~10,000 out of ~18,500 primary care team members (physicians, nurse practitioners, physician assistants, nurses, pharmacists, etc.) have been trained

- 16 percent increase in total PACT encounters in FY 2011 (e.g., face-to-face, phone, group, secure messaging)

- 15 percent increase in same-day access to primary care physicians in FY 2011

- Overall, urgent care visits by primary care patients decreased by 8 percent and admission rates decreased by 4 percent since the implementation of PACT

FOR MORE INFORMATION

Please contact: Richard Stark, MD (richard.stark@va.gov)

CARE DELIVERY PRIORITIES
INTEGRATED CARE—RIGHT CARE, RIGHT SETTING, RIGHT PROVIDER, RIGHT TEAMWORK

CASE Medical Team Training at the Veterans Health Administration

In order to improve the quality and efficiency of surgical procedures at the Veterans Health Administration (VHA), in 2003, the VA National Center for Patient Safety (NCPS) developed and launched a pilot medical team training (MTT) program focusing on patient-centered, checklist-guided briefings and debriefings in operating rooms. Key objectives of this program were to improve communication among clinicians in high-risk situations and to deliver safer care. This program was grounded in aviation's high-reliability crew resource management (CRM) approach. Participation in the training program required— and continues to require—leadership, clinical, and support-service staff participation prior to and following the training (feedback on implementation results and pre-/post-attitudinal data is collected). Success among the pilot sites in both patient care (e.g., increased timeliness of care) and staff satisfaction (e.g., team skills) during the pilot led to a mandatory national roll-out of the program during subsequent years for all facilities with operating rooms. Following the mandatory roll-out, the MTT program became a voluntary, self-enrolled program available to any facility. The success of this initial program led to the expansion of team training and CRM techniques to a wider variety of clinical settings (e.g., inpatient wards, outpatient care, dental clinics, etc.).

RESULTS

- 18 percent decrease in surgical mortality
- 17 percent decrease in surgical morbidity
- 25 percent decrease in operating room adverse events

FOR MORE INFORMATION

Please contact: Robin R. Hemphill, MD, MPH (robin.hemphill@va.gov)

CARE DELIVERY PRIORITIES

✓ **Shared Decision Making**—patient–clinician collaboration on care plans

CASE ThedaCare Collaborative Care Units

To better involve patients in care planning and to eliminate wasteful and contradictory steps that result from having multiple care plans, ThedaCare introduced Collaborative Care, a redesign of inpatient care to focus on those elements of care that add value to the patient experience. It was designed using Lean methods, with patients and caregivers working together to identify the steps in the inpatient care process that are important to care while eliminating the steps that are wasteful. The basic unit of collaborative care is the interdisciplinary team with the patient at the center. On admission, a physician, nurse, discharge planner, and pharmacist jointly meet the patient, and with the patient's input, develop a single plan of care. This unified plan replaces the multiple, sometimes contradictory, plans of care previously maintained separately by physicians, nurses, and ancillary practitioners. The nurse monitors the progression of care using evidenced-based guidelines available in the single care plan, which exists in the electronic health record. When they detect a barrier to the progression, it is the nurse who contacts the team's physician with recommendations, not the other way around.

RESULTS

- 25 percent reduction in direct and indirect costs of inpatient care
- Average length of stay dropped 17 percent
- Elimination of all medication-reconciliation errors and near 100 percent compliance with care protocols
- Patient satisfaction scores rose to 95 percent rating their care as 5 out of 5 (from 68 percent previously)

FOR MORE INFORMATION

Please contact: ThedaCare Center for Healthcare Value (info@createvalue.org)

CASE Lung Transplant Care at Cleveland Clinic

To improve outcomes, lower costs, and enhance the patient experience for lung transplants, Cleveland Clinic initiated a care improvement process that involved mapping all aspects of the procedure and involving patients and their families, cardiothoracic surgery, pulmonary medicine, anesthesia, intensive care, respiratory therapy, nursing, physical therapy, and case management in the care improvement process. In 2010, protocols were developed for ventilator management, blood utilization, respiratory therapy, medication administration, and postoperative patient mobilization. Daily "huddles" with the patient and all caregivers were initiated to inform the patient and family of the expected progress and to develop a consistent plan between caregivers and the patient. Attending physicians were scripted to take a threefold approach with patients: (1) introduction of the attending, in which the attending states that he/she will be responsible for the patient's care; (2) if another attending is assuming care, the current attending announces the change, including the incoming attending's name and states that the incoming attending will review the case with the current attending. The incoming attending then introduces himself/herself to the patient and reviews the discussion with the transferring physician; and (3) on the day of discharge, the attending meets with the patient and family to review the course of the hospitalization, home-going medications, follow-up appointment(s), and who to contact with problems and questions. Follow-up data was obtained after 12 months and compared to pre-protocol implementation.

RESULTS

- Total length of stay reduced by 1.54 days (6.9 percent) with an 1.34-day (18.7 percent) decrease in the ICU length of stay
- 6 percent decrease in costs of care
- 28 percent improvement in patient satisfaction regarding clinician communication
- 30-day survival improved by 3 percent (93.8 to 96.8 percent)

FOR MORE INFORMATION

Please contact: Robert Wyllie, MD (wyllier@ccf.org)

CARE DELIVERY PRIORITIES

✓ **Targeted Services**—tailored community and clinic interventions for resource-intensive patients

CASE   High-Risk Asthma Patient Initiative at Cincinnati Children's Hospital Medical Center

To better focus its resources toward high-risk patients, in October 2003, a primary care independent practice association (Ohio Valley Primary Care Associates, LLC) and a physician–hospital organization (Tri State Child Health Services, Inc.) affiliated with Cincinnati Children's Hospital Medical Center, launched a large-scale asthma-improvement initiative across 38 community-based pediatric practices, impacting nearly 13,000 children with asthma (approximately 40 percent of the pediatric asthma population across the region). This initiative is ongoing, with a significant focus on the following interventions: strong physician leadership at the Board and practice levels; network-level goal setting by the Board (network-level improvement defines success); measurable practice-level quality-improvement participation expectations/requirements (linked to American Board of Pediatrics Maintenance of Certification approval and payer reward programs); multidisciplinary practice quality-improvement teams; web-based registry with all-payer population reconfirmation at regular intervals; real-time patient, practice, and network-level data/reporting; transparent, comparative practice data on process and outcome measures; concurrent use of data collection/decision-support tools at point of care through high-reliability principles/workflow changes (generates disconfirming data at point of care); pay-for-performance/incentive models aligned with improvement objectives; evidence-based care components ("perfect care" composite measure); population segmentation with a significant focus on the "high-risk" cohort; cross-practice communication/shared learning forums to spread successful interventions; integration of multiple administrative/electronic data sources (hospital, practice, regional health information exchange); automated routing of ED/urgent care visit and admission alerts to primary care practices; and network- and practice-level sustainability measurement/interventions.

RESULTS

- 35 percent reduction in both admissions and ED/urgent care visits in the physician–hospital organization vs. comparison group for commercially insured, population-based asthma
- 92 percent of all-payer asthma population receiving "perfect care" (composite measure of severity classification, written management plan, and controller medications [if patient has "persistent" asthma])
- Reduction in commercially insured asthma-related admissions: savings estimated at $322,000 for the most recent 12-month period (92 admissions avoided)
- Reduction in commercially insured asthma-related ED/urgent care visits: savings estimated at $93,000 for the most recent 12-month period (266 ED/urgent care visits avoided)

FOR MORE INFORMATION

Please contact: Uma Kotagal, MBBS, MSc (uma.kotagal@cchmc.org)

CASE   High-Risk Medicare Patient Demonstration Project at Partners

To reduce emergency department visits and readmissions among high-risk Medicare patients, in 2006, Massachusetts General Hospital (MGH), a member of the Partners HealthCare System, participated in a 3-year demonstration project to test strategies to improve the coordination of Medicare services for high-cost, fee-for-service beneficiaries. To help the primary care physicians manage these patients, MGH integrated 12 care managers into their primary care practices. The care managers developed personal relationships with enrolled patients and worked closely with physicians to help identify gaps in patient care, coordinate providers and services, facilitate communication (especially during transitions), and help educate patients and providers. A comprehensive health IT system supports the entire program, which includes electronic health records, patient tracking, and monitoring from home. Since the program's inception, additional patients were added at MGH, and the program was extended to Brigham and Women's Hospital and North Shore Health System.

RESULTS

- Return on investment: $2.65 for every $1 spent
- 20 percent reduction in admissions and 13 percent reduction in emergency department visits
- Total gross savings among enrolled patients of 12 percent (7 percent after accounting for the management fee paid by the Centers for Medicare and Medicaid Services)

FOR MORE INFORMATION

Please contact: Tim Ferris, MD (tferris@partners.org)

CASE   Intensive Outpatient Care Program at Virginia Mason

In order to reduce costs and improve quality for high-cost patients, Virginia Mason (VM), in partnership with Regence Blue Shield of Washington and other health organizations, launched an Intensive Outpatient Care Program (IOCP) in 2007. Patients eligible to be part of the IOCP represented the top 10 percent of predicted spending. VM worked with Regence and the Boeing Company to design, test, and implement the program. Under the program, Boeing aimed to improve quality of care and substantially reduce total spending for the predicted highest-cost quintile of its Puget Sound employees and their adult dependents who participated in Boeing's self-funded, non-HMO medical plans. In addition to Regence, several health care consulting and management groups participated. Boeing incentivized the groups via a monthly per-patient fee to test a new, intensified chronic care model—the "ambulatory intensive caring unit" (A-ICU). Designed to both lower per capita spending and improve quality, the A-ICU model development was based on the experiences of successful primary care innovators. Patients were invited to enroll in the IOCP if they had a severe chronic illness and would likely benefit from intensified primary care. The pilot enrolled more than 740 eligible non-Medicare Boeing patients, approximately 300 of whom were VM patients. The patients were connected to a care team that included a dedicated RN care manager and an IOCP-participating primary care provider. Each IOCP-enrolled patient received a comprehensive intake interview, physical exam, and diagnostic testing. A care plan was developed in partnership with the patient. The plan was executed through intensive in-person, telephonic, and email contacts, including frequent proactive outreach by an RN, education in self-management of chronic conditions, rapid access to and care coordination by the IOCP team, and direct involvement of specialists, including behavioral health specialists when feasible.

RESULTS

- 33 percent reduction in annual per capita claims
- 14.8 percent improvement in patients' physical function; 16.1 percent improvement in mental function
- 17.6 percent improvement in timeliness of care
- 56.5 percent reduction in patients' work-days missed

FOR MORE INFORMATION
Please contact: Ingrid Gerbino, MD (ingrid.gerbino@vmmc.org)

CARE DELIVERY PRIORITIES
TARGETED SERVICES—TAILORED COMMUNITY AND CLINIC INTERVENTIONS FOR
RESOURCE-INTENSIVE PATIENTS

CASE   HIV Care at Kaiser Permanente

To improve care and reduce disparities among its 20,000 patients with HIV, Kaiser Permanente (KP), in conjunction with the President's Advisory Council on HIV/AIDS, the VA, and NCQA, developed and piloted a series of performance measures that will be incorporated into the National HEDIS measures by NCQA. Additionally, early in 2012, KP issued the "HIV Challenge" to all care systems in America in an attempt to stimulate other health care organizations to adopt these practices and to assist them in their efforts. As part of its HIV Challenge effort, KP is sharing best practices and tools for private health care providers and community health clinics to replicate: quality-improvement programs that measure gaps in care; testing, prevention, and treatment guidelines; how to set up multidisciplinary care team models that emphasize the "medical home" so HIV specialists, care managers, clinical pharmacists, and providers work together; and education for both the provider and patient.

RESULTS

Kaiser Permanente demonstrated excellence in HIV clinical care outcomes with:

- 89 percent of its HIV-positive patients are in HIV-specific care within 90 days (compared to 50 percent within 1 year in the United States)
- 94 percent median treatment adherence among patients regularly in care and on antiretroviral therapy
- No disparities among Black and Latino HIV-positive patients for both mortality and medication rates
- 69 percent of all HIV-positive patients have maximal viral control (compared to 19-35 percent nationally)
- HIV mortality rates that are half the national average

FOR MORE INFORMATION

Please contact: Michael Horberg, MD (michael.horberg@kp.org)

RELIABILITY AND FEEDBACK

✓ **Embedded Safeguards**—supports and prompts to reduce injury and infection

CASE Reducing Surgical Site Infections at Cincinnati Children's
Hospital Medical Center

To reduce the incidence of surgical site infections (SSIs), Cincinnati Children's
implemented a bundle of interventions, each designed for reliability and
error reduction. Each surgical division developed a list of procedures for
which antibiotic prophylaxis was required. To ensure timely and appropriate
administration of prophylactic antibiotics, a pediatric-specific list of appropriate
antibiotics was developed. Pediatric dosing time frames, limits, and parameters
for re-dosing were also established. A computerized forced-function was
developed to attach required antibiotics to all procedures within the division-
specific list of evidence-based need for antibiotic prophylaxis. A new file
was added to the computer screen used by surgical schedulers to identify
procedures for which antibiotics are required. This reminder was also printed
on the operating room schedule for nurses, surgeons, and anesthesiologists
to see. For same-day surgery patients, the complete preoperative antibiotic
orders were due before 10:00 a.m. the day before surgery, and an "identify and
mitigate" process was established to identify potential failures. On the day of
surgery, a medication nurse was required to confirm the antibiotic order and
the accuracy of the dose, and to put an orange "antibiotic required" bracelet on
the child as a reminder to the anesthesiologist. Daily data concerning potential
failures at any step critical for success were collected, and team leaders
discussed any failures the next day with the critical providers. Additionally,
a bundle compliance-monitoring form, designed to be completed by nurses,
helped to build quality improvement into daily work.

RESULTS

- Reduced average length of stay per case to 10 days, resulting in an average
  savings of $27,000 per case
- Six-year savings of $6.3 million
- An estimated 233 surgical site infections were prevented in the past 6 years

FOR MORE INFORMATION

Please contact: Uma Kotagal, MBBS, MSc (uma.kotagal@cchmc.org)

RELIABILITY AND FEEDBACK
EMBEDDED SAFEGUARDS—SUPPORTS AND PROMPTS TO REDUCE INJURY AND INFECTION

CASE Reducing Central Line–Associated Bloodstream Infections at HCA

To reduce central line–associated bloodstream infections, HCA conducted a multi-year effort that incorporates the latest evidence-based recommendations, including insertion and maintenance practices, supply standardization of central line kits, and competency training for all HCA physicians as part of their biannual credentialing. By developing and implementing evidence-based central line insertion and maintenance bundles, HCA reduced variation in clinical practice and improved quality and patient outcomes.

RESULTS

- $44,000 in savings per case—$17.5 million saved system-wide annually
- 57.4 percent decrease in hospital-acquired bloodstream infections within the ICU since 2006
- Up to 200 lives saved
- More than 400 fewer infections annually since 2006
- 80 HCA facilities with zero hospital-acquired bloodstream infections

FOR MORE INFORMATION

Please contact: Jason Hickok, RN, MBA (jason.hickok@hcahealthcare.com)

CASE Sepsis Treatment Protocols at Kaiser Permanente

To better diagnose and treat community-acquired sepsis, in July 2009, Kaiser Permanente established early-intervention protocols through its Sepsis Care Performance Initiative. The findings from the Initiative dramatically demonstrated the importance and impact of early intervention on clinical patient outcomes. Kaiser Permanente nursing, physician, informatics, and quality leaders translated existing guidelines into specific competencies, practices, and roles for the care delivery staff. Changes in patient care protocols in the ED and ICU provided early recognition and treatment intervention opportunities. The clinical teams became more proficient in inserting central lines and utilizing hemodynamic monitors for continual monitoring of central venous pressure, oxygenation, and mean arterial pressure through training and simulation. Patients in the early stages of sepsis were identified more quickly through EMR decision support, allowing for targeted therapy to be administered within an hour of diagnosis using resuscitation bundles of broad spectrum antibiotics, fluids, and hemodynamic support during a 6-hour period.

RESULTS

- Sepsis mortality reduced by over half (26 percent to 10 percent)
- ~3-fold increase in the number of sepsis cases diagnosed (now 119.4/1,000 admissions)
- ~3-fold increase in the number of admitted patients with blood culture who had serum lactate drawn in ED (now 97 percent)
- 3.5-day decrease in the length of stay for patients with a principle diagnosis of sepsis
- 93 percent of patients with sepsis treated within 1 hour of diagnosis (19 percent increase)

FOR MORE INFORMATION

Please contact: Ruth Shaber, MD (ruth.shaber@kp.org)

RELIABILITY AND FEEDBACK
EMBEDDED SAFEGUARDS—SUPPORTS AND PROMPTS TO REDUCE INJURY AND INFECTION

CASE Reducing Pharmacy Errors at Partners

To reduce serious medication errors, in 2003 Brigham and Women's Hospital (BWH), a member of the Partners HealthCare System, implemented pharmacy barcoding, in which pharmacists barcode-scan all medications dispensed from the pharmacy to ensure that the medications match physicians' orders (which are entered electronically via computerized physician order entry [CPOE]). In addition, in 2005, BWH implemented electronic medication-administration records (EMAR)/barcoding at the bedside, in which nurses scan medications prior to administration to patients, and are alerted about possible errors.

RESULTS

- $3.3 million in cumulative 5-year savings (costs recouped within first year)
- 31 percent reduction in serious medication-administration errors
- An annual savings of $2.2 million from decreased adverse drug events
- Increased on-time medication availability on nursing units

FOR MORE INFORMATION

Please contact: Tejal Gandhi, MD, MPH (tgandhi@partners.org)

CASE Reducing MRSA at VHA Hospitals

In response to growing concerns about methicillin-resistant Staphylococcus aureus (MRSA) health care–associated infections (HAIs), in 2007 the VHA implemented a MRSA Prevention Initiative to decrease MRSA HAIs in acute care VA hospitals nationwide. The focal point of this initiative consisted of a bundle of evidence-based practices known as the "MRSA Bundle"—universal nasal surveillance for MRSA, implementation of "contact precautions" for patients infected and/or colonized with MRSA, renewed emphasis on hand-hygiene practices, and an institutional culture change in which infection prevention and control became everyone's responsibility. Furthermore, management support was provided for a newly recognized position at each medical center known as the MRSA Prevention Coordinator (MPC), who coordinates local medical center implementation efforts of the initiative with the national MRSA project office. Currently, the MRSA Prevention Initiative is being expanded to become the Multidrug-Resistant Organisms (MDROs) Prevention Initiative and will target other MDROs that contribute to health care–associated infections.

RESULTS

- From October 2007 to June 2010, MRSA HAI rates declined by 62 percent in VHA ICUs nationwide
- During this same period, non-ICU MRSA HAI rates fell by 45 percent
- Approximately 1,000 MRSA HAIs were prevented during this period
- Currently, more than 70 percent of VHA facilities report zero MRSA HAIs monthly

FOR MORE INFORMATION

Please contact: Martin Evans, MD (martin.evans@va.gov)

RELIABILITY AND FEEDBACK

✓ **Internal Transparency**—visible progress in performance, outcomes, and costs

CASE Chronic Disease Patient Registries at Denver Health

To improve population health and reduce variation in practice among primary care providers, in 2006, Denver Health began developing preventive health and chronic disease patient registries for the 100,000 users of their community health center network. A prerequisite for this work is the use of a single-patient identifier to link care from multiple sites to a single patient. Step 1 in the registry development was the selection of high-impact and high-opportunity areas of focus: diabetes care, hypertension care, and cancer screening. Step 2 was the creation of an assignment algorithm so that each user of the primary clinics is assigned to a medical home and a primary care provider (PCP) based on services utilization in the prior 3 years. Step 3 was the development of outreach tools for individual clinicians to manage patients between visits. Step 4 was the creation of performance report cards aggregated across patients and time and populated by nearly real-time data. An essential feature of the report cards is the transparent display (i.e., without blinding) of performance by site of primary care and by PCP, which has driven reduced variation and improved overall performance.

RESULTS

- Colorectal cancer screening rates nearly doubled in 3 years after starting at 32 percent

- Breast cancer screening rates increased by 20 percent in 3 years after many years of flat performance

- Hypertension control rates increased from 60 percent to 72 percent in 3 years

FOR MORE INFORMATION

Please contact: Tom MacKenzie, MD (thomas.mackenzie@dhha.org)

CASE Internal, Non-Blinded Performance Transparency at Cleveland Clinic

To engage providers in quality improvement and waste reduction, Cleveland Clinic implemented web-based business intelligence tools to collect and display provider performance data for a wide variety of metrics. By giving providers transparent access to metrics that identify variations in practice, utilization rates, and performance against internal and external benchmarks, Cleveland Clinic saw dramatic reductions in waste, improved quality, and a sustained change in culture, as practitioners take pride when they do well and foster the desire to change when they recognize the need to improve.

RESULTS

- >40 percent reduction in ICU central line–associated bloodstream infections (CLABSIs)
- 50 percent reduction in ICU urinary tract infections per 1,000 patient days
- Cost avoidance of $30,000 for each CLABSI and $5,000 for each urinary tract infection
- Increased compliance in administration of pneumonia vaccinations to a sustained level near 100 percent
- 13 percent increase in operating room on-time first starts
- 10 percent improvement in transferred patients assigned to a receiving bed within 12 hours or less
- 10 percent reduction in blood units used per 1,000 patient days

FOR MORE INFORMATION

Please contact: Robert Wyllie, MD (wyllier@ccf.org)

APPENDIX II

Identifying Unnecessary Services

The Checklist addresses the systems-level issues central in transitioning to high-value care—care that improves outcomes while reducing costs. Part of the systems-level change necessary requires identifying unnecessary services and engaging individual practitioners to be better stewards of limited resources. Summarized below are examples of recent analyses and inventories that have been developed to identify services that are often overused, unnecessary, or were otherwise wasteful.

National Physicians Alliance [1]

Members of the National Physicians Alliance's Good Stewardship Working Group identified common clinical activities that could lead to higher-quality care and better use of finite clinical resources. These are presented as "top 5" lists for primary care, internal medicine, and pediatrics.

- **Primary care**
  1. Don't do imaging for low back pain within the first 6 weeks unless red flags are present
  2. Don't routinely prescribe antibiotics for acute mild to moderate sinusitis
  3. Don't order annual ECGs for asymptomatic, low-risk patients
  4. Don't perform Pap tests on patients younger than 21 years
  5. Don't use DEXA screening for osteoporosis for women under 65 or men under 70 with no risk factors

- **Internal medicine**
  1. Don't do imaging for low back pain within the first 6 weeks unless red flags are present
  2. Don't obtain blood chemistry panels or urinalysis screenings for asymptomatic, healthy adults
  3. Don't order annual ECGs for asymptomatic, low-risk patients
  4. Use generic statins when initiating lipid-lowering drug therapy
  5. Don't use DEXA screening for osteoporosis for women under 65 or men under 70 with no risk factors

- **Pediatrics**
  1. Don't prescribe antibiotics for pharyngitis unless the patient tests positive for streptococcus
  2. Don't obtain diagnostic images for minor head injuries without loss of consciousness or other risk factors
  3. Don't refer OME early in the course of a problem
  4. Advise patients not to use cough and cold medications
  5. Use inhaled corticosteroids to control asthma appropriately

[1] The Good Stewardship Working Group. 2011. The "Top 5" lists in primary care: Meeting the responsibility of professionalism. *Archives of Internal Medicine* 171(15):1385-1390. Reproduced with permission from the American Medical Association.

American College of Physicians[2]

A working group of the American College of Physicians convened a workgroup of physicians to identify common clinical situations in which screening and diagnostic tests are used in ways that do not reflect high-value care. The 37 situations identified are listed below.

1. Repeating screening ultrasonography for abdominal aortic aneurysm following a negative study

2. Performing coronary angiography in patients with chronic stable angina with well-controlled symptoms on medical therapy or who lack specific high-risk criteria on exercise testing

3. Performing echocardiography in asymptomatic patients with innocent-sounding heart murmurs, most typically grade I to II/VI short systolic, midpeaking murmurs that are audible along the left sternal border

4. Performing routine periodic echocardiography in asymptomatic patients with mild aortic stenosis more frequently than every 3 to 5 years

5. Routinely repeating echocardiography in asymptomatic patients with mild mitral regurgitation and normal left ventricular size and function

6. Obtaining electrocardiograms to screen for cardiac disease in patients at low to average risk for coronary artery disease

7. Obtaining exercise electrocardiograms for screening in low-risk asymptomatic adults

8. Performing an imaging stress test (echocardiographic or nuclear) as the initial diagnostic test in patients with known or suspected coronary artery disease who are able to exercise and have no resting electrocardiographic abnormalities that may interfere with interpretation of test results

9. Measuring brain natriuretic peptide in the initial evaluation of patients with typical findings of heart failure

10. Annual lipid screening for patients not receiving lipid-lowering drug or diet therapy in the absence of reasons for changing lipid profiles

11. Using MRI rather than mammography as the breast cancer screening test of choice for average-risk women

12. In asymptomatic women with previously-treated breast cancer, performing follow-up complete blood counts, blood chemistry studies, tumor marker studies, chest radiography, or imaging studies other than appropriate breast imaging

13. Performing DEXA screening for osteoporosis in women younger than 65 years in the absence of risk factors

14. Screening low-risk individuals for hepatitis B virus infection

15. Screening for cervical cancer in low-risk women aged 65 years or older and in women who have had a total hysterectomy (uterus and cervix) for benign disease

16. Screening for colorectal cancer in adults older than 75 years or in adults with a life expectancy of less than 10 years

17. Repeating colonoscopy within 5 years of an index colonoscopy in asymptomatic patients found to have low-risk adenomas

[2] Qaseem, A., et. al. 2012. Appropriate use of screening and diagnostic tests to foster high-value, cost-conscious care. *Annals of Internal Medicine* 156:147-149. Reproduced with permission from the American College of Physicians.

18. Screening for prostate cancer in men older than 75 years or with a life expectancy of less than 10 years

19. Using CA-125 antigen levels to screen women for ovarian cancer in the absence of increased risk

20. Performing imaging studies in patients with nonspecific low-back pain

21. Performing preoperative chest radiography in the absence of a clinical suspicion for intrathoracic pathology

22. Ordering routine preoperative laboratory tests, including complete blood count, liver chemistry tests, and metabolic profiles, in otherwise healthy patients undergoing elective surgery

23. Performing preoperative coagulation studies in patients without risk factors or predisposing conditions for bleeding and with a negative history of abnormal bleeding

24. Performing serologic testing for suspected early Lyme disease

25. Performing serologic testing for Lyme disease in patients with chronic nonspecific symptoms and no clinical evidence of disseminated Lyme disease

26. Performing sinus imaging studies for patients with acute rhinosinusitis in the absence of predisposing factors for atypical microbial causes

27. Performing imaging studies in patients with recurrent, classic migraine headache and normal findings on neurologic examination

28. Performing brain imaging studies (CT or MRI) to evaluate simple syncope in patients with normal findings on neurologic examination

29. Routinely performing echocardiography in the evaluation of syncope, unless the history, physical examination, and electrocardiogram do not provide a diagnosis or underlying heart disease is suspected

30. Performing predischarge chest radiography for hospitalized patients with community-acquired pneumonia who are making a satisfactory clinical recovery

31. Obtaining CT scans in a patient with pneumonia that is confirmed by chest radiography in the absence of complicating clinical or radiographic features

32. Performing imaging studies, rather than a high-sensitivity D-dimer measurement, as the initial diagnostic test in patients with low pretest probability of venous thromboembolism

33. Measuring D-dimer rather than performing appropriate diagnostic imaging (extremity ultrasonography, CT angiography, or ventilation–perfusion scintigraphy), in patients with intermediate or high probability of venous thromboembolism

34. Performing follow-up imaging studies for incidentally discovered pulmonary nodules >4 mm in low-risk individuals

35. Monitoring patients with asthma or chronic obstructive pulmonary disease by using full pulmonary function testing that includes lung volumes and diffusing capacity, rather than spirometry alone (or peak expiratory flow rate monitoring in asthma)

36. Performing an antinuclear antibody test in patients with nonspecific symptoms, such as fatigue and myalgia, or in patients with fibromyalgia

37. Screening for chronic obstructive pulmonary disease with spirometry in individuals without respiratory symptoms

ABIM Foundation's Choosing Wisely® Campaign[3]

The American Board of Internal Medicine (ABIM) Foundation has worked with various physician specialty societies to identify common tests and procedures that may be overused or unnecessary. Each society developed a list of "5 Things Physicians and Patients Should Question," which contains evidence-based recommendations for physicians and patients to consider when making care decisions. Below are the lists for the initial nine specialty societies. Eight more societies are expected to contribute lists in Fall 2012.

- **American Academy of Allergy, Asthma & Immunology** (AAAAI)

  1. Don't perform unproven diagnostic tests, such as immunoglobulin G (IgG) testing or an indiscriminate battery of immunoglobulin E (IgE) tests, in the evaluation of allergy.

  2. Don't order sinus computed tomography (CT) or indiscriminately prescribe antibiotics for uncomplicated acute rhinosinusitis.

  3. Don't routinely do diagnostic testing in patients with chronic urticaria.

  4. Don't recommend replacement immunoglobulin therapy for recurrent infections unless impaired antibody responses to vaccines are demonstrated.

  5. Don't diagnose or manage asthma without spirometry.

- **American Academy of Family Physicians** (AAFP)

  1. Don't do imaging for low back pain within the first six weeks, unless red flags are present.

  2. Don't routinely prescribe antibiotics for acute mild-to-moderate sinusitis unless symptoms last for seven or more days, or symptoms worsen after initial clinical improvement.

  3. Don't use dual-energy x-ray absorptiometry (DEXA) screening for osteoporosis in women younger than 65 or men younger than 70 with no risk factors.

  4. Don't order annual electrocardiograms (EKGs) or any other cardiac screening for low-risk patients without symptoms.

  5. Don't perform Pap smears on women younger than 21 or who have had a hysterectomy for non-cancer disease.

- **American College of Cardiology** (ACC)

  1. Don't perform stress cardiac imaging or advanced non-invasive imaging in the initial evaluation of patients without cardiac symptoms unless high-risk markers are present.

  2. Don't perform annual stress cardiac imaging or advanced non-invasive imaging as part of routine follow-up in asymptomatic patients.

  3. Don't perform stress cardiac imaging or advanced non-invasive imaging as a pre-operative assessment in patients scheduled to undergo low-risk non-cardiac surgery.

  4. Don't perform echocardiography as routine follow-up for mild, asymptomatic native valve disease in adult patients with no change in signs or symptoms.

[3] Available at http://choosingwisely.org/?page_id=13. Reproduced with permission from the American Board of Internal Medicine Foundation.

5. Don't perform stenting of non-culprit lesions during percutaneous coronary intervention (PCI) for uncomplicated hemodynamically stable ST-segment elevation myocardial infarction (STEMI).

- **American College of Physicians** (ACP)
  1. Don't obtain screening exercise electrocardiogram testing in individuals who are asymptomatic and at low risk for coronary heart disease.
  2. Don't obtain imaging studies in patients with non-specific low back pain.
  3. In the evaluation of simple syncope and a normal neurological examination, don't obtain brain imaging studies (CT or MRI).
  4. In patients with low pretest probability of venous thromboembolism (VTE), obtain a high-sensitive D-dimer measurement as the initial diagnostic test; don't obtain imaging studies as the initial diagnostic test.
  5. Don't obtain preoperative chest radiography in the absence of a clinical suspicion for intrathoracic pathology.

- **American College of Radiology** (ACR)
  1. Don't do imaging for uncomplicated headache.
  2. Don't image for suspected pulmonary embolism (PE) without moderate or high pre-test probability.
  3. Avoid admission or preoperative chest x-rays for ambulatory patients with unremarkable history and physical exam.
  4. Don't do computed tomography (CT) for the evaluation of suspected appendicitis in children until after ultrasound has been considered as an option.
  5. Don't recommend follow-up imaging for clinically inconsequential adnexal cysts.

- **American Gastroenterological Association** (AGA)
  1. For pharmacological treatment of patients with gastroesophageal reflux disease (GERD), long-term acid suppression therapy (proton pump inhibitors or histamine2 receptor antagonists) should be titrated to the lowest effective dose needed to achieve therapeutic goals.
  2. Do not repeat colorectal cancer screening (by any method) for 10 years after a high-quality colonoscopy is negative in average-risk individuals.
  3. Do not repeat colonoscopy for at least five years for patients who have one or two small (< 1 cm) adenomatous polyps, without high-grade dysplasia, completely removed via a high-quality colonoscopy.
  4. For a patient who is diagnosed with Barrett's esophagus, who has undergone a second endoscopy that confirms the absence of dysplasia on biopsy, a follow-up surveillance examination should not be performed in less than three years as per published guidelines.
  5. For a patient with functional abdominal pain syndrome (as per ROME III criteria) computed tomography (CT) scans should not be repeated unless there is a major change in clinical findings or symptoms.

- **American Society of Clinical Oncology** (ASCO)
  1. Don't use cancer-directed therapy for solid tumor patients with the following characteristics: low performance status (3 or 4), no benefit from prior evidence-based interventions, not eligible for a clinical trial, and no strong evidence supporting the clinical value of further anti-cancer treatment.
  2. Don't perform PET, CT, and radionuclide bone scans in the staging of early prostate cancer at low risk for metastasis.
  3. Don't perform PET, CT, and radionuclide bone scans in the staging of early breast cancer at low risk for metastasis.
  4. Don't perform surveillance testing (biomarkers) or imaging (PET, CT, and radionuclide bone scans) for asymptomatic individuals who have been treated for breast cancer with curative intent.
  5. Don't use white cell stimulating factors for primary prevention of febrile neutropenia for patients with less than 20 percent risk for this complication.

- **American Society of Nephrology** (ASN)
  1. Don't perform routine cancer screening for dialysis patients with limited life expectancies without signs or symptoms.
  2. Don't administer erythropoiesis-stimulating agents (ESAs) to chronic kidney disease (CKD) patients with hemoglobin levels greater than or equal to 10 g/dL without symptoms of anemia.
  3. Avoid nonsteroidal anti-inflammatory drugs (NSAIDS) in individuals with hypertension or heart failure or CKD of all causes, including diabetes.
  4. Don't place peripherally inserted central catheters (PICC) in stage III–V CKD patients without consulting nephrology.
  5. Don't initiate chronic dialysis without ensuring a shared decision-making process between patients, their families, and their physicians.

- **American Society of Nuclear Cardiology** (ASNC)
  1. Don't perform stress cardiac imaging or coronary angiography in patients without cardiac symptoms unless high-risk markers are present.
  2. Don't perform cardiac imaging for patients who are at low risk.
  3. Don't perform radionuclide imaging as part of routine follow-up in asymptomatic patients.
  4. Don't perform cardiac imaging as a pre-operative assessment in patients scheduled to undergo low- or intermediate-risk non-cardiac surgery.
  5. Use methods to reduce radiation exposure in cardiac imaging, whenever possible, including not performing such tests when limited benefits are likely.

Appendix C

ACA Provisions with Implications for a Learning Health Care System*

QUALITY AND EFFECTIVENESS

Quality Measurement

- Extends the *Physician Quality Reporting Initiative*, a program that makes incentive payments to physicians who report quality measures data to Medicare.
- Requires the HHS Secretary to develop a *National Strategy to Improve Health Care Quality* to improve health outcomes and efficiency, identify areas for improvement, address gaps in comparative effectiveness information and data gathering, and improve research and dissemination of best practices. The national strategy must be updated annually, with the initial report submitted to Congress by January 1, 2011. A draft report was released on September 9, 2010.
- Requires AHRQ and CMS to develop quality measures that conform to the *National Strategy*, and requires the HHS Secretary to develop and periodically update provider-level outcome measures for hospitals and physicians, including 10 outcome measurements

---

*Reproduced with permission from the Institute of Medicine Roundtable on Value & Science-Driven Health Care. Available at http://www.iom.edu/vsrt (accessed February 27, 2012).

for acute and chronic diseases by March 2012 and 10 outcome measurements for primary and preventive care by March 2013.

- Establishes the *Medicaid Quality Measurement Program*, which requires state Medicaid plans to report on state-specific health quality measures, as determined by the HHS Secretary, and requires the HHS Secretary to test, validate, and develop the quality measures, and to publish annual recommendations on changes to the core set of measures. The ACA appropriates $60 million per year for fiscal years 2010 through 2014 to the *Medicaid Quality Measurement Program* for a total appropriation of $300 million.
- Creates a quality measures reporting system for long-term care hospitals, inpatient rehabilitation facilities, cancer hospitals, and hospice programs.
- Creates an *Interagency Working Group on Health Care Quality* to coordinate quality activities across 23 federal departments.
- Creates a website, *HealthCare.gov*, to educate consumers about the Affordable Care Act, including insurance coverage options and information on health care quality and preventive care.

Comparative Effectiveness Research

- Establishes the *Patient-Centered Outcomes Research Institute*, a nonprofit Board consisting of the directors of AHRQ and NIH, as well as 19 members appointed by the U.S. Government Accountability Office (GAO), that will conduct research comparing the clinical effectiveness and appropriateness of medical treatments and procedures. The Institute's research is aimed to assist patients, providers, purchasers, and policy makers in making informed health decisions.
- Directs the HHS Secretary to make standardized extracts of Medicare claims data available to qualified entities, as determined by the HHS Secretary, for analysis of provider and supplier performance on quality, efficiency, and effectiveness. Qualified entities must release their evaluations to the public, and reports must include descriptions of the metrics used.

Care Continuity

- Establishes the *Community-Based Care Transitions Program* to improve home-based chronic care management for Medicare beneficiaries with multiple chronic conditions.

- Creates the *Community First Choice Option*, which gives states the ability to offer home and community-based attendant services to certain Medicaid beneficiaries.
- Establishes the *Community-Based Collaborative Care Network Program* to support groups of providers that coordinate care for low-income and underinsured populations.
- Establishes interdisciplinary community health teams, created by grants and contracts to eligible organizations from the HHS Secretary, to facilitate collaboration between primary care providers and community-based prevention, patient education, and other resources.
- Creates the *Federal Coordinated Health Care Office*, a new office within the Centers for Medicare and Medicaid Services to improve coordination of care for dual eligibles.

Condition-Specific Care Improvement

- Creates a *National Congenital Heart Disease Surveillance System* to track epidemiological data on heart disease and identify areas for prevention and outreach.
- Establishes *Centers of Excellence for Depression*, a network of organizations that will develop and implement evidence-based treatment and prevention standards, foster communication with stakeholders, leverage community resources, and promote the use of electronic health records to coordinate and manage treatment of depressive disorders.
- Creates a *National Diabetes Report Card*, a biennial, publically-available report of aggregate prevention, quality of care, risk factors, and outcomes data for diabetic patients.

VALUE

Payment Reform

- Establishes a pilot program to test value-based purchasing programs in long-term care hospitals, inpatient rehabilitation facilities, cancer hospitals, and hospice programs.
- Prohibits Medicaid from paying costs associated with health care-acquired conditions.

Medicare-Specific Initiatives

- Establishes a national pilot program to improve patient care and reduce Medicare costs by bundling payments for episodes of care.
- Promotes value-based purchasing in Medicare by paying hospitals based on their performance on quality measures for common and high-cost conditions, including acute myocardial infarction, heart failure, pneumonia, surgeries, and health care–associated infections. Value-based incentive payments begin for discharges on or after October 1, 2012.
- Extends the *Medicare Hospital Gainsharing Demonstration*, which evaluates arrangements between hospitals and providers aimed at improving utilization of inpatient hospital resources.
- Modifies the Medicare physician fee schedule to incorporate payments that vary based on the quality of care provided, as measured by quality of care measures established by the HHS Secretary. The HHS Secretary must publish the quality measures and announce the effective date of payment modification by January 1, 2012. The modifier will be applicable to specific physicians and physician groups, as determined by HHS, beginning January 1, 2015, and will apply to all physicians and physician groups starting January 1, 2017.
- Reduces Medicare payments to hospitals for hospital-acquired conditions and preventable readmissions; imposes monetary penalty on hospitals with the worst rates of hospital-acquired conditions.
- Establishes an *Independent Payment Advisory Board*, a Board of 15 members appointed by the President and confirmed by the Senate that will recommend to Congress ways to slow the rate of growth in national health expenditures while preserving quality of care. Beginning January 15, 2014, in years when the CMS Chief Actuary projects Medicare spending growth to exceed the target growth rate for the year, the Board must submit to Congress and the President a proposal to reduce Medicare spending. The Board's proposals will be binding unless Congress passes an alternative measure that achieves the same level of savings. In years when the Board is not required to submit a proposal, it must still submit an advisory report on the Medicare program. The Board must also produce an annual public report on systemwide health care costs, access to care, utilization, and quality, and an annual advisory report with recommendations to slow growth in health care costs while maintaining quality.

- Allows *accountable care organizations* (ACOs), groups of Medicare providers that voluntarily meet quality thresholds, to share in cost savings; establishes a demonstration project for pediatric ACOs.
- Creates an *Independence at Home* demonstration program to provide home primary care services for high-need Medicare patients and allow providers to share in cost savings.

State Initiatives

- Requires health plans to report their medical loss ratios and provide rebates to consumers if less than 85 percent of their premium (for large group market plans) and 80 percent (for individual and small group markets) is spent on clinical services and quality improvement. On November 22, 2010, HHS issued an interim final rule implementing the ACA's medical loss ratio requirements, based on recommendations from the National Association of Insurance Commissioners (NAIC).
- Requires HHS and state health insurance commissions to establish a process for reviewing health plan premium increases; requires plans to justify increases; requires states to report on trends in premium increases and recommend whether plans should be excluded from Exchanges due to unjustified increases. The ACA appropriates $250 million to the HHS Secretary for grants to states of $1 million to $5 million between 2010 and 2014.

Fraud Elimination

- Seeks to reduce fraud in federal programs through enhanced oversight and screening by the HHS Office of the Inspector General for providers and suppliers participating in Medicare and by states for providers and suppliers participating in Medicaid, including licensure checks, criminal background checks, fingerprinting, unannounced site visits, and database checks. Establishes enrollment moratoria for providers and suppliers in categories at elevated risk of fraud, and requires providers and suppliers to establish claim submission compliance programs. The ACA appropriates a total of $350 million in fiscal years 2011 through 2020 to the Health Care Fraud and Abuse Control Fund for these and other fraud-fighting measures.

PUBLIC HEALTH/WELLNESS

Leadership

- Establishes the *National Prevention, Health Promotion and Public Health Council* to coordinate federal public health activities, fund prevention and public health programs, and develop evidence-based recommendations on the use of clinical and community preventive services.
- Establishes an *Office of Women's Health* and an *Office of Minority Health*.
- Establishes a *Regular Corps* and a *Ready Reserve Corps* to serve in national emergencies.

Capacity

- Establishes a *Prevention and Public Health Fund* (PPHF) to invest in prevention and public health programs and slow the rate of growth in health care costs. The ACA appropriates $500 million to the PPHF in fiscal year 2010, $750 million in 2011, $1 billion in 2012, $1.25 billion in 2013, $1.5 billion in 2014, and $2 billion in 2015 and each fiscal year thereafter.
- Eliminates cost-sharing in Medicare and Medicaid for preventive services defined as effective by the Preventive Services Task Force.
- Provides access to annual wellness visits, comprehensive risk assessments, and personalized prevention plans for Medicare beneficiaries.
- Awards grants to states for programs that incentivize Medicaid beneficiary participation in tobacco cessation, weight control, and other health promotion programs to help prevent or manage chronic disease. The ACA appropriates $100 million for 5 years beginning in 2011.
- Creates a Medicaid demonstration program requiring states to reimburse qualified mental health care institutions for services to stabilize Medicaid beneficiaries experiencing an emergency psychiatric condition.
- Requires non-profit hospitals to conduct community needs assessments, taking into account input from the community served by the hospital, and adopt implementation strategies to meet identified needs.
- Promotes employer-based wellness programs through assessment, technical support on implementation, and grants to small employers.

- Increases funding for the *National Health Service Corps*, community health centers, school-based health centers, and nurse-managed clinics.
- Supports *Aging and Disability Resource Centers* aimed at streamlining access to long-term care for the elderly and people with physical, mental, or developmental disabilities.
- Creates an evidence-based national education campaign to increase awareness about breast cancer.

CROSS-CUTTING

Innovation

- Creates a new *Center for Medicare & Medicaid Innovation* (CMMI) within CMS to test and evaluate payment and service delivery models that reduce costs and maintain or improve quality of care. CMMI was formally established on November 16, 2010, with Richard Gilfillan, M.D., named as Acting Innovation Center Director. In Phase I of CMMI's operation, CMMI will test payment and service delivery models for their effect on public expenditures and quality of care. Models to be evaluated include

— Promoting patient-centered medical homes in primary care
— Contracting directly with providers, services, and suppliers
— Utilizing geriatric assessments and comprehensive care plans to coordinate care for patients with multiple chronic conditions
— Promoting care coordination between providers and suppliers to transition away from fee-for-service reimbursement and toward salary-based payment
— Supporting care coordination for chronically ill patients through the use of health IT-enabled provider networks, including care coordinators, a chronic disease registry, and home tele-health technology
— Varying payment to physicians ordering advanced diagnostic imaging services according to the appropriateness of the service ordered
— Utilizing medication therapy management services
— Establishing community-based health teams by assisting primary care providers in chronic care management
— Assisting patients in making informed health care choices by paying providers for using patient decision-support tools
— Allowing states to test and evaluate integration of care for dual eligibles

— Allowing states to test and evaluate systems of all-payer payment reform
— Aligning evidence-based guidelines of cancer care with payment incentives for treatment planning and follow-up care
— Improving post-acute care through continuing-care hospitals, long-term care hospitals, home health, and skilled nursing care
— Funding home health providers of chronic care management services
— Developing a collaborative of health care institutions responsible for developing, documenting, and disseminating best practices, implementing best practices within institutions to demonstrate improved quality and efficiency, and proving assistance to other health care institutions on how to employ best practices and proven care methods
— Facilitating inpatient care of hospitalized patients through use of electronic monitoring by specialists
— Promoting efficiency and access to outpatient services though models that do not require a provider's referral to the service
— Establishing payments to Healthcare Innovation Zones— teaching hospitals, groups of providers, and other clinical entities that, through their structure, deliver integrated and comprehensive health services while incorporating innovative methods for the clinical training of future health care professionals

In Phase II of CMMI's operation, the HHS Secretary may expand the duration and scope of a model being tested, if the model meets certain criteria. Successful models will be implemented in Medicare, Medicaid, and CHIP. Beginning in 2012, the HHS Secretary is required to report to Congress every other year on CMMI's activities. The ACA appropriates $5 million for CMMI's design, implementation, and evaluation of models during fiscal year 2010. The law also appropriates funding for CMMI indefinitely, with a $10 billion appropriation for fiscal years 2011 through 2019, and $10 billion more for each subsequent 10 fiscal year period.

• Provides an *Encouraging Investment in New Therapies* tax credit to encourage investments in new therapies to prevent and diagnose acute and chronic diseases. The tax credit, which covers 50 percent of an eligible taxpayer's investment on a therapeutic discovery project, is temporary for tax years 2009 and 2010 and is subject to a cap of $1 billion.
• Establishes the *Cures Acceleration Network* in the Office of the Director of NIH that will award grants and contracts to accelerate

the development of products and therapies to cure certain high-need conditions.

- Directs the HHS Assistant Secretary for Preparedness and Response (ASPR) to award grants to pilot projects that design, implement, and evaluate new models for emergency care. Funds emergency medicine research, pediatric emergency medicine research, and directs the HHS Secretary to award grants to states to improve trauma center capacity.

- Authorizes the HHS Patient Safety Research Center (PSRC) to award grants and contracts to implement collaborative medication management services, where pharmacists and other providers would formulate treatment plans, prevent adverse drug interactions, and educate patients and caregivers on the management of chronic diseases.

- Establishes a formal licensing process for approving biosimilar therapeutics, with data exclusivity periods established to encourage creation of new biologics.

- Awards 5-year demonstration grants to states to develop, evaluate, and implement alternatives to current medical malpractice litigation, with preference given to states that consult relevant stakeholders and propose alternatives likely to reduce medical errors and improve patient safety.

Transparency

- Creates *Physician Compare*, a Web-accessible database of performance, effectiveness, safety, and other assessments of providers who participate in the *Medicare Physician Quality Reporting Initiative*.

- Requires disclosure of financial relationships between hospitals, providers, and manufacturers and distributors of drugs and devices.

- Requires Medicare and Medicaid nursing facilities to disclose ownership, expenditure, and certification information; creates a website allowing beneficiaries to compare facilities.

- Increases disclosure requirements for providers and suppliers enrolling in federal health programs.

- Requires states to keep accountings of state health insurance exchange expenditures, and authorizes audits by the HHS Secretary and Inspector General to prevent and detect fraud.

Data Resources

- Requires enhanced collection and reporting of data on race, ethnicity, sex, primary language, and disability status in all federally conducted or supported health care or public health programs. Such data will be used for statistical analysis, including analysis of geographic health disparities.
- Creates a database to share fraud data across federal and state health programs.

Information Technology

American Recovery and Reinvestment Act reforms:

- Formally establishes the *Office of the National Coordinator for Health Information Technology* to oversee development of a national health information network.
- Strengthens health information privacy and security standards.
- Authorizes grants to assist state and local governments and health care providers in adopting and using health IT.
- Provides financial incentives under Medicare and Medicaid to encourage hospitals, physicians, and health professionals to become meaningful users of health IT by using certified electronic health record technology in ways that allow the electronic exchange of information to improve health care quality.
- Encourages state Medicaid agencies to adopt a meaningful use incentive program similar to the federal program.

Workforce

- Establishes a *National Health Care Workforce Commission* of 15 members, appointed by the U.S. Government Accountability Office, to develop a national workforce strategy. The Commission will serve as a resource for Congress and the President, communicate and coordinate with the Departments of Health and Human Services, Labor, Veterans Affairs, Homeland Security, and Education, evaluate education and training activities in relation to demand, identify barriers to improved coordination between federal, state, and local levels, and encourage innovations to address population needs, changes in technology, and other environmental factors.
- Increases the nurse workforce though training programs, loan repayment, and retention grants.

- Redistributes unused Graduate Medical Education training positions toward primary care, general surgery, and medically underserved geographic areas.
- Provides bonus payments and grants for recruitment and training of providers to serve in rural and underserved areas.
- Supports development of training programs focused on prevention, public health, primary care, medical homes, team management of disease, and integration of mental and physical health services.

Appendix D

Biosketches of Committee Members and Staff

Mark D. Smith, M.D., M.B.A. (*Chair*) is president and CEO of the California HealthCare Foundation. The Foundation is an independent philanthropy, headquartered in Oakland, California, dedicated to improving the health of the people of California through its three program areas: Innovations for the Underserved, Better Chronic Disease Care, and Market and Policy Monitor. A board-certified internist, Dr. Smith is a member of the clinical faculty at the University of California, San Francisco, and an attending physician at the Positive Health Program for AIDS care at San Francisco General Hospital. He is a member of the Institute of Medicine (IOM) and serves on the board of the National Business Group on Health. Prior to joining the California HealthCare Foundation, Dr. Smith was executive vice president of the Henry J. Kaiser Family Foundation and previously served as associate director of the AIDS Service and assistant professor of medicine and of health policy and management at Johns Hopkins University. He has served on the Performance Measurement Committee of the National Committee for Quality Assurance and the editorial board of the *Annals of Internal Medicine*. Dr. Smith received a B.A. in Afro-American Studies from Harvard College, an M.D. from the School of Medicine at the University of North Carolina at Chapel Hill, and an M.B.A. with a concentration in health care administration from the Wharton School at the University of Pennsylvania.

James P. Bagian, M.D., P.E., is a professor of engineering and director of the Center for Health Engineering and Patient Safety at the University of Michigan. Previously, he served as the first director of the Department

401

of Veterans Affairs' (VA's) National Center for Patient Safety (NCPS) and as the VA's first chief patient safety officer from 1999 to 2010. As NCPS director, he was responsible for the development and implementation of techniques designed to reduce avoidable injuries and deaths among patients throughout the VA's 154 medical centers and associated clinics and long-term care facilities. From 1980 to 1995, Dr. Bagian served as a NASA astronaut; he is a veteran of two space flights (STS-29 in 1989 and STS-40 in 1991). He took part in both the planning and provision of emergency medical and rescue support for the first six space shuttle flights. In 1986, Dr. Bagian served as an investigator for the Space Shuttle Challenger accident and as the astronaut on-scene adviser for the salvage operations of the Space Shuttle Challenger crew module; he was the individual who dove and made the positive identification of the Challenger crew module debris on the ocean floor. Subsequently, he was responsible for the development and implementation of the pressure suit used for crew escape and other crew survival and escape equipment used on Shuttle missions. He was also selected in 2003 to be chief flight surgeon and medical advisor for the Space Shuttle Columbia Accident Investigation Board. Dr. Bagian is an adjunct assistant professor of military and emergency medicine at the Uniformed Services University of Health Sciences at F. Edward Hebert School of Medicine and a clinical associate professor of preventive medicine and community health at the University of Texas Medical Branch. In addition, he is a colonel in the U.S. Air Force Reserve and serves on the Trauma and Injury Subcommittee of the Defense Health Board for the Department of Defense. He received a B.S. degree in mechanical engineering from Drexel University and his M.D. degree from Thomas Jefferson University. He is a diplomate of the American Board of Preventive Medicine, with a subspecialty in aerospace medicine. Dr. Bagian was elected to the National Academy of Engineering in 2000 and to the IOM in 2003.

Anthony S. Bryk, Ed.D., is the ninth president of The Carnegie Foundation for the Advancement of Teaching. He held the Spencer Chair in Organizational Studies in the School of Education and the Graduate School of Business at Stanford University from 2004 until assuming Carnegie's presidency in September 2008. Previously, he held the Marshall Field IV Professor of Education post in the sociology department at the University of Chicago. There he founded the Center for Urban School Improvement, which supports reform efforts in the Chicago Public Schools. Dr. Bryk also founded the Consortium on Chicago School Research, which has produced a range of studies to advance and assess urban school reform. In addition, he has made contributions to the development of new statistical methods in educational research. At Carnegie, he is leading work on strengthening the research and development infrastructure for improving teaching and learning. Dr. Bryk holds a B.S. from Boston College and an Ed.D. from Harvard University, and was recently honored by Boston College with an honorary doctorate for his contributions to education reform.

Gail H. Cassell, Ph.D., retired as vice president, Scientific Affairs and Distinguished Lilly Research Scholar for Infectious Diseases, Eli Lilly and Company, in October 2010. She is former Charles H. McCauley professor and chair of the Department of Microbiology at the University of Alabama Schools of Medicine and Dentistry at Birmingham, a department that ranked first in research funding from the National Institutes of Health (NIH) during the decade of her leadership. She obtained her bachelor's degree from the University of Alabama in Tuscaloosa and in 1993 was selected as one of the top 31 female graduates of the twentieth century. Dr. Cassell obtained her doctorate in microbiology from the University of Alabama at Birmingham and was selected as its 2003 distinguished alumnus. She is a past president of the American Society for Microbiology and was a member of the NIH director's advisory committee and of the advisory council of the National Institute of Allergy and Infectious Diseases. She was named to the original Board of Scientific Councilors of the Center for Infectious Diseases, Centers for Disease Control, and served as chair of the board and a member of the advisory board of the director of the Centers for Disease Control and Prevention. After the terrorist attacks of 2001, she was appointed to the Secretary of Health and Human Services Advisory Council on Public Health Preparedness. As a member of the Science Board of the federal Food and Drug Administration, Advisory Committee to the Commissioner, she received a Commissioner's Citation Award for authoring the 2007 report *FDA: Science and Mission at Risk*. Since 1996, she has been a member of the U.S.-Japan Cooperative Medical Science Program, responsible for advising the respective governments on joint research agendas. Dr. Cassell has served on several editorial boards of scientific journals and has authored more than 250 articles and book chapters. She has received national and international awards and an honorary degree for her research in infectious diseases. She is a member of the IOM and is currently serving a second term on the IOM Council. Dr. Cassell has been intimately involved in the establishment of science policy and legislation related to biomedical research and public health. For 9 years she was chair of the Public and Scientific Affairs Board of the American Society for Microbiology. She has served as an adviser on infectious diseases and indirect costs of research to the White House Office of Science and Technology Policy, and she has been an invited participant in numerous congressional hearings and briefings related to infectious diseases, antimicrobial resistance, and biomedical research. She has served two terms on the Liaison Committee on Medical Education, the accrediting body for U.S. medical schools, as well as other national committees involved in establishing policies on training in the biomedical sciences. She is a past member of the board of directors of the Burroughs Wellcome Fund, Research!America, the leadership council of the School of Public Health of Harvard University, and the Advisory Council of the School of Nursing of Johns Hopkins. She is currently a member of the NIH Science Management Review Board and a member of the advisory council of NIH's Fogarty International Center, the executive committee of the Visiting Board of the School of Medicine of Columbia University, the board of advisors of the School of Public Health of the University of North Carolina at Chapel Hill, and the board of trustees of Moorehouse School of Medicine.

James B. Conway, M.S., is an adjunct lecturer at the Harvard School of Public Health, principal of the Governance and Leadership Group of Pascal Metrics in Washington, DC, and a senior fellow at the Institute for Healthcare Improvement (IHI). From 2006 to 2009, he was senior president of IHI, and from 2005-2006, he was senior fellow. During 1995-2005, Mr. Conway was executive vice president and chief operating officer of Dana-Farber Cancer Institute (DFCI) in Boston. Prior to joining DFCI, he had a 27-year career at Children's Hospital, Boston, in radiology administration and finance and as assistant hospital director. His areas of expertise and interest include governance and executive leadership, patient safety, change management, and patient-/family-centered care. He holds an M.S. degree from Lesley College, Cambridge, Massachusetts. Mr. Conway has received numerous awards, including the 1999 Association for Continuing Higher Education Massachusetts Regents Award and the 2001 first Individual Leadership Award in Patient Safety from the Joint Commission on Accreditation of Healthcare Organizations and the National Committee for Quality Assurance. In 2008, he received the Picker Award for Excellence in the Advancement of Patient Centered Care and in 2009 the Mary Davis Barber Heart of Hospice Award from the Massachusetts Hospice and Palliative Care Federation. A fellow of the American College of Healthcare Executives, Mr. Conway is a member of the Clinical Issues Advisory Council of the Massachusetts Hospital Association and is a distinguished advisor to the Lucian Leape Institute for the National Patient Safety Foundation. He has served as board chair, The Partnership for Healthcare Excellence; board member, Winchester Hospital; board member, the American Cancer Society, New England Region; and board member, Medically Induced Trauma Support Services. He also served as a member of the Commonwealth of Massachusetts Quality and Cost Council, 2006-2010.

Helen B. Darling, M.A., is president and CEO of the National Business Group on Health, a nonprofit membership organization devoted exclusively to providing solutions to its employer-members' most important health care problems and representing large employers on health policy issues. The organization's 303 members, including 64 of the Fortune 100 companies in 2010, purchase health benefits for more than 50 million employees, retirees, and dependents. Dr. Darling received WorldatWork's prestigious Keystone Award for sustained contributions to the field of human resources in 2009 and the President's Award from the American College of Occupational and Environmental Medicine in 2010. She serves on the Committee on Performance Measurement (National Committee for Quality Assurance) (co-chair for 10 years); the Medical Advisory Panel, Technology Evaluation Center (Blue Cross Blue Shield Association); the Medicare Coverage Advisory Committee; and the boards of the National Quality Forum and the Reagan-Udall Foundation. Previously, she directed the purchasing of health and disability benefits at Xerox Corporation. Ms. Darling was health advisor to Senator David Durenberger on the Senate Finance Committee. She directed three studies at the IOM. She received a master's degree in demography/sociology and a B.S. degree in history/english, cum laude, from the University of Memphis.

T. Bruce Ferguson, Jr., M.D., is professor and inaugural chairman of the Department of Cardiovascular Sciences at the East Carolina Heart Institute and the Brody School of Medicine at East Carolina University (ECU). He is a board-certified cardiothoracic surgeon who specializes in adult cardiothoracic surgery. He came to North Carolina from Louisiana, where he was chief of cardiac surgery at Louisiana State University (LSU) Health Sciences Center in New Orleans prior to Hurricane Katrina. While in Louisiana, he received funding from the Agency for Healthcare Research and Quality's (AHRQ's) Transforming Healthcare Quality through Information Technology program to begin development of a longitudinal cardiovascular information system for the statewide Charity Hospital System population. He served for 6 years as inaugural chair of The Society of Thoracic Surgeons' (STS') Council on Quality, Research, and Patient Safety, which oversees all aspects of the Society's national database efforts, in collaboration with the Duke Clinical Research Institute. He was principal investigator for the Society's two clinical trials in quality improvement from 1999 through 2007, funded by AHRQ. Dr. Ferguson is currently co-principal investigator for the combined Duke-ECU clinical site for the National Heart, Lung, and Blood Institute Cardiac Surgical Network and is principal investigator for the Clinical Research Skills Development Core. He is a fellow of the American Heart Association; a member of the Informatics Committee and the Surgical Council for the American College of Cardiology; and chair of the STS Workforce on Health Policy, Reform and Advocacy. He received his degree in chemistry from Williams College and his M.D. from Washington

University in St. Louis. He completed his training in general surgery and cardiothoracic surgery at Duke University Medical Center.

Ginger L. Graham, M.B.A., is a senior lecturer at Harvard Business School, president and CEO of Two Trees Consulting, and a public speaker and health care consultant. She is the former president and CEO of Amylin Pharmaceuticals, a biopharmaceutical company based in San Diego, California, focused on diabetes and obesity. During Ms. Graham's tenure at Amylin, the company launched two first-in-class medicines for people with diabetes, was listed on the Nasdaq 100, and was rated as one of the top 10 places in the industry for scientists to work. Prior to her time at Amylin, she was group chairman, Office of the President, for Guidant Corporation, a major cardiovascular medical device manufacturer based in Indianapolis. During her tenure at Guidant, the company launched the world's leading stent platform, was listed as a Fortune 500 company, was recognized by *Fortune* magazine as one of the best companies to work for in America, and was included among *Industry Week* magazine's 100 best managed companies in the world. Ms. Graham has received numerous awards and honors, including being named as Emerging Company Executive of the Year by the Global Health Council in 2005, a finalist for Marketwatch's CEO of the Year in 2006, and the American Diabetes Association's Woman of Valor award in 2006. She was included on Pharma VOICE's "100 of the Most Inspiring People" list in 2006, and *World Pharmaceuticals* magazine named her number 10 on a list of the 40 most influential people in the industry in 2007. Ms. Graham serves on the boards of directors for Walgreen Co.; Genomic Health, Inc.; Proteus Biomedical Pharmaceutical Systems Division; ICAT Managers; Praline Holdings, Ltd.; and the American Diabetes Association Research Foundation, where she serves as vice chair. She is a member of the Harvard Business School Health Industry Alumni Advisory Board, the University of Arkansas chancellor's board of advisors, and the University of Colorado Initiative for Molecular Biotechnology. She also serves on the advisory boards for the Kellogg Center for Executive Women and the Women Business Leaders of the US Health Care Industry Foundation. She serves as well on the editorial advisory board for the *Journal of Life Sciences*, frequently speaks at business schools, and has written for *Harvard Business Review*. She received a B.S. in agricultural economics from the University of Arkansas and holds an M.B.A. from Harvard University.

George C. Halvorson, is chairman and CEO of Kaiser Permanente, headquartered in Oakland, California. Kaiser Permanente is the nation's largest nonprofit health plan and hospital system, serving about 8.6 million members and generating $42 billion in annual revenue. It has been investing heavily in electronic medical records and physician support systems over the past 5 years. Kaiser Permanente also is a leader in electronic connectivity between doctors and patients, with patients choosing more than 6 million "e-visits" this year instead of face-to-face clinical visits. Mr. Halvorson serves on the IOM's Roundtable on Value & Science-Driven Health Care, the American Hospital Association's Advisory Committee on Health Reform, and the Commonwealth Fund Commission on a High Performance Health System. He also serves on the boards of America's Health Insurance Plans and the Alliance of Community Health Plans. He chairs the International Federation of Health Plans and co-chairs IHI's Annual National Forum on Quality Improvement in Health Care. In 2009, he chaired the World Economic Forum's Health Governors meetings in Davos. Mr. Halvorson has received the Modern Healthcare/Health Information and Management Systems Society CEO IT Achievement Award, and the Workgroup for Electronic Data Interchange awarded him the 2009 Louis Sullivan Award for leadership and achievements in advancing health care quality. He has written several books on health care reform, including the recently released *Health Care Will Not Reform Itself: A User's Guide to Refocusing and Reforming American Health Care*. He also wrote *Health Care Reform Now!*, *Health Care Co-ops in Uganda*, *Strong Medicine*, and *Epidemic of Care* as guidebooks for health care reform. Mr. Halvorson has served as an advisor to the governments of Uganda, Great Britain, Jamaica, and Russia on issues of health policy and financing. His strong commitment to diversity and interethnic healing has led him to his current writing project, a book about racial prejudice around the world. Prior to joining Kaiser Permanente, Mr. Halvorson was president and CEO of HealthPartners, headquartered in Minneapolis. With more than 30 years of health care management experience, he has also held several senior management positions with Blue Cross and Blue Shield of Minnesota.

Brent C. James, M.D., M.Stat., is chief quality officer and executive director of the Institute for Health Care Delivery Research at Intermountain Healthcare in Salt Lake City. For more than 20 years, Dr. James has championed the standardization of clinical care through data collection and analysis on a wide variety of treatment protocols and complex care processes. In the tradition of medical pioneers such as Florence Nightingale, Abraham Flexner, and William Osler, he has devoted himself to using quality improvement tools to better understand the cause-and-effect relationships among various practice and environmental factors. In addition to his duties at Intermountain Health Care, Dr. James is adjunct professor at the University of Utah School of Medicine, Department of Family and Preventive Medicine. He also holds a visiting lectureship in the Department of Health Policy and Management at the Harvard School of Public Health. In

addition, he has served with a number of national task forces and committees that examine health care quality and cost control, as well as AHRQ,
and was recently appointed by the federal comptroller to an advisory group
on making American health care more accessible and affordable. Dr. James
has received numerous national awards recognizing his vision and energy
in making the U.S. health care system better.

Craig A. Jones, M.D., is director of the Vermont Blueprint for Health, a
program established by the State of Vermont under the leadership of its
governor, legislature, and bipartisan Health Care Reform Commission. The
Blueprint was developed to guide a statewide transformation resulting in
seamless and well-coordinated health services for all citizens, with an emphasis on prevention. It is intended to improve health care for individuals,
improve the health of the population, and result in more affordable health
care. Previously, Dr. Jones was an assistant professor in the Department
of Pediatrics at the Keck School of Medicine, University of Southern California, and director of the Division of Allergy/Immunology and director
of the Allergy/Immunology Residency Training Program in the Department of Pediatrics at the Los Angeles County + University of Southern
California (LAC+USC) Medical Center. He was director, in charge of the
design, implementation, and management, of the Breathmobile Program,
a program using mobile clinics, team-based care, and health information
technology to deliver ongoing preventive care to inner-city children with
asthma at their schools and at county clinics. The program evolved from
community outreach to provide more fully integrated pediatric asthma
disease management for the Los Angeles County Department of Health
Services and has spread to several other communities across the country.
Dr. Jones has published papers, abstracts, and textbook chapters on topics
related to health services, health outcomes, and allergy and immunology in
*Pediatric Research, Pediatrics, Journal of Pediatrics, Pediatrics in Review,
Journal of Clinical Immunology, Journal of Allergy and Clinical Immunol-
ogy, Annals of Allergy, Asthma and Immunology, CHEST,* and *Disease
Management.* He served as executive committee and board member for
the Southern California Chapter of the Asthma and Allergy Foundation of
America, as well chapter president. He is a past president of the Los Angeles
Society of Allergy, Asthma and Clinical Immunology, and a past president
and a member of the board of directors for the California Society of Allergy
Asthma, and Immunology. Dr. Jones received his undergraduate degree at
the University of California, San Diego, and his M.D. degree from the University of Texas Health Science Center in San Antonio. He completed his
internship and residency in pediatrics at LAC+USC Medical Center, where
he also completed his fellowship in allergy and clinical immunology.

Gary S. Kaplan, M.D., has served as chairman and CEO of the Virginia Mason Health System since 2000. He received his medical degree from the University of Michigan and is board certified in internal medicine. Since Dr. Kaplan became chairman and CEO, Virginia Mason has received significant national and international recognition, including being recognized as one of 37 hospitals and 8 children's hospitals designated as top hospitals in the nation by the Leapfrog Group for the fourth consecutive year. Virginia Mason is also a national leader in deploying the Virginia Mason Production System—reducing the high costs of health care while improving quality, safety, and efficiency. In addition to his patient-care duties and position as CEO, Dr. Kaplan is a clinical professor at the University of Washington. He has been recognized for his service and contribution to many regional and national boards. He currently serves on the boards of IHI, the American Medical Group Association, the Medical Group Management Association, the Washington Healthcare Forum, the Special Olympics, and the Greater Seattle Chamber of Commerce. He also is current chair of the National Patient Safety Foundation Board. In 2007, Dr. Kaplan was designated a fellow in the American College of Physician Executives. He was recently named one of the 50 most powerful physician executives in health care by *Modern Healthcare* and *Modern Physician* magazines. In 2009, he was named the 16th most influential U.S. physician leader in health care by *Modern Healthcare* magazine. In 2009, Dr. Kaplan received the John M. Eisenberg Award from the National Quality Forum and the Joint Commission for Individual Achievement at the national level for his outstanding work and commitment to patient safety and quality. Additionally, he was recognized by the Medical Group Management Association and the American College of Medical Practice Executives as the recipient of the Harry J. Harwick Lifetime Achievement Award, which recognizes outstanding national contributions to health care administration, delivery, and education while advancing the field of medical practice management.

Arthur A. Levin, M.P.H., is director of the Center for Medical Consumers. He served as the consumer representative on the U.S. Food and Drug Administration (FDA) Drug Safety and Risk Management Advisory Committee from its establishment in 2003 through May 2007. He continues to participate as a consumer expert on FDA advisory panels by invitation. Mr. Levin is the only consumer member of the New York State Department of Health Healthcare Acquired Infection Reporting Workgroup and co-wrote the original legislation that mandated public reporting of hospital-acquired infections in the state. From 1998 to 2000, he served on the IOM's Committee on the Quality of Health Care in America. That committee issued the landmark report *To Err Is Human*, which garnered international attention for its depiction of medical errors as a leading cause of preventable death and injury in the United States, as well as *Crossing the Quality Chasm*, which set goals for reforming the nation's health care system. Mr. Levin subsequently served on IOM committees that assessed federal government efforts to improve patient safety in the health systems it manages, reported on the performance of the Office of the National Coordinator for Health Information Technology, and recommended national standards for systematic evidence reviews and clinical guidelines. In 2009, he was a member of the IOM committee advising the Secretary of Health and Human Services on how to allocate $400 million in stimulus money targeted for comparative effectiveness research. Mr. Levin serves as chair of the National Quality Forum's Consensus Standards Approval Committee and co-chair of the National Committee for Quality Assurance's Committee on Performance Measurement. He is a board member of the IOM, Board on Health Care Services; the Foundation for Informed Medical Decision Making; the Citizens Advocacy Center; THINC, a regional health information project in the mid-Hudson Valley; and the New York eHealth Collaborative. He is also the consumer representative on the steering committee of the Centers for Education and Research on Therapeutics.

Eugene Litvak, Ph.D., is president and CEO of the Institute for Healthcare Optimization. He is also an adjunct professor in operations management in the Department of Health Policy & Management at the Harvard School of Public Health, where he teaches the course "Operations Management in Service Delivery Organizations." Previously, he was co-founder (with Michael C. Long, M.D.) and director of the Program for the Management of Variability in Health Care Delivery at the Boston University (BU) Health Policy Institute and a professor at the BU School of Management. Before joining BU, Dr. Litvak was a faculty member at the Harvard Center for Risk Analysis. His research interests include operations management in health care delivery organizations and operations research. He is the author of more than 60 publications in these areas. Since 1995 he has led the development and practical application of the innovative variability methodology (which he introduced together with Dr. Long) for cost reduction and quality improvement in health care delivery systems. This methodology has resulted in significant quality improvement and multimillion dollar improvements in the margins for every hospital that has applied it. Dr. Litvak was a member of the IOM Committee on the Future of Emergency Care in the United States Health System. He is a member of the National Advisory Committee to the American Hospital Association for Improving Quality, Patient Safety and Performance and is principal investigator for many hospital operations improvement projects. Dr. Litvak frequently presents as an invited lecturer at national and international meetings. He also serves as a consultant on operations improvement to several major hospitals.

David O. Meltzer, M.D., Ph.D., is an associate professor in the Department of Medicine and an associated faculty member in the Harris School and the Department of Economics at the University of Chicago. His research explores problems in health economics and public policy, with a focus on the theoretical foundations of medical cost-effectiveness analysis and the determinants of the cost and quality of care, especially in teaching hospitals. Dr. Meltzer has conducted several studies comparing the use of doctors who specialize in inpatient care ("hospitalists") with the use of traditional physicians in academic medical centers and exploring the economic forces that have led to the growing use of hospitalists in the United States. His work in cost-effectiveness analysis has included the use of value-of-information analysis to inform research priorities and studies of the value of individualized care. Dr. Meltzer received his M.D. and Ph.D. in economics from the University of Chicago and completed his residency in internal medicine at Brigham and Women's Hospital in Boston. He is chief of the section of Hospital Medicine, director of the Center for Health and the Social Sciences, and chair of the Committee on Clinical and Translational Science at the University of Chicago, where he also directs the M.D./Ph.D. program in the social sciences. He is the recipient of numerous awards, including the NIH Medical Scientist Training Program Fellowship, the National Science Foundation Graduate Fellowship in Economics, the University of Chicago Searle Fellowship, the Lee Lusted Prize of the Society for Medical Decision Making, the Health Care Research Award of the National Institute for Health Care Management, the Eugene Garfield Award from Research America, and the Robert Wood Johnson Generalist Physician Award. Dr. Meltzer is a research associate of the National Bureau of Economic Research, elected member of the American Society for Clinical Investigation, and past president of the Society for Medical Decision Making. He has served on panels examining the future of Medicare for the National Academy of Social Insurance and the Department of Health and Human Services (HHS), and U.S. organ allocation policy for the IOM. He recently served on an IOM panel examining the effectiveness of the U.S. drug safety system and currently serves on the HHS Secretary's Advisory Committee on Healthy People 2020, which aims to establish health objectives for the U.S. population.

Mary D. Naylor, Ph.D., RN, is Marian S. Ware professor in gerontology and director of the NewCourtland Center for Transitions and Health at the University of Pennsylvania School of Nursing. Since 1990, she has led a multidisciplinary program of research designed to improve health and quality-of-life outcomes, decrease unnecessary hospitalizations, and reduce health care costs among chronically ill older adults. Dr. Naylor also is national program director for the Robert Wood Johnson Foundation program

Interdisciplinary Nursing Quality Research Initiative. She was elected to the IOM in 2005. She also is a member of the RAND Health Advisory Board and the National Quality Forum's board of directors and chairs the board of the Long Term Quality Alliance. In 2010, Dr. Naylor was appointed to the Medicare Payment Advisory Commission.

Rita F. Redberg, M.D., M.Sc., has been professor of medicine and director of women's cardiovascular services in the division of cardiology at the University of California, San Francisco (UCSF) Medical Center since 1990. She is chief editor of the *Archives of Internal Medicine* and recently added the *Less is More* series to this journal to explore how more health care is not always better. Dr. Redberg earned her B.A. degree from Cornell University and her M.D. degree from University of Pennsylvania Medical School. She was awarded a Thouron Fellowship, which allowed her to complete an M.S. degree in health policy and administration from the London School of Economics in 1980. After completing her medical residency and cardiology fellowship at Columbia-Presbyterian Hospital, Dr. Redberg joined the faculty at Mount Sinai Medical Center in New York before moving to UCSF. She helped develop and was co-director of UCSF's National Center of Excellence in Women's Health, a designation awarded by the Office of Women's Health in 1997. She has been the director of a successful annual American College of Cardiology (ACC) Extramural Program on Heart Disease in Women since 1997, and she started a national committee on Women in Cardiology for the American Heart Association (AHA) in 1994. Dr. Redberg has had a long-standing passion for politics and health policy and was a Robert Wood Johnson Health Policy Fellow. She serves on the California Technology Assessment Forum, is a member of the FDA Cardiovascular Device Expert Panel and the American College of Cardiology Quality Committee, and chaired the AHA Communications Committee. She also chaired the ACC/AHA Writing Committee on Performance Measures for Primary Prevention of Cardiovascular Disease. Dr. Redberg is a champion for physical activity and healthy eating and chairs the AHA's Scientific Advisory Board for the Choose To Move program. Her main research interests have been the evidence base for new medical technology and how it relates to FDA approval and coverage by the Centers for Medicare & Medicaid Services. She lectures nationally in the areas of diagnostic testing and screening for coronary artery disease, technology assessment, and preventive cardiology.

Paul C. Tang, M.D., M.S., is an internist; vice president, chief innovation and technology officer at the Palo Alto Medical Foundation (PAMF); and consulting associate professor of medicine (biomedical informatics) at Stanford University. Dr. Tang is vice chair of the federal Health Information

Technology Policy Committee and chair of its Meaningful Use Work Group. Established under the 2009 American Recovery and Reinvestment Act (ARRA), the group advises the Department of Health and Human Services on policies related to health information technology. An elected member of the IOM, Dr. Tang chaired an IOM committee on patient safety that published reports in 2003-2004: *Patient Safety: A New Standard for Care* and *Key Capabilities of an Electronic Health Record System*. He is also a member of the IOM Board on Health Care Services. He chairs the National Quality Forum's Health Information Technology Advisory Committee and is a member of the Forum's Consensus Standards Approval Committee. Dr. Tang is a past chair of the board for the American Medical Informatics Association. He is a member of the National Committee on Vital and Health Statistics (NCVHS) and co-chair of the NCVHS Quality Subcommittee. He co-chairs the Measurement Implementation Strategy work group of the Quality Alliance Steering Committee and chairs the Robert Wood Johnson Foundation's National Advisory Council for ProjectHealth Design. He has published numerous papers in medical informatics, especially related to electronic health records, personal health records, and quality, and has delivered more than 280 invited presentations to national and international organizations and associations. Dr. Tang is a fellow of the American College of Medical Informatics, the American College of Physicians, the College of Healthcare Information Management Executives, and the Healthcare Information and Management Systems Society.

STUDY STAFF

Robert Saunders, Ph.D., program officer and study director, received a B.S. in physics from the College of William and Mary in 2000 and a Ph.D. in physics from Duke University in 2006. His graduate research focused on quality measures of medical imaging systems, specifically evaluating breast imaging systems for their performance in breast cancer detection. After his graduate work, Dr. Saunders continued his research as a postdoctoral fellow in the Duke University Medical Center Department of Radiology, where he also taught public speaking courses in the medical physics department. In 2008, he was selected as Guenther Congressional Science Fellow, serving in the office of Rep. Rush Holt (New Jersey). Upon completing his fellowship, he was hired as a legislative assistant for Rep. Holt, dealing with health care reform, Medicare and Medicaid, small business, the Congressional Biomedical Research Caucus, and budget policy. In addition to these activities, he has served on the board of trustees of Duke University and is a current member of the William and Mary Graduate Studies Advisory Board.

Leigh Stuckhardt, J.D., program associate, received a B.S. in biological sciences with an additional major in philosophy from Carnegie Mellon University in 2007. In 2010, she received her J.D. with a concentration in health care law from the University of Pittsburgh School of Law, where her research focused on bioethics and issues of access to care, including a critique of the legal framework for the resolution of custody disputes over frozen embryos and analysis of the accessibility of mental health care following the passage of mental health parity and health care reform legislation. During law school, Ms. Stuckhardt also explored public health, health care law, and public policy issues firsthand through internships at the University of Pittsburgh Medical Center and the Veterans Health Administration National Center for Ethics in Health Care and in the office of Rep. Anthony Weiner (New York).

Julia Sanders, senior program assistant, graduated from Brown University in December 2010 with an Sc.B. in human biology. Her studies focused on human health and disease, culminating in a senior research project dedicated to ameliorating the current HIV/AIDS epidemic among Philadelphia's African American population. Ms. Sanders supplemented her academic pursuits with an internship at the Rhode Island Health Center Association, where she researched, organized, and catalogued pending legislation related to health center operations and surveyed Rhode Island's health centers regarding available behavioral health services. In fall 2008, she took a leave of absence from Brown to work as a field organizer on President Obama's campaign for office, later serving as a White House Intern for the Obama Administration in summer 2009.

Brian W. Powers, senior program assistant, received a B.A. in history from Bowdoin College (magna cum laude), where he also concentrated in biology and chemistry. Within the field of U.S. history, Mr. Powers focused on Civil War–era African American history, undertaking a project on the Reconstruction era Ku Klux Klan as well as an honors thesis on the professional experience of early black physicians. Mr. Powers' work in history was supplemented by a sustained engagement in the natural sciences; he spent time in both chemistry and biology laboratories examining the effects of various neurotransmitters on cardiac function in the American lobster. Outside of the classroom, he performed outcomes research on colorectal cancer treatment during an internship at the Washington University School of Medicine and expanded his knowledge of the health care delivery system during time at Piedmont Health Services, a Community Health Center in Carrboro, North Carolina.

Valerie Rohrbach, senior program assistant, graduated from the Pennsylvania State University in December 2009 as a Schreyer Honors Scholar with a bachelor's degree in international politics. Her honors thesis examined the various methods by which countries address the human rights violations of their past. While working on her thesis, she interned at the Center for Strategic and International Studies and the Woodrow Wilson Center in Washington, DC. From January to August 2010, she interned with Congressman Patrick Murphy (Pennsylvania) and became well versed in the Patient Protection and Affordable Care Act of 2010, recent reforms to Medicare, and other topics pertaining to national health policy. She then worked on the re-election campaign of Congressman Murphy as a field organizer.

Claudia Grossmann, Ph.D., senior program officer, received a B.A. in biology with concentrations in molecular biology and microbiology from Washington University in St. Louis in 2000 and a Ph.D. in biomedical sciences from the University of California, San Francisco (UCSF) in 2007. At UCSF, her dissertation focused on the exploitation of the innate immune system by the Kaposi's Sarcoma Associated Herpesvirus, a human virus that causes Kaposi's sarcoma as well as other rare neoplastic, inflammatory diseases. During her graduate studies, Dr. Grossmann spent the summer of 2005 as a science and technology policy fellow at the National Academies, where she worked on the first congressionally mandated evaluation of the President's Emergency Program for AIDS Relief (PEPFAR). Before joining the Roundtable on Value & Science-Driven Health Care, she served as program evaluator, directing evaluation and strategic planning efforts at the California Breast Cancer Research Program, the largest state-funded research effort in the nation. She remains committed to working toward the improvement of human health through the real-world application of research.

Isabelle Von Kohorn, M.D., Ph.D., program officer, received an A.B. from the Woodrow Wilson School of Public and International Affairs at Princeton University in 1998 and her M.D. from the University of Pennsylvania in 2003. She completed her residency and chief residency in pediatrics at UCSF, where she received the UCSF Medical Center Exceptional Physician Award in 2007. She then moved to Yale University, where she finished her fellowship in neonatology in 2010 and received her Ph.D. in investigative medicine in 2011. Dr. Von Kohorn has used qualitative and epidemiologic research methods in her work. Her dissertation research focused on helping mothers who quit smoking avoid relapse after pregnancy. In her approach to health care and policy, she is committed to the fundamental right of every human being to enjoy the highest attainable standard of health.

J. Michael McGinnis, M.D., M.P.P., executive director, is a physician and epidemiologist who lives and works in Washington, DC. Through his writing, government service, and work in philanthropy, he has been a long-time contributor to field leadership in health and medicine. Currently senior scholar and executive director of the IOM's Roundtable on Value & Science-Driven Health Care, he previously served as founding director of the Robert Wood Johnson Foundation's (RWJF's) Health Group, the World Health Organization's Office for Health Reconstruction in Bosnia, the federal Office of Research Integrity, and the federal Office of Disease Prevention and Health Promotion. In a tenure unusual for political and policy posts, Dr. McGinnis held continuous appointment through the Carter, Reagan, Bush, and Clinton Administrations at HHS, with policy responsibilities for disease prevention and health promotion (1977-1995). Programs and policies conceived and launched at his initiative include the Healthy People process for setting national health goals and objectives (1979-present), the U.S. Preventive Services Task Force (1984-present), the Dietary Guidelines for Americans (with the U.S. Department of Agriculture, 1980-present), the multilevel Public Health Functions Steering Group and the Ten Essential Services of Public Health (1994-present), the RWJF Active Living family of programs (2000-present), the RWJF Young Epidemiology Scholars Program (2001-present), the RWJF Health and Society Scholars Program (2002-present), and the current Learning Health System initiative of the IOM. Internationally, he served in Bosnia (1995-1996) as chair of the joint World Bank/European Commission Task Force on Reconstruction of the Health and Human Services Sector and in India (1974-1975) as epidemiologist and state director for the World Health Organization's successful smallpox eradication program. Dr. McGinnis's research has been widely cited and focuses on the multiple determinants of health and the rational allocation of social resources. He is an elected member of the IOM.